Live Like Nobody Is Watching

Relational Autonomy in the Age of Artificial Intelligence Health Monitoring

ANITA HO

OXFORD
UNIVERSITY PRESS

OXFORD
UNIVERSITY PRESS

Oxford University Press is a department of the University of Oxford. It furthers the University's objective of excellence in research, scholarship, and education by publishing worldwide. Oxford is a registered trade mark of Oxford University Press in the UK and certain other countries.

Published in the United States of America by Oxford University Press
198 Madison Avenue, New York, NY 10016, United States of America.

CIP data is on file at the Library of Congress

ISBN 978–0–19–755626–9

DOI: 10.1093/med/9780197556269.001.0001

Printed by Integrated Books International, United States of America

Contents

Preface

At a social gathering in San Francisco shortly before the beginning of the COVID-19 pandemic, I mentioned this book to a friend, whom I will call "Jon." As the conversation turned to artificial intelligence (AI) health monitoring for older adults, he shared a story.[1] Jon's elderly mother—whom I will call "Diane"—has early-stage dementia and was wondering why things were constantly being moved around in her assisted living apartment. She thought that Jon or her property manager might have entered her apartment and reorganized her belongings (they had not). The incongruence was causing Diane tremendous stress and anxiety, and she resisted any suggestion that she was the culprit and had simply forgotten that she had rearranged the items herself. Diane's geriatrician indicated that it is not unusual for people with dementia to suspect intruders, and they recommended a "simple" solution: Jon could place a smart video camera at his mother's apartment so that he could later play back the footage and prove to her that it was she—and not an intruder—who had rearranged things. The camera could also reveal if Diane was exhibiting behavior that indicated other forms of cognitive or functional decline.

Given that this suggestion of surveillance came from a health care provider, Jon's story brought up interesting and even troubling questions of whether or how privacy and consent norms are changing in the contemporary social and health care spaces, and what choices people truly have regarding (not) being monitored in an environment of growing surveillance. The general Western bioethical requirement of respect for autonomy indicates that personal and health monitoring is ethically permissible only if the person provides explicit consent, and that due care is necessary in protecting people's privacy and confidentiality to uphold their autonomy and prevent harm. But how might consent apply in Diane's situation? While Jon is her power of attorney and designated health care agent in the event she loses decisional capacity, he was understandably concerned about recording his mother in her private space without her consent or knowledge. Moreover, even if Jon were to ask for Diane's consent, she might not understand why she needed to be monitored or what she was agreeing to, or she might not remember giving permission for continuous monitoring. She might not even remember seeing the footage afterward, just as she did not recall moving the objects in her apartment. Jon also worried that his mother would feel humiliated that others doubted her account of events, and that it could be psychologically damaging to show Diane that she was performing acts that she could not remember, especially when there is no cure for this neurodegenerative condition.

Because it was her primary care doctor who recommended such monitoring, its implementation might be interpreted as a benevolent medical strategy, turning Diane's home into a therapeutic care environment. This raises other ethical questions regarding the status of monitoring data and expectations of data security and privacy. Would the video data become personal health data that could be used for health care management and protected by regulations that govern other forms of health data? Who would be able to access the footage? Jon? The primary care doctor? Other health care professionals? The device company? Moreover, how would the data be transmitted (e.g., secured vs. unsecured transmission) and stored? And who owns the data or has the right to share identifiable or anonymized data for research or commercial purposes?

As we will see throughout this book, health monitoring in the broader social context of hyperconnectivity, data mining, public health surveillance, and the expanding spaces of care provision is drastically changing normative meanings and expectations about maintaining our health and privacy in the evolving technological landscape. E-commerce, cloud computing, digital streaming, social media, and other internet service companies continue to harvest and trade data on people's online activities. Internet users and consumers of connected devices are continuously tracked—with or without cameras—with their data being used and sold to data brokers and advertisers, often in the name of providing more user-tailored experiences. For example, learning from consumers' online messaging and search activities, AI can filter spam emails and highlight important messages, predict what people are searching for, connect and introduce friends on social media, and advise consumers about what to buy, watch, or read, generally based on data of their past consumption and behavioral patterns.

Though privacy experts and advocates have raised concerns about such AI monitoring technologies, many consumers in industrialized countries such as the United States continue to actively seek out or at least passively accept these services out of convenience or other perceived benefits. Headline news regarding data mismanagement or breaches of presumably private and secured networks notwithstanding, many gleefully share their images and videos online for all to see. Instead of shunning data tracking, Americans are using more AI-powered applications and products that monitor and share their information than ever before. Not only do consumers accept product or dating recommendations based on algorithmic analysis of their internet activities, despite generally not knowing how their data have been collected or how the algorithms reach decisions on what to present to users. More notably, there is an increasing interest in and consumption of monitoring technologies that explicitly track people's continuous information for convenience and safety, indicating that significant social and cultural changes in privacy expectations may be under way.

Take, for example, the expanding market for AI-enabled home security and monitoring systems that integrate with consumer video cameras and audio recordings. Data from a market research firm showed that sales of smart doorbells in the United States increased by 58 percent from January 2019 to January 2020.[2] Using facial and voice recognition functionalities, the AI system analyzes detected objects and sounds in video and audio recordings against previously uploaded and preapproved images and sound clips. The system can then distinguish an intruder from a resident and trigger alerts accordingly. Data from continuous monitoring and incoming alerts can also be further analyzed to improve system accuracy. These systems are increasingly integrated with other home automation devices to iteratively learn the behaviors and preferences of residents, automatically adjusting settings to accommodate residents' inclinations and habits (e.g., room temperature, lighting). Some companies are also partnering with law enforcement agencies by sharing video footage to aid various types of investigations or courting them to help promote these products in the name of home safety and neighborhood security. These companies also share videos on social and news media for marketing purposes, disguised as entertainment or safety alerts.[3]

Our homes were traditionally considered to be private spaces for ourselves and intimate, trusted others. They stood in stark contrast to health care institutions, where people are constantly monitored by unknown professionals and anonymous technologies. However, as consumer and health technologies converge, and as health care monitoring increasingly moves out of the clinic and hospitals and into people's homes, particularly for long-term elder care and mental health care (a trend that has been further accelerated by the COVID-19 pandemic), automated monitoring in our everyday lives may be affecting how people think about continuous and algorithmic health tracking and data sharing. The home is now increasingly a place for health monitoring and care delivery, carried out by oneself and both informal (e.g., family) and professional caregivers, blurring the distinction between private and health care spaces.

Echoing the broader adoption of internet- and AI-powered technologies in other parts of our lives, community care and health monitoring are increasingly delivered with the assistance of remote technologies, some of which are AI-enabled. From direct-to-consumer (DTC) health tracking devices to home health monitoring technologies, AI is progressively utilized to collect, analyze, and interpret health monitoring data and provide predictive analytics. There is great hope that these automated and continuous health monitoring technologies can help to assess users' health risks and facilitate self-management and early intervention. AI-powered algorithms and clinical decision support are already being used to detect cancer in radiology images and to identify atrial fibrillation (irregular heart rhythm). Enthusiasts believe that if these predictive technologies can be deployed outside of the hospital setting, AI health monitoring that can suggest real-time preventive measures or other actionable interventions will lead to better health outcomes, help avoid or delay institutional care,[4] and lower health care costs,[5] thereby promoting high-value care.

The need for some form of remote monitoring and care is undeniable. While the COVID-19 pandemic is not the main focus of this book, lingering concerns of viral spread have highlighted the need for health systems to consider alternatives to in-person care monitoring and delivery, expanding digital health monitoring at both the individual and population levels during the pandemic. Many clinics and hospitals around the world have had to postpone or cancel elective procedures, and virtual visits for non-urgent concerns and ongoing care have become the norm. Likewise, to control rampant viral transmission among staff and residents in assisted living and nursing homes, in-person care in many facilities, such as where Diane resided, has become severely limited. The ongoing battle against COVID-19 raises questions of whether AI-powered health monitoring may better serve our general, and particularly older, populations and become the new standard even beyond the pandemic.

Nonetheless, as respect for patient autonomy and data privacy is generally accepted as one of the foundational Western bioethical values, questions abound about how AI health monitoring may change the way we define or understand consent, what counts as recreational versus health data, and who should have access to such data and for what purpose. As our society embraces expanding forms of personal and health monitoring, particularly in the context of an aging population and the increasing prevalence of chronic diseases, how can we strike a balance between users' physical safety and their autonomy? And to what extent should we allow individuals to forgo continuous health monitoring, even if such monitoring may help to minimize injury risks, confer health benefits, and lower health care costs? Some of these questions are longstanding bioethical and health policy concerns. Nonetheless, advancing health monitoring technologies and computational methods in the era of big data are bringing forth new ethical considerations of not only autonomy and privacy but also how we can promote responsive and respectful care relationships. In particular, there are ethical concerns that being continuously watched by connected devices and being expected to self-monitor through electronic and algorithmic devices may ironically render patients more isolated and their data more exposed than ever.

Drawing on different use cases of AI health monitoring and focusing on the American context, this book explores the socio-relational contexts that are framing the development and promotion of AI health monitoring for patients and the mass public, as well as the potential consequences of such monitoring for people's autonomy. It argues that the evaluation, design, and implementation of AI health monitoring should be guided by a relational conception of autonomy, which addresses both people's capacity to exercise their agency and broader issues of power asymmetry and social justice. It explores how interpersonal and socio-systemic conditions intersect and shape the cultural meanings of personal responsibility, healthy living/aging, trust, and caregiving. These norms in turn structure the ethical space within which AI health monitoring decisions and care management occur. This book also examines how intersecting norms and expectations regarding predictive analytics, risk tolerance, privacy, self-care, and trust relationships are expressed in the evolving social, technological, and health care landscape, bringing into focus various social and systemic powers that may affect or even control how stakeholders in different social locations may perceive the utility and burdens of AI health monitoring. As Jon's conflict regarding whether to remotely monitor his mother suggests, the decision to decline a monitoring option that may help provide "objective" evidence, especially when recommended by a clinician, involves complex ethical considerations and power dynamics. Through an analysis of home health monitoring for older and disabled adults, DTC health monitoring devices, and medication adherence monitoring, this book proposes ethical strategies at both the professional and systemic levels that can help preserve and promote people's relational autonomy in the digital era.

Notes

1. Permission granted by my friend to share this story.
2. John Herrman, "Who's Watching Your Porch?" *New York Times*, January 19, 2020, https://www.nytimes.com/2020/01/19/style/ring-video-doorbell-home-security.html.
3. Herrman, "Who's Watching Your Porch?"
4. E. Ray Dorsey et al., "Moving Parkinson Care to the Home," *Movement Disorders* 31, no. 9 (September 2016): 1258–62, https://doi.org/10.1002/mds.26744.
5. Josephine McMurray et al., "The Importance of Trust in the Adoption and Use of Intelligent Assistive Technology by Older Adults to Support Aging in Place: Scoping Review Protocol," *JMIR Research Protocols* 6, no. 11 (November 2017): e218, https://doi.org/10.2196/resprot.8772.

Acknowledgments

On most of my writing days, I questioned if I should simply swap AIs and replace Anita's intelligence with artificial intelligence. When I received emails from strangers offering to write or publish "intelligible" books for me, I wondered, how did they know about my own doubts? Have they been watching me or using algorithms to scour through my keystrokes and social media posts, and predicted that I was still writing, writing, and writing?

I am indebted to many who have supported and encouraged me throughout this journey. First and foremost, my parents, especially my late father, who first sowed the idea that propelled me to embark on this journey. I'm also grateful for my editor, Lucy Randall, whose tremendous patience and unfailing encouragement have kept me grounded (and not to give up). I also thank Alison Howard, Wendy Walker, Brent Matheny, and Shanmuga Priya for their most helpful editorial and production work, and Paul Fogarty for friendly discussions of his experiences.

A special gratitude is due to Scott Anderson, Richard Bedell, Daniel Buchman, Stacy Carter, Amy Kim, Catherine Mills, Joseph Robert Perry, Oliver Quick, David Unger, anonymous reviewers, as well as participants at the McGill Biomedical Ethics Unit Seminar and the Centre for Advancing Responsible and Ethical Artificial Intelligence (CARE-AI) Seminar. Their thoughtful comments on earlier versions and related articles have helped me develop and refine my ideas. I am also grateful for research and fellowship funding from the Canadian Institutes of Health Research and Emerson Collective, which have allowed me to deeply learn about this topic.

Finally, my great appreciation for Matthew Radisch, without whose love, patience, and unwavering support for Anita's intelligence this project could not have been undertaken.

Abbreviations

AGI	artificial general intelligence
AI	artificial intelligence
ANI	artificial narrow intelligence
CDC	Centers for Disease Control and Prevention
CNMP	chronic non-malignant pain
DL	deep learning
EHR	electronic health record
FDA	U.S. Food and Drug Administration
FTC	Federal Trade Commission
HIPAA	Health Insurance Portability and Accountability Act
IoT	Internet of Things
IRB	institutional review board
ML	machine learning

Introduction

In recent years, artificial intelligence (AI) has garnered tremendous attention across a range of sectors, including health care. AI is a comprehensive term, broadly defined as computational machines making decisions and performing tasks that previously required human intelligence or cognition.[1] There are high expectations of what AI can do; enthusiasts sometimes refer to it as a central pillar of the Fourth Industrial Revolution, with an impact on humanity as profound as that of the steam engine or electricity.[2] Building on the Third Industrial Revolution (or Digital Revolution) that began in the middle of the twentieth century and was characterized by the spread of automation and digitization through the use of electronics, computers, and communication technologies (e.g., the internet), the Fourth Industrial Revolution is characterized by a fusion of advancing technologies in AI, robotics, the Internet of Things (IoT), genetic engineering, and quantum computing. These technologies blend physical production and operations with smart digital technologies, promising to transform the operation, management, and governance of every industry, including health care.[3]

From clinical uses in diagnostics and treatment, to biomedical research and drug discovery, to operational and administrative tasks, AI has the potential to solve problems in almost all areas of health care provision and management. The health sector relies on various forms of information and data to prevent diseases or illness progression, diagnose a wide array of conditions, and provide/organize care delivery. With rapidly advancing computational capacities and vastly expanding data availability, AI-guided analytical approaches are heavily promoted as being more objective, more accurate, and more efficient than our inherently complex human processes, with the promise of facilitating greater precision, standardization, and automation in health care delivery. As the long-term challenges of aging populations, workforce shortages, and growing health spending are exacerbated by the ongoing COVID-19 pandemic, testing the capacity and responsiveness of health systems across the world, there is high hope that AI can help promote better resilience and emergency preparedness, enhancing health systems' and societies' capacity to respond to not only disease outbreaks but also changing demographics.[4]

Most AI health applications are still in the research and developmental stages, and the use of AI in formal health care delivery and administration settings is currently very limited due to questions about the quality of available health data and the robustness of algorithms in the real world. Nonetheless, the number of potential applications is rapidly expanding. In addition to using AI algorithms that aim to facilitate disease diagnosis and screening in hospitals, clinics, and laboratories, there is a burgeoning market for home health monitoring technologies and direct-to-consumer (DTC) devices that continually collect and analyze users' health, wellness, and other behavioral data. These products target people like Diane (see Preface), who may experience gradual cognitive or functional changes that are not formally monitored or recorded by health care professionals and may not appear obvious to untrained family members. Such health monitoring technologies purport to provide tailored health-related recommendations based on users' longitudinal and real-time data. In the area of medication safety, particularly in the context of the ongoing opioid and mental health crises in the United States, there has also been increasing enthusiasm for AI that monitors and predicts patients' medication adherence, using automated reminders and timely interventions to prevent costly adverse events that result when patients deviate from prescribed regimens.

Given the additional challenges to in-person health monitoring and care delivery due to the ongoing COVID-19 pandemic, many technologists and policymakers express hopes that remote AI technologies can transform health systems management, strengthen health research, assist with clinical care, and facilitate self-management and preventive care, which will in turn improve health care access and health outcomes. High-income governments around the world and venture capitalists are increasing their research investment in these technologies,[5] expressing substantial optimism in AI's ability to detect early problems, provide proactive predictions and recommendations, and help manage emerging concerns, thereby minimizing unnecessary visits to emergency rooms or clinics. Many technology and e-commerce companies are also expanding their presence in the health care market by either developing health apps (e.g., Apple) or acquiring other health-related companies (e.g., Amazon).

However, despite rapid development in the field of AI, the levels of accuracy, utility, and oversight of different types of AI health monitoring technologies for individual and institutional adoption remain variable, raising ethical concerns about how these technologies are promoted, implemented, and regulated. For example, despite broad claims even in peer-reviewed literature that various medical AI systems outperform clinical experts, there have been very few controlled trials for these systems, and the quality of existing studies of nontransparent algorithms is often questionable.[6] As the COVID-19 pandemic further accelerates the development and utilization of remote, automated, and continuous predictive health monitoring, it is necessary to carefully consider the broader ethical implications of utilizing and promoting these technologies, most of which have not been proven to have meaningful clinical value due to methodological flaws and/or underlying biases.[7]

Even as these technologies iteratively improve and advance with more high-quality data and computational power, expanding the implementation of AI health monitoring may have other ethical implications. In addition to its long-term effects on how we perform diagnostic and preventive care, provide and receive formal and informal care, and access and share medical and personal data, promotion of AI technologies to continuously monitor people's health may also affect asymptomatic individuals' self-identity and perception of their health status, their therapeutic relationship with health care providers, their social relationship with intimate others and informal caregivers, and their experiential relationship with or within their personal space (e.g., the home). Thus, while AI holds tremendous potential for more accurate, efficient, and equitable care, this book seeks to address the tension between that potential and the technical and ethical challenges posed by the implementation of AI in the domain of health monitoring. In particular, it focuses on how emerging AI health monitoring technologies that continuously track people's activities and physiological data outside of clinics and hospitals may affect prospective users' autonomy in the name of health maintenance and improvement.

This chapter introduces the key concepts and technologies driving health-related AI today, as well as the ethical quandaries that accompany those technologies. Section 1 provides a brief primer on the origins of AI and why there is increasing excitement surrounding its development and deployment in health care and health monitoring. Section 2 explains how the promises of AI in health care are tempered by growing ethical concerns as implementation of these technologies expands: Are the data used to train algorithms biased? How do algorithms arrive at their conclusions and make health recommendations, and are those processes valid and reliable? How is patient information shared, and with whom? Section 3 introduces the concept of relational autonomy, which will ground the ethical analysis of various emerging AI health monitoring practices. I conclude with a brief outline of the subsequent chapters.

1. Artificial Intelligence in Health Care: What Is It, and Why Should We Care?

Despite its association with futuristic science fiction, AI is nothing new. Simple programmable computers that could solve linear equations appeared in the late 1930s and 1940s, and by 1950, British mathematician Alan Turing had proposed his eponymous "Turing test" or "imitation game"—a means of determining whether a computer could sufficiently mimic human thinking and actions to the point that a judge would not be able to distinguish between human and machine.[8] Just six years later, in 1956, the term AI was coined at an academic conference devoted to exploring whether computing machines could be taught to simulate human beings by using language, abstract forms, and concepts to reason, solve problems, and make decisions. It was here that the first computer program specially engineered to emulate the problem-solving skills of a human being, Logic Theorist, was presented.[9]

Creating AI that can pass the Turing test continues to be a central, long-term vision for many researchers today. This is the version of AI that has captured the popular imagination, with most media defaulting to depictions of artificial *general* intelligence (AGI)—powerful machines that can mimic humans to generalize and abstract learning across various cognitive functions or solve any multifaceted problem, only faster, more accurately, and more consistently. Similar publicity has also surfaced in health care. One company, Isabel, which has developed differential diagnostic tools and symptom checkers based on natural language algorithms, claims to have "all the concepts required to be considered as a step towards" AGI.[10] Hyperboles in promotional claims and aspirational goals notwithstanding, most technologists in AI development acknowledge that we are far from developing machines with complex sensory-perception capabilities, fine motor skills, creativity, social and emotional understanding and engagement, natural language understanding, common sense, or contextual knowledge.[11]

To date, most breakthroughs in AI have taken the form of artificial *narrow* intelligence (ANI), such as custom-built smart machines that operate within a predefined context and perform specific reasoning tasks based on previously curated data from a specific setting. These algorithms cannot generalize outside the boundaries within which the model was trained. Everyday examples include weather forecast algorithms, computer programs that can play chess, and translation algorithms. In health care, ANI examples include automating computers to analyze radiological images[12] or predict the probability of specific disease outcomes using electronic health records (EHRs).[13] Medical ANI research has predominantly focused on a few disease types, such as cancer, nervous system disease, and cardiovascular disease,[14] although in recent years we have witnessed accelerating research in other areas, including an algorithm that uses data from EHRs to predict the progression from prediabetes to type 2 diabetes.[15] Given the narrow and specific focus of most algorithms, for the remainder of this book AI will refer to ANI, except when otherwise noted.

With the expanding volume and types of health care data and the rapid development of new analytical methods, there are high hopes that AI-powered machines and applications can enhance or even replace certain human health monitoring tasks in ways that will lead to quicker detection and prediction of health problems, more precise diagnoses, more customized treatments, higher patient experience or satisfaction, better health outcomes, and lower costs. Nonetheless, as developers, researchers, marketers, and health systems increasingly embrace AI solutionism—that is, the belief that AI is the technological solution to most or all health problems—the distinction or technological distance between AGI and ANI is often glossed over or downplayed. As we will see through various use cases in subsequent chapters, such overhyped promise is a form of epistemic injustice that can exacerbate power asymmetry in health care delivery and compromise patients' relational autonomy.

Early medical problem-solving algorithms included data-driven expert systems, which employ knowledge about their application domain and use logical reasoning rules or inferences to solve problems that would otherwise require human expertise.[16] These systems first emerged in the early 1950s and achieved broader application in health care and other sectors in subsequent decades. Expert medical systems rely on a stored repository of curated medical knowledge and heuristic knowledge (i.e., rules of thumb) provided by experts. They use robust logical rules, such as if-then rules and decision trees, to provide sequential processing of the input data and derive the most appropriate answer from an expert-determined set of possible responses. For example, an expert diagnostic system can process a knowledge database containing information on diseases, patient findings, and the correlations between these elements. Clinicians can then input new patients' symptoms, medical history, and laboratory test results to combine their knowledge with information or suggestions provided by the expert system to generate a differential diagnosis to guide treatment plans.[17]

While expert systems may provide efficient answers for a particular problem and offer consistent solutions,[18] maintenance and improvement of these systems require human experts to provide ongoing updates based on new research, which can be labor-intensive and time-consuming.[19] Early expert system models were also only capable of processing limited input data and finite decisional steps to manage complex medical problems, and there was a lack of satisfactory techniques for responding to new data or reasoning with uncertainty.[20] Moreover, there was professional resistance towards these machines due to fears that these systems may threaten experts' autonomy in their own practices and worries of liability when adopting the recommendation of a system with imperfect explainability.[21]

In the last decade, the expanding quantity and quality of data, improvements in computing power and storage, and advancing algorithms have led to a rapid transformation in big data analytical methods. As clinicians, hospitals, and health systems increasingly adopt EHRs,[22] public and private health care datasets are becoming more widely available, allowing cross-referencing of historical clinical data collected during patients' health care or clinical research encounters. There is now a growing repository of patient-reported symptoms, blood types, medication lists, lab results, clinical notes, radiology images, and genomic data in EHRs, providing clinicians more comprehensive information about their patients than ever before.

In addition to traditional types of medical information collected in formal health care settings, entire new streams of multimodal health and personal data are amassed by private corporations as health monitoring expands into consumer markets and reaches into people's homes and personal devices. These include data from wearable and ambient sensors, mobile devices that track activities and pathophysiological information, and the IoT, which refers to a vast network of physical devices (e.g., "smart home" appliances) embedded with processability, software, or other technologies that gather, transmit, and exchange data with other devices and systems over the internet or other communications networks. As a broad array of factors can influence one's physiology, demographic data and other digital information from social media, internet searches, online purchasing, etc. are also gradually being used to provide additional insight into an individual's health status or concerns and discover correlations between different behaviors and health outcomes. Companies that are not engaged in health care may nonetheless collect, use, and sell consumer data to technology developers that will utilize such data to build, train, and test AI models.

Given this proliferation of big data, medical professionals and decision-makers require more advanced analytical tools to help them harness the power of those data. A newer and disruptive computational technique, machine learning (ML), had led to a paradigm shift in AI capabilities and applications. ML is defined by the capacity of a computer algorithm to utilize data to determine or modify decision-making rules or behavioral structure during operation autonomously.[23] Instead of having predefined logical rules that instruct the machine to perform fixed and sequential stepwise decision-making, ML constructs data analytical algorithms using statistical techniques to teach the computer system to identify patterns in the input data that will help make outcome predictions beyond the training data.[24] By inputting large volumes of high-quality data, the machine can learn to discover relationships between the variables over time and improve task performance or outcome accuracy.

ML algorithms may be categorized as either supervised or unsupervised. In supervised ML, the algorithm is presented with a large number of labeled training cases. For example, patients' EHRs, which contain multiple input variables such as patient characteristics (e.g., age, sex, medical history) and disease-specific data (e.g., symptoms, medications, laboratory results), are now commonly used in training ML algorithms. The algorithm then analyzes the relationship between these input variables and their corresponding output of interest, such as the probability of not taking medications as prescribed or hospital readmission. The learning is "supervised" in the sense that the data is manually labeled to indicate the target outcome value (e.g., taking x number of doses as prescribed, readmission within 30 days). The goal of using labeled data to train the algorithm is to approximate the matching function so that the machine can automatically and accurately predict the output value given new input variables.

For example, in training or supervising a machine to monitor the gait and predict the fall risk of an older adult with Parkinson's disease, we may present the ML algorithm a training dataset of past patient reports that include input variables such as the patient's age, family history, symptoms reports, medications, etc. The programmers may also present prelabeled output events, such as falling when unassisted, as proxies to indicate disease progression. After the initial training, the learning algorithm can be given a testing input dataset of other patients with similar characteristics for validation, calculating the accuracy, sensitivity, and specificity of the algorithm before implementing it in real-world settings. Sensitivity is the ability of the predictive classification or diagnostic model to correctly identify those with the output event, such as true-positive examples of monitored subjects who experienced a fall event. Specificity, conversely, is the ability of the algorithm to correctly identify those without the output event, such as true-negative examples of monitored individuals who did not suffer a fall.[25] An ideal algorithm has high sensitivity and specificity, as false positives and overdiagnosis can prompt unnecessary follow-up testing that may result in overtreatment, and false negatives may delay pertinent diagnosis and postpone medical interventions, potentially leading to harmful outcomes. Under ML, if the predictive model is incorrect, the algorithm can be updated to iteratively improve forecast of disease progression. Once successfully trained and validated, the algorithm can be used in real-world situations of similar contexts and populations to make reliable projections from new data.[26]

In health care, one of the most developed areas for supervised ML is radiology, where AI-powered applications seek to recognize unusual patterns that may suggest malignant tumors. ML has also been utilized to develop predictive models for breast cancer diagnoses, using labeled descriptions of nuclei sampled from breast masses to detect cancerous tumors.[27] Other use cases include a supervised ML study using labeled images of skin cancer to teach an algorithm to distinguish benign from malignant skin lesions. In this study, the machine was reportedly able to classify skin cancer with a level of accuracy comparable to that of a trained dermatologist.[28] If the algorithm is accurate for different populations and affordable for the health system,[29] these predictive technologies may be particularly helpful in rural or lower-resource settings that have a shortage of specialized personnel and diagnostic equipment. They may provide decision support for primary care clinicians to promote more effective preventive, diagnostic, and clinical care for patients worldwide, thereby facilitating more equitable domestic and global health.

It is worth noting that ML algorithms do not function in isolation. Data labeling or annotation in supervised learning requires humans to be involved in a continuous cycle in which they train and test a particular algorithm. Under this approach, sometimes referred to as human-in-the-loop, researchers finetune the algorithm to enhance machine performance.[30] Data labeling is critical to providing greater context, quality, and usability to the dataset for ML training purposes. However, data labeling for complex datasets with numerous variables requires first filtering and cleaning the data by stratifying population cohorts and segmenting the data to extract the region of interest for machine interpretation. This process is often difficult, costly, time-consuming, and prone to human coding biases or manual entry errors, raising clinical and ethical questions as to whether ML algorithms are inherently more objective and accurate, as is commonly presumed, and the impact of overconfidence in these algorithms on therapeutic relationships. Data labeling is particularly complex for large datasets that require meticulous identification of each relevant data point, such as different types or features of skin lesions.[31] Multiple human annotators are often required to label the same data points, score data and outputs to cross-check for quality control, and correct misclassified predictions accordingly.[32]

Since labels are selected by humans, as we will see throughout this book, there are also concerns of label choice bias, whereby biased proxies can lead to biased outcomes. For example, a 2019 study explored a widely used high-risk care management algorithm for allocating "extra help" health care services to patients with the most complex chronic conditions, with the aim of reducing complications and hospital admissions. The algorithm used the most readily available data—health care costs—rather than illnesses as a proxy to identify the sickest patients.[33] However, the American society spends less on Black patients than equally sick and similarly insured White patients, possibly due to substantial barriers Black patients experience in accessing health care due to transportation barriers, competing job or childcare demands, or lack of knowledge of reasons to seek care. The algorithm did not account for these factors for lower access and health spending, and thus understated the former's true health needs and assigned them lower risk scores, thereby perpetuating the underspending on Black patients. The researchers estimated that only 17.7 percent of patients that the algorithm flagged for extra help were Black, when the proportion should have been 46.5 percent if based on true illness severity.

Unsupervised ML can avoid some of these drawbacks and is particularly useful for extracting features or discovering hidden patterns within the data.[34] With unsupervised ML, no manual prelabeling is required. There is no target outcome value to dictate the correct output, and no predetermined relationship or correlation between the unlabeled data. Without being explicitly programmed or supervised by humans, the machine determines its own output by using exploratory techniques, defining for itself best-fit models to make sense of a set of inputs.[35] It observes various elements in the vast number of input data points to discover or model the structure in the datasets, such as identifying subgroups of patients with heart failure using telehealth services in the home health setting.[36] Unsupervised machines iteratively learn to recognize similarities and differences contained in the data and gain valuable insights on their own regarding which features to select and which existing features can be combined.

One key unsupervised ML technique is clustering, which was used in the aforementioned heart failure example. The algorithms can segment or partition the raw data by discovering similar patterns and making meaningful groupings accordingly. The algorithm then learns by defining rules to determine how new inputs will be clustered.[37] Clustering can reveal subgroups within heterogeneous data so that each individual cluster has greater homogeneity than the whole.[38] For example, clustering techniques have been used to segment health care utilization patterns among "super-utilizers,"[39] who incur high medical costs from frequent inpatient or emergency department visits, often because of complex physical, behavioral, and social needs. Unsupervised clustering techniques have also been used by learning algorithms to detect resemblances that allow the machine to find patterns across patients with Alzheimer's disease (AD) that may be too complex for individual practitioners to discern.[40]

Another promising feature of unsupervised ML is its ability to discover relationships between variables inside the dataset, such as recognizing features that underlie the conversion from early-stage AD to advanced AD. Such techniques may help to predict patients' illness trajectory and guide follow-up observations and treatment plans accordingly. Similar methods have been utilized to facilitate the diagnosis of breast cancer, Parkinson's disease, mental health and psychiatric disorders, cardiac and diabetic diseases, and Huntington's disease.[41] If accurate, the ability to identify subgroups and their correlating risk factors may be particularly helpful in developing targeted resources and support measures for underserved populations to promote better health outcomes and equity.

However, as mentioned before, the sheer volume, diversity, and complexity of these health-related datasets require increasingly sophisticated data processing methods in order to apply relevant learning to health care delivery. In recent years, deep learning (DL) has become a popular technique for fulfilling that need. DL utilizes multilayer artificial neural networks (ANNs), which are loosely modeled on the structure and function of the human brain.[42] "Deep" nets contain anywhere from three to hundreds of hidden layer combinations of prespecified functions that analyze the input data with a logical structure similar to how humans would reason and reach conclusions.[43]

In this complex layered computing system, interconnected artificial neurons imitate organic neurons by responding to external input data and transmitting information to other network neurons, combining lower-level features into a unified and compact representation. Mimicking neuroscientific models of cognition,[44] DL continually scrutinizes vast quantities of multiple types of data, such as sound (e.g., voice recordings), images (e.g., radiology images), and text (e.g., clinical notes).[45] It does this through a hierarchy of interconnected layers in the training neural network, which capture complex nonlinear relationships between input variables and an outcome.[46] Starting from the raw input data, each processing layer of a DL system produces a representation of the observed patterns, gradually transforming the representation into a higher, slightly more abstract level with each progressive layer.[47] The first layer of digital neurons (i.e., nodes) receives raw inputs, such as pixels in a radiology image of tumors. It mixes and scores these inputs according to simple mathematical rules, then passes the outputs to the next layer of nodes.[48] Part of the DL process involves estimating the weights through input and outcome data so as to minimize potential prediction error.[49] In learning the deep structures and generalizable representations based on multilayer processing of the input data, the last layer distills these neural activities into a final prediction, such as whether the radiology image shown is one of a malignant versus a benign tumor.

The multiple types of health care and related data used in ML/DL can be either structured or unstructured. Structured data are presented in a specific, standardized, or consistent format, usually in the quantitative form of numbers and values. They generally fit neatly within fixed fields and columns in spreadsheets and can be easily harnessed and understood by supervised ML. Everyday examples of structured data include demographic information, such as patients' names, birthdates, addresses, educational levels, and geolocations. In health care, running massive structured datasets through analytical tools to explore the past health care utilization of a population with various demographic characteristics can help uncover patterns and trends to predict individual- and population-level utilization. For example, a DL algorithm may analyze the frequency of clinic and hospital visits, diagnoses, medication history, laboratory values, interventions (e.g., surgeries), and lengths of hospital stays in the EHRs to predict how people with different conditions and socioeconomic statuses may seek various types of health care in the future under distinct circumstances. These AI-powered technologies may help clinics, hospitals, health systems, and social service organizations anticipate staffing needs and service demand so that they can make informed hiring, training, scheduling, utilization management, and patient education decisions.

Unstructured data are generally qualitative data, which often contain rich and more in-depth information about a person or a phenomenon being explored, and may provide valuable contextual information about a patient's functional and health status. Raw unstructured data in everyday life include text, audio, photo, or video files, such as those that are posted on social media or run through chatbots and virtual assistants. Examples of unstructured health care data include nursing notes, dictation notes, radiology images, sensor data, and free text in patient correspondence or clinic visit notes. With the proliferation of AI home health technologies and health care apps, two use cases that will be explored further in subsequent chapters, patients are producing and recording more visual, audio, and textual data than ever. The expanding plethora of unstructured data generally cannot be processed or analyzed using conventional quantitative data tools and methods because they lack a predefined data model. These data need to be converted to a machine-understandable format before the computer can extract features for analysis.[50] By inputting unstructured data through multiple layers of neural networks, DL can learn to identify and categorize the person's behavior, intent, or concerns and explore the associations among the different datapoints to help make health care predictions and decisions accordingly. As we will see in subsequent chapters, the conversion and reduction of rich qualitative experiential data into machine-compatible formats raises various ethical concerns around whether or how ML in health monitoring may distort people's embodied and psychosocial experience, and impose recommendations that conflict with their practical identity (i.e., a person's self-conception regarding how they want to live and what actions or decisions they deem worth undertaking).[51]

As sophisticated DL algorithms can process large and diverse datasets efficiently, they may be able to harness multimodal wellness, clinical, home monitoring, and/or genomics data to provide a more comprehensive picture of a person's health and functional status, and then translate these data into actionable insights to predict, prevent, and/or solve complex health care problems. The breakthrough innovation of DL is driving the AI boom, especially as the flexibility of unsupervised learning allows multilayer neural networks to outperform other simpler forms of ML. If an initial prediction is incorrect, the self-learning, evolving neural network can iteratively tweak the links between nodes, steering the system closer to the right result for future forecast.[52] Once trained and refined, a DL algorithm can identify relevant patterns from previously unconnected datasets, detect correlations among datasets and attributes, and categorize information that may be too complex for manual detection, analysis, and interpretation.[53]

The current AI applications with the greatest potential to enhance clinical care and health care delivery include computer vision systems, audio and speech recognition systems, natural language processing (NLP) systems, text mining platforms, bioinformatics systems, and medical image analysis systems. A number of these systems are poised to augment clinicians' ability to accurately diagnose patients' conditions,[54] reliably determine the risk of disease onset and forecast disease progression,[55] and tailor self-management and treatment recommendations in a timely manner.[56] Promising platforms include a "deep patient" algorithm, which uses EHR data spanning twelve years, from 76,214 test patients, comprising seventy-eight diseases from diverse clinical domains and temporal windows.[57] The algorithm can reportedly predict with high accuracy whether a patient will develop severe diabetes, schizophrenia, and various cancers within a year, months before a doctor would make the call.[58] Other successful algorithms include a model for diagnosing congenital cataract disease through learning ocular images,[59] another diagnostic model that can classify skin cancer from clinical images,[60] and a DL algorithm for detecting referable diabetic retinopathy through retinal fundus photographs.[61] Given the early successes of these algorithms, the excitement surrounding AI use in health monitoring is understandable. AI holds tremendous promise for timely disease detection, improved efficiency and accuracy in health care delivery, and greater health equity. What remains underdiscussed, however, are the accompanying risks and ethical quandaries posed by these emerging technologies.

2. Artificial Intelligence and Health Monitoring: A Technological-Ethical Juncture

Based on the examples above, it is apparent that even before the first case of COVID-19 was discovered, there was already substantial interest among technologists, health care providers, insurance companies, and health systems to utilize AI technologies for health monitoring at both individual and population levels. The pandemic has further propelled investment and development in remote and automated monitoring that can be used outside of hospitals and clinics. Patients with chronic and intensive long-term care needs are more susceptible to various diseases, including severe illness from COVID-19 infection, such that reducing unnecessary clinic and hospital visits may help to minimize their exposure to other patients and infectious conditions. For patients who have contracted COVID-19 but have not (yet) developed severe symptoms, AI-enabled wearable thermometers and pulse oximeters allow them to rest, track, and forecast their disease progression at home unless AI-indicated for further medical attention, enhancing patients' well-being while also preserving scarce health care resources for those requiring higher levels of care. Pulse oximeters monitor patients' arterial oxygen saturation levels to determine if they may be at risk of hypoxemia (low oxygen saturation) and require supplemental oxygen. As public health agencies around the world encourage people who may be infected with COVID-19 to self-monitor and isolate at home, a mobile phone app has also been developed to detect COVID-19 infection in people's voices. Its developers claim in a preprint article that the AI model is more accurate (89 percent) than some of the lateral flow and rapid antigen tests in identifying infected individuals.[62]

AI-assisted health monitoring is expected to stay even after the pandemic is over, potentially expanding opportunities for further remote and AI-assisted monitoring. Aligning themselves with the foundational Western bioethical focus on individual autonomy and patient well-being, AI promoters promise that the growing array of automated health monitoring technologies can facilitate not only early discovery and anticipation of health decline, accurate and timely diagnosis, and continuity of care between clinic visits, but also patient engagement and self-management in the safety and comfort of their personal environments, thereby promoting patient autonomy and high-quality care.[63] At the health system level, if accurate algorithms are implemented properly, they may help clinicians to triage patients based on the acuity and urgency of their needs, enhance clinical decision-making, and prevent acute deteriorations or serious injuries, which in turn will promote better health outcomes and delay or avoid undesired and costly institutional care.[64]

Many enthusiasts insist that AI-powered technologies are more objective than human judgment and will bring more reliable and personalized care in the long run, thereby enhancing patient safety and quality improvement efforts.[65] AI-powered remote health monitoring may be especially useful for democratizing health information and keeping patients out of hospitals, particularly in the context of an aging population and the growing prevalence of chronic conditions. These technologies can be crucial resources when in-person care is unavailable or restricted, as is the case for non-urgent care needs during the COVID-19 pandemic, or when mobility challenges or the lack of family or social support renders it difficult for patients to seek in-person clinical consultation. If AI health monitoring can facilitate more convenient and effective preventive, diagnostic, and support care for hard-to-reach populations as well as areas with less specialists, these technologies may also promote justice and health equity.

Nonetheless, while existing AI/DL models demonstrate great *promise* for harnessing multimodal and complex data for predictive analysis and discovery, many technical challenges remain in making appropriate and full use of complex biomedical and other ancillary data. Large datasets often include a high volume of heterogeneous types of data with numerous traits (i.e., high-dimensional data). Countless streams of personal and health data are now generated or collected at an unprecedented speed by diverse networks and platforms, posing challenges for multimodal data fusion (i.e., the process of integrating multiple data sources to produce consistent, accurate, and useful information).[66] Even when these datasets are used, non-representativeness, sparsity, and irregularity in the data raise further concerns regarding accuracy and quality.

Moreover, DL algorithms are often opaque "black boxes" that offer few clues as to how the hidden multilayer neural networks connect the numerous input variables to arrive at their conclusions,[67] especially when these predictions are combined probabilistically in complex ways.[68] These challenges raise questions about how users can ensure or verify an algorithm's validity or reliability and make informed decisions about whether to utilize these technologies.[69] While these neural networks are loosely modeled after the human brain, researchers often discover (after numerous inaccurate predictions) that ML-powered machines learn differently from humans in complex situations.

The high-profile example of IBM—which partnered with large health systems after its supercomputer, Watson, won *Jeopardy!* in 2011—offers a cautionary tale for anyone presuming that algorithms designed for narrow purposes can work comparatively well in complex health care contexts. On the quiz show, Watson used NLP to parse complicated wordplay clues, mine millions of text sources, decipher relationships among these sources, and provide automated question answering. Over the next few years, IBM invested billions of dollars into promoting Watson as a benevolent AI assistant for other industries, including forming the Watson Health division in 2015 and acquiring four health data companies for $4 billion in mid-2016.[70] The company sought out major medical centers where researchers work with massive amounts of health and genetic data, as well as thousands of medical research papers, with the high hopes that Watson could mine and derive advanced insights from all that medical information to improve diagnosis, treatment, and health outcomes. Nonetheless, bearing in mind the distinction between AGI and ANI, a technology that was specifically engineered to identify word patterns and predict correct answers for a trivia game did not transfer well to the complex arena of medicine, where incongruent data points in medical records and local variabilities abound. Despite being able to analyze massive sets of EHRs, official medical guidelines, and the outcomes of published medical studies, Watson's "evidence-based" recommendations could not match the expertise of trained oncologists, who draw on not only external guidelines but also their prior experiences and insights with patients, treatments, and outcomes when they devise a holistic strategy for a new patient and/or navigate ambiguities.[71] The problem may have also been partly that the AI model was overfitting—that is, it learned statistical irregularities specific to the data on which it was trained, such as missing data in EHRs.

To make matters worse, the diagnostic information came from experts at the specific partnering institutions and therefore consisted of only certain subsets of patients (e.g., wealthy patients with access to major academic centers). In particular, Watson for Oncology, a collaboration with the Memorial Sloan Kettering Cancer Center, was trained using hypothetical cases, or synthetic data, developed by the physicians at that center. Thus, the model was unable to generalize to other input data to accurately discover hidden patterns in new clinical situations, populations, and contexts.[72] When the model was tested with colon cancer patients in South Korea, researchers found only 49 percent concordance between the algorithm-derived treatment recommendations and the local oncologists' recommendations.[73] In Thailand, the model showed a 76 percent concordance for patients with breast cancer.[74] In China, different cancer types had wildly different concordances with the Watson model, ranging from only 12 percent for gastric cancer, to 64 percent for colon and cervical cancers, to 96 percent for ovarian cancer.[75] Such discordance raises questions of how applicable or acceptable these algorithmic recommendations are in different treatment contexts, which can be affected by incidence, cost, insurance requirements, drug availabilities, as well as patient and physician preference. While IBM made almost fifty announcements about partnerships to develop new AI-enabled tools for medicine, most did not lead to successful commercial products.[76] MD Anderson Cancer Center canceled its Oncology Expert Advisor project in 2016 after reportedly spending $62 million in only two years.[77] IBM also discontinued Watson for Genomics in 2020, a project that grew out of joint research with the University of North Carolina, as well as the aforementioned Watson for Oncology.[78] In 2022, IBM sold Watson Health's data and analytics assets to an investment firm for a price reportedly in the $1 billion range—a small fraction of the company's investment.[79]

IBM Watson and countless other examples of failed ambitious enterprises from even the most resourceful institutions have shown that, while DL has tremendous potential to facilitate efficient and effective processing of big datasets and thereby guide clinical decisions, some of the advantages of DL techniques, including continuous learning, are accompanied by other problems. For example, since neural nets program themselves and evolve without human supervision, they do not require the same level of human resources for training as supervised networks. This means that even the computer engineers who design the algorithm may not completely understand how DL combines or processes the input variables to make the final decisions or predictions, or where in the hidden layers something takes an unexpected turn.[80] In addition, even if the algorithm underwent exemplary development and rigorous initial evaluation, if the training data do not match the new input patient data, such as when the algorithm is applied to a population with higher disease prevalence than the training population data, a distributional shift may occur, whereby the algorithmic outputs adapt to the new data environment and draw inaccurate conclusions.[81] These problems were illustrated in the IBM Watson journey. Moreover, proprietary algorithms, and the datasets used to train them, are notoriously inaccessible to outsiders, rendering scrutiny of these algorithms or algorithmic decisions difficult. It is often only when blatant biases, repeated errors, and adverse health consequences have occurred in real-time medical settings that the problems are revealed and addressed.

Such concerns are exacerbated when the datasets used for training or testing are not representative of the intended users, or when flawed assumptions and biases of the humans that generated and labeled the data are disguised and reinforced by the power of data anonymization and aggregation.[82] Whether it is facial recognition,[83] criminal risk assessment, skin cancer diagnosis, or pulse oximeters, we have seen how biased historical data or homogeneous training datasets from only certain population groups may reflect and amplify mistakes of the past, thereby exacerbating harm and injustice.[84] For example, as mentioned earlier, DL algorithms for skin lesions have been developed to assist dermatologists in diagnosing skin cancer. However, if the training data come from primarily light-skinned people due to a lack of diversity in clinical trials, lesions on patients with darker skin may be less likely to be diagnosed correctly, provoking efficacy, safety, and equity concerns for these underserved populations.[85]

Similar problems have been documented for pulse oximeters. Both hospital-based and DTC versions of these devices have been widely utilized during the COVID-19 pandemic because of the way the virus interferes with the body's natural ability to process oxygen.[86] However, a recent study in the United States revealed that Black patients had nearly three times the frequency of occult hypoxemia not detected by pulse oximetry as White patients.[87] The exact reasons for such differences are unclear; these technologies were originally developed in non-diverse populations, with no concerted effort to study whether or why there may be population differences for historically underserved groups. Nonetheless, the U.S. Food and Drug Administration (FDA) warned two months after the publication of the aforementioned study that skin pigmentation and skin thickness may be among the multiple factors that can affect the accuracy of pulse oximeter readings.[88] Given such data biases or limitations, reliance on pulse oximeters to triage diverse patients and adjust supplemental oxygen levels without integrating other clinical and patient-reported data may place Black patients at increased risk for hypoxemia.[89] The disparate impact of potentially biased health monitoring algorithms, which can provide inaccurate results for some populations, may spill over to other areas of health care for these historically marginalized groups, reinforcing distrust and perpetuating their reluctance to seek medically necessary care or follow clinical advice, thereby exacerbating health inequities.

The use of big datasets for DL reveals other ethical concerns around algorithmic and operational transparency. Health systems, including tax-funded academic health centers, are increasingly working with commercial partners to build algorithms to enhance patient care, as was the case for the IBM Watson collaborations. These joint public–private ventures raise questions of what data sharing agreements need to be in place to ensure data privacy and security, how to ensure that data collected with infrastructure built by public dollars is used for public benefits, who should retain control over the data, and whether or what types of patient consent should be required for sharing EHRs and implementing new technologies in these collaborative efforts.[90] In addition, vast amounts of intimate and detailed personal and medical information about individuals continue to be collected and shared by IoT and AI-powered platforms, sometimes "consented to" through complex and incomprehensible agreements that most users quickly click through without reading or understanding their content. For those who take the time to review the information, there is generally no mechanism to seek further clarification on the agreement or the algorithm. Users often have to agree to *all* terms in order to access *any* service being offered by the technology. The nontransparency of some DL models and their data usage or sharing practices stands in sharp contrast to the "open book" subjects that many ordinary patients and citizens have inadvertently become in the era of big data. For example, one study assessing data sharing and privacy practices of smartphone apps for depression and smoking cessation found that only 69 percent of these apps had *any* privacy policies, even though 92 percent of them shared data with third-party companies, mostly for advertising and marketing analytical purposes.[91] This raises important ethical questions of how health care systems and providers should manage the opacity and assess the validity and reliability of health monitoring algorithms in patient care, whether individual consent in the context of nontransparent algorithms and data sharing practices is meaningful in upholding users' autonomy, and who should be held accountable for algorithmic and data sharing decisions that may have adverse impacts on patients and users. For example, as private companies offer an expanding array of unregulated wellness applications to monitor and predict users' health status, questions abound as to whether a "buyer beware" mindset versus a more protective approach would be more appropriate in upholding users' meaningful autonomy and well-being.

As individuals whose data are being collected, shared, linked, and processed by black box algorithms are subjected to automated recommendations or predictions, the lack of transparency provokes urgent epistemological and ethical questions about the power bestowed on AI platforms and those who utilize these algorithms in organizing, delivering, and financing care. Because decisions to fund or adopt AI health monitoring technologies generally happen at the health system or institutional level, individual consumers and patients often have minimal to no power to choose other data collection and monitoring options, regardless of their own priorities, preferences, and goals, especially if funding models or financial incentives are tied to the use of these technologies at individual and health system levels. As we will see in Chapter 3, even in the case of DTC devices, pervasive social expectations of self-monitoring by technologies are potentially affecting users' autonomy by restructuring their motivations regarding how or whether they want their activities and health status to be continuously tracked.

Moreover, the development and utilization of AI-powered technologies influence personal, social, and professional relationships in small yet significant ways. Despite the traditional dyadic models of provider–patient relationship, which focus on in-person monitoring and care for people with illnesses and injuries, AI technologies are gradually changing the wellness and health care landscape, reflecting and simultaneously affecting professional and informal care relationships and expectations. In the United States, individually identifiable health information collected by health plans and health care providers is protected under the Health Insurance Portability and Accountability Act of 1996 (HIPAA), which requires covered entities to abide by various regulations around sharing personal information to protect patient privacy. The Common Rule (i.e., *The Federal Policy for the Protection of Human Subjects*), promulgated in 1991 and updated in 2018, also sets forth requirements for federal agencies and federally funded research involving human participants.[92] But as AI health monitoring is increasingly developed by private entrepreneurs and moves outside of formal health institutions into patients' homes and consumer devices, the rights, obligations, and boundaries for different stakeholders become blurry. In this rapidly advancing technological space that is increasingly occupied by actors outside of the health systems, it is often unclear when and whether consent is required for data collection, who can collect health versus personal information, what types of information cannot be collected or shared, what constitutes health advice versus recreational information, who can provide such advice, and who is accountable or liable for adverse events or outcomes from faulty algorithmic outputs. There are also questions of how the broader sociocultural and systemic contexts within which AI technologies are conceptualized, developed, promoted, financed, and utilized may impose disparate impacts on different populations and exacerbate various forms of inequities.

3. AI Health Monitoring: A Relational Labyrinth

As we can see, health monitoring at the dawn of AI is not just technologically complicated. More importantly, it is also socio-relationally complex, reflecting and reinforcing various social norms and power hierarchies in health care.[93] The potential impact of these emerging technologies and related practices calls for anticipation and evaluation of challenges if we hope to achieve ethical development, implementation, and governance. As AI finds its way into the very fabric of health care and people's own health management, automating health monitoring without necessarily enhancing in-person care management, this book will explore the ethical implications of three broad use cases of AI health monitoring that target different populations with varying degrees of vulnerability: (1) home health monitoring for older or disabled adults, (2) DTC health and wellness tracking products, and (3) medication adherence monitoring. Given pertinent questions of how various bioethical values may manifest and intersect in the context of AI health monitoring, we need to determine the most ethical processes and strategies for incorporating these values into AI technologies' design and implementation plans.

Exploring the intersection of Western liberal respect for autonomy with foundational bioethical values like non-maleficence, beneficence, and justice, this book will focus on whether or how the expanding development and implementation of AI health monitoring may affect people's ability to make health monitoring decisions that promote their goals and well-being. Chapter 1 examines how the liberal conceptualization of autonomy has fueled pledges to democratize health information in the converging private, commercial, wellness, and health care spaces, but falls short of truly promoting people's autonomous agency and decision-making. New predictive health monitoring technologies and data sharing practices are touted as tools to balance power asymmetry and promote more choices for patients and consumers. Nonetheless, while proponents of these practices presume that AI technologies will promote individual autonomy by giving users more information and choices, they neglect how much power and control *other* individuals and entities hold over monitored individuals as AI and health maintenance converge in the hyperconnected digital era.

Informed by the feminist conception of relational autonomy, which goes beyond the rhetoric of consumer sovereignty and self-regulating markets to attend to human vulnerability, (inter)dependency, and power asymmetry in health care,[94] this chapter argues for situating the promotion and utilization of AI health monitoring in a wider socio-relational context. It examines how interpersonal and socio-systemic conditions shaping the cultural meanings of personal responsibility, adherence, healthy living/aging, trust, and caregiving may affect people's self-governance, self-determination, and self-authorization, which are important in navigating available health monitoring options. It explores how the changing technological environment may structure people's decisional contexts and subsequent choices to forgo (some levels of) human monitoring for AI health tracking, regardless of their own goals and priorities. In considering what external conditions are required for moral agents—including patients and caregivers—to have de facto power and authority over decisions significant to the direction of their lives and care pathways, this chapter will argue for a constitutively relational approach to autonomy that considers interpersonal or social conditions as crucial to autonomous agency. By understanding autonomy relationally, we can bring into focus various social and systemic powers that may predetermine how individuals and their support networks will perceive the utility and burdens of AI health monitoring, as well as their freedom and opportunities to accept or decline such monitoring.

The lens of relational autonomy can help us explore critically the ways in which the promotion of AI health monitoring may influence how we define and facilitate healthy aging. AI home health monitoring for older adults and people with disabilities,[95] which is the focus of Chapter 2, reflects and simultaneously propels sociocultural changes in how we conceptualize healthy aging and independent living, and how we may organize health monitoring and care work accordingly. Against the backdrop of the growing prevalence of chronic and degenerative conditions among older adults, AI home health monitoring is increasingly touted as a cost-effective alternative to or enhancement of personal monitoring. Nonetheless, while these technologies are often promoted as empowering means to enhance independent living and personal privacy, the lens of relational autonomy reveals that, as technological practices and funding decisions often predetermine available health monitoring options, people who are deemed by others as requiring ongoing monitoring often have little to no freedom or opportunity to decide whether or how health monitoring should take place. It is noteworthy that the technological shift in health monitoring may impose care work on targeted individuals and family caregivers while masking system inadequacies, further compromising older and disabled adults' ability to make health monitoring and care decisions according to their practical identities and well-being. Moreover, there are important ethical questions regarding how we can uphold the autonomy of people with declining cognitive capacity, who may lack the capacity to provide meaningful consent or informed refusal due to their inability to fully comprehend the benefits and burdens of continuous and automated monitoring.

As AI health monitoring moves into people's homes and consumer markets, these technologies are increasingly commercialized in the name of democratizing health information and empowering people to become more informed and engaged in their own care. Many private companies are developing self-monitoring applications and devices that provide users access to certain physiological information whenever and wherever they want, an area that will be explored in detail in Chapter 3. In addition to monitoring various chronic conditions, commercial developers are increasingly targeting asymptomatic and presymptomatic populations with DTC AI health monitoring products that collect wellness data (e.g., physical activity, diet) and other health information (e.g., blood pressure, heart monitoring). These products and their marketing messages often blur the distinctions between recreational and health products, technologists and health care providers, and consumers and patients. This is particularly true for companies that produce both prescription and DTC versions of their technologies, or that make opaque health claims. Such muddling has ethical and regulatory implications, as these intentionally chosen categories and promotional strategies affect whether device companies must follow the same stringent rules regarding safety, accuracy, efficacy, and privacy, and whether any therapeutic and fiduciary responsibilities such as informed consent and non-maleficence can be expected and enforced. Moreover, many of these devices collect and convert users' rich embodied and psychosocial experience into oversimplified and quantified outputs without transparent explanation of the analytical process, changing people's relationship to their bodies and identities. These technologies may give the veneer of promoting user understanding of and control over their health while subtly disciplining users into adopting certain behaviors via ongoing monitoring and nudging, raising questions of whether these technologies may compromise rather than enhance users' autonomy in other ways.[96]

Another area of AI health monitoring that has gained increasing interest in the name of patient safety is the use of medication adherence algorithms, a use case that will be discussed in Chapter 4.[97] In the United States, medication nonadherence contributes to 125,000 deaths and more than $100 billion in health care costs annually.[98] Some of these technologies are designed to look at the life cycle of treatment in order to see when and how nonadherence takes place (e.g., did not fill/pick up the prescription, did not take the medication as directed) and predict barriers to such adherence (e.g., side effects, work schedule).

AI enthusiasts believe that, when coupled with patient-centered case management, automated medication monitoring systems can help to ensure that prescriptions are taken as instructed and facilitate timely follow-up in cases of nonadherence. However, in the context of pharmaco-vigilance for various drug classes and patients with certain diagnoses, questions abound as to whether targeted patients will have the freedom to decline automated monitoring, which may further stigmatize patients and perpetuate distrust among those who are already wary of the therapeutic space.[99] For productive healing relationships, patients need to be able to see themselves as someone who can be trusted in their own judgments and actions.[100] Focusing on the contentious arena of mental health and pain conditions, this chapter explores how AI medication monitoring, particularly when deployed as a form of surveillance to manage distrust of patients' credibility and/or competency, may further compromise patients' self-governance, self-determination, and self-authorization.[101] Since one of the prerequisite components for self-authorization is self-trust, this chapter considers whether medication monitoring algorithms, which inherently question the veracity or trustworthiness of the patient's self-report, may reinforce medical power and compromise patients' relational autonomy.[102]

Incorporating discussions from previous chapters, Chapter 5 tackles three intersecting socio-relational layers of the ethical issues with AI health monitoring: the individual-familial level, the professional-institutional level, and the systemic-structural level. It examines the blurring of private and therapeutic spaces, the impact of automated and predictive health monitoring on familial care relationships and professional therapeutic relationships, and the pressure of health system inadequacies on how stakeholders in different social locations think about AI health monitoring. Recalling different use cases discussed throughout the book, this chapter explores how to ensure that the increasing digitization of patient experiences and algorithmic practices will not inadvertently further isolate patients and erode trust relationships. Against the backdrop of patients gradually becoming quantified entities through the use of AI and other electronic health technologies, this chapter considers how we can preserve patients' relational identities and enhance therapeutic relationships in the evolving digital age. It argues that, to truly democratize health information, the use of AI health monitoring must be accompanied by broader efforts to promote health and digital literacy as well as a system reorganization that can further align patients' and families' health priorities and overall values.

Notes

1. Alexander L. Fogel and Joseph C. Kvedar, "Artificial Intelligence Powers Digital Medicine," *npj Digital Medicine* 1 (2018), article 5, https://doi.org/10.1038/s41746-017-0012-2.
2. Organization for Economic Cooperation and Development, *Trustworthy AI in Health: Background Paper for the G20 AI Dialogue, Digital Economy Task Force*, April 2020, https://www.oecd.org/health/trustworthy-artificial-intelligence-in-health.pdf.
3. Klaus Schwab, "The Fourth Industrial Revolution: What It Means and How to Respond," World Economic Forum, January 14, 2016, https://www.weforum.org/agenda/2016/01/the-fourth-industrial-revolution-what-it-means-and-how-to-respond/.
4. Organization for Economic Cooperation and Development, *Trustworthy AI in Health.*
5. For example, in 2020 the Australian government announced it would invest AU$19 million over three years into AI-based health research projects designed to prevent, diagnose, and treat a range of health conditions. See https://www.zdnet.com/article/australian-government-sinks-au19-million-into-ai-health-research-projects/.
6. Konstantin Genin and Thomas Grote, "Randomized Controlled Trials in Medical AI: A Methodological Critique," *Philosophy of Medicine* 2, no. 1 (2021), https://doi.org/10.5195/philmed.2021.27.
7. Michael Roberts et al., "Common Pitfalls and Recommendations for Using Machine Learning to Detect and Prognosticate for COVID-19 Using Chest Radiographs and CT Scans," *Nature Machine Intelligence* 3 (2021): 199–217, https://doi.org/10.1038/s42256-021-00307-0.
8. Rebecca Reynoso, "A Complete History of Artificial Intelligence," G2, May 25, 2021, https://www.g2.com/articles/history-of-artificial-intelligence.
9. Rockwell Anyoha, "The History of Artificial Intelligence," Science in the News, Harvard University, August 28, 2017, https://sitn.hms.harvard.edu/flash/2017/history-artificial-intelligence/.

10. Mandy Tomlinson, "Artificial General Intelligence (AGI) and Healthcare Adaptation," Isabel, February 17, 2016, https://info.isabelhealthcare.com/blog/artificial-general-intelligence-agi-and-healthcare-adaptation.
11. Federico Berruti, Pieter Nel, and Rob Whiteman, "An Executive Primer on Artificial General Intelligence," McKinsey, April 29, 2020, https://www.mckinsey.com/business-functions/operations/our-insights/an-executive-primer-on-artificial-general-intelligence.
12. Alejandro Rodriguez-Ruiz et al., "Stand-Alone Artificial Intelligence for Breast Cancer Detection in Mammography: Comparison with 101 Radiologists," *Journal of the National Cancer Institute* 111, no. 9 (2019): 916–22, https://doi.org/10.1093/jnci/djy222.
13. Alison M. Darcy, Alan K. Louie, and Laura Weiss Roberts, "Machine Learning and the Profession of Medicine," *Journal of the American Medical Association* 315, no. 6 (2016): 551–52, https://doi.org/10.1001/jama.2015.18421.
14. Fei Jiang et al., "Artificial Intelligence in Healthcare: Past, Present and Future," *Stroke and Vascular Neurology* 2, no. 4 (2017), https://doi.org/10.1136/svn-2017-000101.
15. Jeffrey P. Anderson et al., "Reverse Engineering and Evaluation of Prediction Models for Progression to Type 2 Diabetes: An Application of Machine Learning Using Electronic Health Records," *Journal of Diabetes Science and Technology* 10, no. 1 (2015): 6–18, https://doi.org/10.1177/1932296815620200.
16. Jay E. Aronson, "Expert Systems," in *Encyclopedia of Information Systems*, ed. Hossein Bidgoli (Cambridge, MA: Academic Press, 2003), 277–89, https://doi.org/10.1016/B0-12-227240-4/00067-8.
17. K. S. Metaxiotis, J.-E. Samouilidis, and J. E. Psarras, "Expert Systems in Medicine: Academic Illusion or Real Power?" *Journal of Innovation in Health Informatics* 9, no. 1 (February 2000): 3–8, https://doi.org/10.14236/jhi.v9i1.228.
18. Arvind Kumar Yadav, Rohit Shukla, and Tiratha Raj Singh, "Machine Learning in Expert Systems for Disease Diagnostics in Human Healthcare," in *Machine Learning, Big Data, and IoT for Medical Informatics*, ed. Pardeep Kumar, Yugal Kumar, and Mohamed A. Tawhid (Cambridge, MA: Academic Press, 2021), 179–200, https://doi.org/10.1016/B978-0-12-821777-1.00022-7.
19. Anitha Kannan, "The Science of Assisting Medical Diagnosis: From Expert Systems to Machine-Learned Models," Medium, April 15, 2019, https://medium.com/curai-tech/the-science-of-assisting-medical-diagnosis-from-expert-systems-to-machine-learned-models-cc2ef0b03098.

20. Heather Heathfield, "The Rise and 'Fall' of Expert Systems in Medicine," *Expert Systems* 16, no. 3 (1999): 183–88, https://doi.org/10.1111/1468-0394.00107.
21. Reed T. Sutton et al., "An Overview of Clinical Decision Support Systems: Benefits, Risks, and Strategies for Success," *npj Digital Medicine* 3 (February 2020), article 17, https://doi.org/10.1038/s41746-020-0221-y.
22. Jenni A. M. Sidey-Gibbons and Chris J. Sidey-Gibbons, "Machine Learning in Medicine: A Practical Introduction," *BMC Medical Research Methodology* 19 (2019), https://doi.org/10.1186/s12874-019-0681-4.
23. Brent Daniel Mittelstadt et al., "The Ethics of Algorithms: Mapping the Debate," *Big Data & Society* 3, no. 2 (December 2016): 2053951716679679, https://doi.org/10.1177/2053951716679679.
24. Jiang et al., "Artificial Intelligence in Healthcare."
25. Kai Ming Ting, "Sensitivity and Specificity," in *Encyclopedia of Machine Learning*, ed. Claude Sammut and Geoffrey I. Webb (Boston: Springer, 2011), 901–2, https://doi.org/10.1007/978-0-387-30164-8_752.
26. As we will see later, one concern in algorithmic development and implementation is the use of algorithms in more diverse populations or settings than those of the original training and testing datasets.
27. Sidey-Gibbons and Sidey-Gibbons, "Machine Learning in Medicine"; Scott Mayer McKinney et al., "International Evaluation of an AI System for Breast Cancer Screening," *Nature* 577 (2020): 89–94, https://doi.org/10.1038/s41586-019-1799-6.
28. Andre Esteva et al., "Dermatologist-Level Classification of Skin Cancer with Deep Neural Networks," *Nature* 542 (2017): 115–18, https://doi.org/10.1038/nature21056.
29. As we will see shortly, biases in skin lesion algorithms have raised questions of whether these technologies can benefit different populations equitably, as they may be less accurate in underserved populations due to a lack of data representation for training and testing.
30. Vikram Singh Bisen, "What is Human in the Loop Machine Learning: Why and How Used in AI?" Medium, May 20, 2020, https://medium.com/vsinghbisen/what-is-human-in-the-loop-machine-learning-why-how-used-in-ai-60c7b44eb2c0.
31. Hany Alashwal et al., "The Application of Unsupervised Clustering Methods to Alzheimer's Disease," *Frontiers in Computational Neuroscience* 13 (2019), https://doi.org/10.3389/fncom.2019.00031.
32. Jennifer Prendki, "Are You Spending Too Much Money Labeling Data?" Towards Data Science, March 24, 2020, https://towardsdatascience.com/are-you-spending-too-much-money-labeling-data-70a712123df1.

33. Ziad Obermeyer et al., "Dissecting Racial Bias in an Algorithm Used to Manage the Health of Populations," *Science* 366, no. 6464 (October 2019): 447–53, https://doi.org/10.1126/science.aax2342.
34. Jiang et al., "Artificial Intelligence in Healthcare."
35. Mittelstadt et al., "Ethics of Algorithms."
36. Eliezer Bose and Kavita Radhakrishnan, "Using Unsupervised Machine Learning to Identify Subgroups among Home Health Patients with Heart Failure Using Telehealth," *Computers, Informatics, Nursing* 36, no. 5 (2018): 242–48, https://doi.org/10.1097/CIN.0000000000000423.
37. Mittelstadt et al., "Ethics of Algorithms."
38. Alashwal et al., "Application of Unsupervised Clustering."
39. J. Madison Hyer et al., "Assessment of Utilization Efficiency Using Machine Learning Techniques: A Study of Heterogeneity in Preoperative Healthcare Utilization among Super-Utilizers," *American Journal of Surgery* 220, no. 3 (2020): 714–20, https://doi.org/10.1016/j.amjsurg.2020.01.043.
40. Alashwal et al., "Application of Unsupervised Clustering."
41. Alashwal et al., "Application of Unsupervised Clustering."
42. Daniele Ravì et al., "Deep Learning for Health Informatics," *IEEE Journal of Biomedical and Health Informatics* 21, no. 1 (January 2017): 4–21, https://doi.org/10.1109/JBHI.2016.2636665.
43. Jiang et al., "Artificial Intelligence in Healthcare."
44. Riccardo Miotto et al., "Deep Patient: An Unsupervised Representation to Predict the Future of Patients from the Electronic Health Records," *Scientific Reports* 6 (2016), https://doi.org/10.1038/srep26094.
45. Sidey-Gibbons and Sidey-Gibbons, "Machine Learning in Medicine."
46. Ian Goodfellow, Yoshua Bengio, and Aaron Courville, *Deep Learning*, 1st ed. (Cambridge, MA: MIT Press, 2016).
47. Riccardo Miotto et al., "Deep Learning for Healthcare: Review, Opportunities and Challenges," *Briefings in Bioinformatics* 19, no. 6 (2018): 1236–46, https://doi.org/10.1093/bib/bbx044.
48. Ariel Bleicher, "Demystifying the Black Box That Is AI," *Scientific American*, August 9, 2017, https://www.scientificamerican.com/article/demystifying-the-black-box-that-is-ai/.
49. Jiang et al., "Artificial Intelligence in Healthcare."
50. Jiang et al., "Artificial Intelligence in Healthcare."
51. Christine Korsgaard, *The Sources of Normativity* (Cambridge: Cambridge University Press, 1996); Christine Korsgaard, *Self-Constitution: Agency, Identity, and Integrity* (Oxford: Oxford University Press, 2009).
52. Bleicher, "Demystifying the Black Box."

53. Miotto et al., "Deep Learning for Healthcare"; "Machine Learning Tools Unlock the Most Critical Insights from Unstructured Health Data," Health Catalyst, December 6, 2019, https://www.healthcatalyst.com/insights/healthcare-machine-learning-unlocks-unstructured-data.
54. Fiona J. Gilbert et al., "Single Reading with Computer-Aided Detection for Screening Mammography," *New England Journal of Medicine* 359, no. 16 (October 2008): 1675–84, https://doi.org/10.1056/NEJMoa0803545.
55. Alvin Rajkomar et al., "Scalable and Accurate Deep Learning with Electronic Health Records," *npj Digital Medicine* 1 (2018), article 18, https://doi.org/10.1038/s41746-018-0029-1.
56. Igor F. Tsigelny, "Artificial Intelligence in Drug Combination Therapy," *Briefings in Bioinformatics* 20, no. 4 (2018): 1434–48, https://doi.org/10.1093/bib/bby004.
57. Bleicher, "Demystifying the Black Box."
58. Miotto et al., "Deep Patient."
59. Erping Long et al., "An Artificial Intelligence Platform for the Multihospital Collaborative Management of Congenital Cataracts," *Nature Biomedical Engineering* 1 (2017), https://doi.org/10.1038/s41551-016-0024.
60. Esteva et al., "Dermatologist-Level Classification."
61. Varun Gulshan et al., "Development and Validation of a Deep Learning Algorithm for Detection of Diabetic Retinopathy in Retinal Fundus Photographs," *Journal of the American Medical Association* 316, no. 22 (2016): 2402–10, https://doi.org/10.1001/jama.2016.17216.
62. Wafaa Aljbawi, Sami O. Simmons, and Visara Urovi, "Developing a Multi-Variate Prediction Model for the Detection of COVID-19 from Crowd-Sourced Respiratory Voice Data," arXiv (preprint, September 8, 2022), https://arxiv.org/abs/2209.03727.
63. Ronald C. Merrell, "Geriatric Telemedicine: Background and Evidence for Telemedicine as a Way to Address the Challenges of Geriatrics," *Healthcare Informatics Research* 21, no. 4 (2015): 223–29, https://doi.org/10.4258/hir.2015.21.4.223.
64. Josephine McMurray et al., "The Importance of Trust in the Adoption and Use of Intelligent Assistive Technology by Older Adults to Support Aging in Place: Scoping Review Protocol," *JMIR Research Protocols* 6, no. 11 (2017): e218, https://doi.org/10.2196/resprot.8772; E. Ray Dorsey et al., "Moving Parkinson Care to the Home," *Movement Disorders* 31, no. 9 (2016): 1258–62, https://doi.org/10.1002/mds.26744.
65. Anita Ho and Oliver Quick, "Leaving Patients to Their Own Devices? Smart Technology, Safety and Therapeutic Relationships," *BMC Medical Ethics* 19 (2018), article 18, https://doi.org/10.1186/s12910-018-0255-8.

66. Jing Gao et al., "A Survey on Deep Learning for Multimodal Data Fusion," *Neural Computation* 32, no. 5 (2020): 829–64, https://doi.org/10.1162/neco_a_01273.
67. Cynthia Rudin and Joanna Radin,"Why Are We Using Black Box Models in AI When We Don't Need To? A Lesson from an Explainable AI Competition," *Harvard Data Science Review* 1, no. 2 (Fall 2019), https://doi.org/10.1162/99608f92.5a8a3a3d.
68. Mittelstadt et al., "Ethics of Algorithms."
69. Juan Manuel Durán and Karin Rolanda Jongsma, "Who is Afraid of Black Box Algorithms? On the Epistemological and Ethical Basis of Trust in Medical AI," *Journal of Medical Ethics* 47, no. 5 (2021): 329–35, https://doi.org/10.1136/medethics-2020-106820.
70. Eliza Strickland, "IBM Watson, Heal Thyself: How IBM Overpromised and Underdelivered on AI Health Care," *IEEE Spectrum* 56, no. 4 (April 2019): 24–31, https://doi.org/10.1109/MSPEC.2019.8678513.
71. Strickland, "IBM Watson, Heal Thyself."
72. Organization for Economic Cooperation and Development, *Trustworthy AI in Health*.
73. Won-Suk Lee et al., "Assessing Concordance with Watson for Oncology, a Cognitive Computing Decision Support System for Colon Cancer Treatment in Korea," *JCO Clinical Cancer Informatics* 2 (December 2018): 1–8, https://doi.org/10.1200/CCI.17.00109.
74. Suthida Suwanvecho et al., "Concordance Assessment of a Cognitive Computing System in Thailand," *Journal of Clinical Oncology* 35, no. 15_suppl (May 2017): 6589, https://doi.org/10.1200/JCO.2017.35.15_suppl.6589.
75. Na Zhou et al., "Concordance Study between IBM Watson for Oncology and Clinical Practice for Patients with Cancer in China," *The Oncologist* 24, no. 6 (June 2019): 812–19, https://doi.org/10.1634/theoncologist.2018-0255.
76. Strickland, "IBM Watson, Heal Thyself."
77. Strickland, "IBM Watson, Heal Thyself."
78. Steve Lohr, "What Ever Happened to IBM's Watson?," *New York Times*, July 17, 2021, https://www.nytimes.com/2021/07/16/technology/what-happened-ibm-watson.html.
79. Heather Landi, "IBM Sells Watson Health Assets to Investment Firm Francisco Partners," Fierce Healthcare, January 21, 2022, https://www.fiercehealthcare.com/tech/ibm-sells-watson-health-assets-to-investment-firm-francisco-partners.
80. Durán and Jongsma, "Who is Afraid of Black Box Algorithms?"

81. Danton S. Char, Michael D. Abràmoff, and Chris Feudtner, "Identifying Ethical Considerations for Machine Learning Healthcare Applications," *American Journal of Bioethics* 20, no. 11 (November 2020): 7–17, https://doi.org/10.1080/15265161.2020.1819469.
82. Shannon Vallor, *Technology and the Virtues: A Philosophical Guide to a Future Worth Wanting* (New York: Oxford University Press, 2016).
83. Richard Van Noorden, "The Ethical Questions That Haunt Facial-Recognition Research," *Nature* 587, no. 7834 (November 2020): 354–58, https://doi.org/10.1038/d41586-020-03187-3.
84. Karen Hao, "AI Is Sending People to Jail—and Getting It Wrong," *MIT Technology Review*, January 21, 2019, https://www.technologyreview.com/2019/01/21/137783/algorithms-criminal-justice-ai/.
85. Adewole S. Adamson and Avery Smith, "Machine Learning and Health Care Disparities in Dermatology," *JAMA Dermatology* 154, no. 11 (2018): 1247–48, https://doi.org/10.1001/jamadermatol.2018.2348.
86. Erin Brodwin and Nicholas St. Fleur, "FDA Issues Alert on 'Limitations' of Pulse Oximeters, Without Explicit Mention of Racial Bias," STAT, February 19, 2021, https://www.statnews.com/2021/02/19/fda-issues-alert-on-limitations-of-pulse-oximeters-without-explicit-mention-of-racial-bi/.
87. Michael W. Sjoding et al., "Racial Bias in Pulse Oximetry Measurement," *New England Journal of Medicine* 383, no. 25 (2020): 2477–78, https://doi.org/10.1056/NEJMc2029240.
88. U.S. Food and Drug Administration, "Pulse Oximeter Accuracy and Limitations: FDA Safety Communication," February 19, 2021, https://www.fda.gov/medical-devices/safety-communications/pulse-oximeter-accuracy-and-limitations-fda-safety-communication.
89. Sjoding et al., "Racial Bias in Pulse Oximetry Measurement."
90. Casey Ross, "At Mayo Clinic, Sharing Patient Data with Companies Fuels AI Innovation—and Concerns about Consent," STAT, June 3, 2020, https://www.statnews.com/2020/06/03/mayo-clinic-patient-data-fuels-artificial-intelligence-consent-concerns/.
91. Kit Huckvale, John Torous, and Mark E. Larsen, "Assessment of the Data Sharing and Privacy Practices of Smartphone Apps for Depression and Smoking Cessation," *JAMA Network Open* 2, no. 4 (April 2019): e192542, https://doi.org/10.1001/jamanetworkopen.2019.2542.
92. U.S. Department for Health and Human Services. "Federal Policy for the Protection of Human Subjects ('Common Rule'). 2018. https://www.hhs.gov/ohrp/regulations-and-policy/regulations/common-rule/index.html

93. Anita Ho, "Deep Ethical Learning: Taking the Interplay of Human and Artificial Intelligence Seriously," *Hastings Center Report* 49, no. 1 (2019): 38–41, https://doi.org/10.1002/hast.977.
94. Catriona Mackenzie, "Feminist Innovation in Philosophy: Relational Autonomy and Social Justice," *Women's Studies International Forum* 72 (2019): 144–51, https://doi.org/10.1016/j.wsif.2018.05.003.
95. I use the phrases "people with disabilities" and "disabled people" interchangeably throughout this book. While the term "people with disabilities" is generally preferable because it emphasizes the person rather than the impairment, some people considered themselves "disabled," not by something inherent in them, but by a world that is not equipped to allow them to participate and flourish. Mary Ann McColl, *Appreciative Disability Studies* (Concord, Ontario: Captus Press, 2019).
96. Deborah Lupton and Annemarie Jutel, "'It's Like Having a Physician in Your Pocket!' A Critical Analysis of Self-Diagnosis Smartphone Apps," *Social Science & Medicine* 133 (2015): 128–35, https://doi.org/10.1016/j.socscimed.2015.04.004; Annemarie Jutel and Deborah Lupton, "Digitizing Diagnosis: A Review of Mobile Applications in the Diagnostic Process," *Diagnosis* 2, no. 2 (2015): 89–96, https://doi.org/10.1515/dx-2014-0068.
97. Daniel L. Labovitz et al., "Using Artificial Intelligence to Reduce the Risk of Nonadherence in Patients on Anticoagulation Therapy," *Stroke* 48, no. 5 (2017): 1416–19, https://doi.org/10.1161/STROKEAHA.116.016281.
98. Fogel and Kvedar, "Artificial Intelligence Powers Digital Medicine"; Aurel O. Iuga and Maura J. McGuire, "Adherence and Health Care Costs," *Risk Management and Healthcare Policy* 7 (2014): 35–44, https://doi.org/10.2147/RMHP.S19801; Meera Viswanathan et al., "Interventions to Improve Adherence to Self-Administered Medications for Chronic Diseases in the United States: A Systematic Review," *Annals of Internal Medicine* 157, no. 11 (2012): 785–95, https://doi.org/10.7326/0003-4819-157-11-201212040-00538.
99. Daniel Z. Buchman, Anita Ho, and Judy Illes, "You Present Like a Drug Addict: Patient and Clinician Perspectives on Trust and Trustworthiness in Chronic Pain Management," *Pain Medicine* 17, no. 8 (2016): 1394–406, https://doi.org/10.1093/pm/pnv083.
100. Thomas Nys, "Autonomy, Trust, and Respect," *Journal of Medicine and Philosophy* 41, no. 1 (2016): 10–24.
101. Simone Lee Joannou, "Toward an Account of Relational Autonomy in Healthcare and Treatment Settings," *Essays in the Philosophy of Humanism* 24, no. 1 (2016): 1–20.

102. Carolyn McLeod and Susan Sherwin, "Relational Autonomy, Self-Trust, and Health Care for Patients Who Are Oppressed," in *Relational Autonomy: Feminist Perspectives on Autonomy, Agency, and the Social Self*, ed. Catriona Mackenzie and Natalie Stoljar (New York: Oxford University Press, 2000), 259–79, https://ir.lib.uwo.ca/philosophypub/345.

1

Artificial Autonomy or Relational Intelligence

How Relationality Matters in Health Monitoring

As we saw in the Preface and Introduction, artificial intelligence (AI) health monitoring is not a morally neutral technological endeavor.[1] Intersecting standards and expectations regarding predictive analytics, risk tolerance, personal and data privacy, and self-care are expressed in the evolving social, technological, and health care landscape. The ability of AI technologies to continuously monitor, analyze, and predict people's behavior and health is changing how we diagnose diseases, forecast health decline, and deliver care. These advancing technological capabilities can affect not only users' health status but also their ability to make autonomous decisions and challenge algorithmic outputs. They raise the important bioethical question of how we can ensure responsible and responsive AI health monitoring practices that can equitably promote the autonomy and well-being of prospective users.

A liberal conception of autonomy, which has generally been the foundational Western bioethical value used to justify informed consent requirements and promote other forms of patient engagement in health care, is sometimes utilized both explicitly and implicitly to support the development and adoption of AI health monitoring. As we will see, via various use cases throughout this book, in popular portrayal of AI development, prospective users of continuous and automated monitoring are promised access to and control of their health data, and that these technologies will help them live freer and more independent lives. In this chapter, I begin by explaining how this liberal account of autonomy, which largely focuses on self-determination in terms of an individual's capacity and authenticity in making choices that align with their values, is too individualistic and narrow to adequately capture the impact of the rapid proliferation of AI health monitoring technologies on people's ability to determine how they would like health monitoring to take place, who should have access to their data, and how collected data can be used. To fully consider these matters, I follow Catriona Mackenzie's tripartite conceptualization of autonomy, which consists of three distinct but causally interdependent axes of autonomy: self-governance, self-determination, and self-authorization.[2] I argue for a constitutively relational approach to autonomy that emphasizes interpersonal, social, and structural conditions as crucial to these three intertwining dimensions of autonomy, and problematize the rapid development and adoption of AI health monitoring technologies through this relational lens. This conceptualization moves relationships and the power asymmetries within these relationships from the periphery to the center of bioethical analysis and practice; it underscores the integral role relationships play in promoting or curbing people's ability to develop and exercise autonomy.[3]

In the context of AI health monitoring, a relational approach to autonomy underscores external socio-relational and opportunity conditions, including available health monitoring options, personal care and professional therapeutic relationships, and health care delivery practices, which are necessary for agents to have de facto power and authority over decisions significant to the direction of their lives. This framework highlights how social domination, oppression, stigmatization, and injustice can thwart individual autonomy, and how increasing optimism towards emerging AI health monitoring technologies and related data practices may restructure interpersonal and professional relations that can affect people's ability to truly form and live according to their reflective self-concepts. A relational lens also helps us to consider possible solutions, such as what types of constructive social and therapeutic relationships, institutional practices, or governance or regulatory structures are necessary to promote people's autonomy in the realm of health monitoring, regardless of whether AI technologies are adopted. Without the relevant social, professional, institutional, and systemic conditions that support people's ability to determine how they would like their health to be monitored and whether they can trust the integrity of the governance structure for these technological processes, people's opportunities and capacity to exercise their autonomy about AI or other health monitoring modalities will be unduly constrained.

1. The Liberal Conception of Autonomy: An Individualist Focus

In most Western societies, particularly since the Enlightenment, respect for individual autonomy has been a foundational principle of liberal and democratic theories. This "cardinal moral value" demands respect for people's interests and normative authority in living their lives according to their own conception of the good.[4] While this principle has also shaped discussions in contemporary Western bioethics across the life cycle, from reproductive matters to end-of-life care, until the second half of the twentieth century, conscientious physicians were actually trained to act paternalistically towards their patients.[5] Prior to that, lay patients were presumed to have minimal to no understanding of medical procedures and practices; they were mostly considered passive recipients of medical care, which was directed by physicians who were uniquely qualified and authorized to properly identify and understand symptoms, draw useful conclusions, and provide treatments according to the physician's own judgment about what would be best for their patients. Patients' own perspectives or preferences were considered irrelevant or unnecessary in determining the most appropriate treatment.

Social attitudes towards physician expertise in the United States began to shift in the second half of the century. While scientific and therapeutic progress further extended the clinical powers of medical professionals,[6] reinforcing the tendency of physicians to assume that they were better able than the patient to judge what was in the latter's best interest,[7] the public began to question how much authority doctors should have on health care decisions. Even though expanding arrays of advancing health care options and powerful drugs provided new hope for curing various conditions, controlling symptoms that accompany various conditions, and extending life expectancy, these treatments came with different levels and types of risks, benefits, and uncertainties. For example, many insurance plans in the United States adopt a step therapy approach, whereby insurers obligate patients to try a less costly treatment and "fail first" with that before covering another, more costly treatment.[8] Depending on the stringency of these policies and how they define ineffectiveness, patients may have to weigh the tradeoffs between a more expensive treatment with fewer side effects and a covered treatment that requires longer recovery time and more unpleasant effects. Patients who suffer from catastrophic accidents or illnesses—or their families—may also need to weigh the benefits and burdens of invasive life-sustaining treatments. Health care decisions often involve intimate and central aspects of a patient's life, including not only matters of health, illness, and death, but also reproduction, bodily integrity, lifestyle, self-image, as well as financial and psychological well-being.[9] As physicians who were well versed in clinical factors might nonetheless be ignorant of patients' broader non-clinical goals and concerns, there was an increasing recognition that patients were uniquely qualified to weigh these competing clinical and non-clinical priorities in making health care decisions.

Historical events and political movements in this era also worked to secure entitlements and rights, to increase equity and equality in the distribution of health care resources, and to dissolve power-oriented hierarchies in therapeutic relationships.[10] The Nuremberg Medical Trial (1946–1947) exposed the international need for more professional standards to prevent research and medical ethics transgressions. In addition to convicting twenty-three leading German physicians and administrators of war crimes and crimes against humanity for their roles in cruel and often lethal concentration camp medical experiments, the court also articulated a ten-point set of research ethics rules, known as the Nuremberg Code.[11] And in the 1960s, partly as a result of simmering public opposition to the U.S. war in Vietnam and the civil rights movement, there was a growing suspicion of institutional authorities and a higher emphasis on individual rights in an increasingly pluralistic society. The recognition that people of diverse backgrounds and realities may hold different conceptions of the good that frame their life goals and health care priorities was accompanied by a rising movement of consumer and patient empowerment, supported by various court decisions. U.S. courts, such as in the case of *Salgo v. Leland Stanford Jr. University Board of Trustees* (1957), began to recognize that physicians' unilateral decisions could lead to results that diverge from patients' own interests and goals.[12] In this case, Martin Salgo awoke paralyzed in his lower extremities after an aortography, in which dye was injected into the aorta to determine if it was blocked. He had never been informed that such a risk existed. The court determined that failure to disclose risks and alternatives was cause for legal action on its own. It announced a new legal doctrine—informed consent—that required physicians to provide patients with all relevant information about their health status and available treatment alternatives, and to allow *patients* to decide how to balance the risks and benefits associated with any particular procedure or treatment. The field of bioethics also emerged in the United States in the late 1960s, placing the rights and interests of patients and research participants at the center of its theorizing,[13] challenging the "doctors know best" attitude that may usurp patients' autonomy. Legislations, regulations, and professional practices continued to evolve to address medical paternalism and prevent potential abuses of power that may arise in these asymmetrical relationships marked by epistemic and social hierarchies.

1.1 Internal and External Conditions for Autonomy

As treatment options continue to expand in technologically advancing societies, there is now a general acceptance of the liberal conception of autonomy in health care, whereby informed patients have the right to reject other people's undue influence and to make health care decisions based on their own goals and values. This conception of autonomy often focuses on the internal and external conditions for autonomy. *Internal* conditions include an individual's competency and authenticity conditions, while external conditions highlight the freedom conditions that allow an individual to carry out their goals and wishes.

Competency denotes one's decision-making capacity. Humans are agents who can develop and exercise their skills and capacities to reflect and form a self-conception that embodies their sense of self-identity, motives, values, or priorities, and then deliberate upon these desires and circumstances to make decisions accordingly.[14] We are capable of normative self-governance by virtue of our ability to explain or justify our actions and decisions.[15] The Kantian principle of respect for autonomy, for example, espouses the idea that persons are rational agents with the internal capacity to determine their own ends or goals; this capacity is the locus and origin of one's absolute inner worth or unconditional value as a moral agent.[16] This substantive account of autonomy focused on the ability of self-governing agents to deliberate and self-determine moral laws under the guidance of practical reason.[17] *Authenticity* conditions specify what it means to be self-governing with respect to one's motivational structure.[18] An authentic individual identifies with their enduring and stable psychological elements such as beliefs, values, and desires—ones that the person would endorse or accept upon critical and informed self-reflection.[19] In contemporary Western bioethics, liberal accounts of autonomy have provided grounds for rejecting or at least constraining medical paternalism. It is now generally accepted that patients are capable of forming their own global conception of a good life and making various domain-specific decisions that align with that self-conception, such that they should be allowed to do so without undue pressure from others.

Intersecting with the internal conditions are *external* conditions for autonomy, which involve having the actual ability to carry out one's goals and wishes. Even for moral agents who have the capacity to form their own self-conception and discern what follows from their corresponding values and desires, their practical ability to act accordingly depends on whether they have the freedom to make and enact relevant choices based on their practical identity.[20]

External freedom conditions consist of both negative and positive conditions for individual autonomy. *Negative freedom conditions* are the social, institutional, and political constraints that interfere with the exercise of self-determination.[21] For example, legislations and institutional practices that restrict access to various forms of reproductive control services (e.g., abortion, pre-implantation genetic diagnosis) or end-of-life interventions (e.g., physician-assisted dying) are often cited by critics as examples of illegitimate curtailment of people's liberty to pursue their personal and health goals. *Positive freedom conditions* are the political and personal liberties that enable people with decisional capacity to exercise autonomy, such as legislations and professional practices that protect or promote freedom of expression, religion, privacy, and confidentiality. The development of advance directives and growing legislations decriminalizing assisted dying, patients' bills of rights, and the rise of bioethics consultations and ombudspersons who educate patients regarding their rights are some examples of provisions that can enhance patients' positive freedom. Regulatory protections that ensure patient confidentiality and appropriate sharing of patient data are other examples, as legislations such as the Health Insurance Portability and Accountability Act (HIPAA) allow patients to feel freer to disclose their health concerns to facilitate appropriate care plans without fear of discrimination by external parties.[22]

Considering internal and external conditions for autonomy, a liberal conception of autonomy generally demands that patients who are capable of forming and reflecting critically on their desires and beliefs be allowed the freedom to act according to their own goals and intentions, without coercive or manipulative influence by other individuals or institutions. In medical research and clinical care delivery, respect for autonomy requires that potential research participants and patients with decisional capacity be informed of relevant research and health care matters and be allowed to decide whether they will accept or refuse various clinical trial opportunities or treatment recommendations.[23] Even if a patient is potentially making unwise decisions regarding their own health, their standing as a moral agent, capable of forming opinions and acting according to their practical identity, requires that their health care providers afford them the right to accept and refuse various recommendations as they see fit. Respect for individual autonomy also stipulates that people will not be made worse off (e.g., lose access to services) if they reject these opportunities or recommendations.

In the context of AI health monitoring, the application of a liberal conception of autonomy would require that moral agents be allowed to decide how and where they would like their health and well-being to be monitored, by whom or by what method, and on what temporal basis. It would demand that health care providers, hospitals, insurance companies, and related entities explicitly notify patients that AI (or the particular algorithmic method) is being piloted, used, or offered in health monitoring; elucidate why such monitoring is recommended or adopted; explain to patients what this means regarding the collection and utilization of their health and ancillary data, and the potential risks and benefits of utilizing the recommended monitoring technology; and respect patients' liberty to agree or refuse to utilize the recommended technologies. If patients do not have the choice to opt out in situations where the adoption of AI processes is decided on an institutional or health system level,[24] other communication strategies to inform patients about the operational implications and impacts on patient care may be required. For example, knowing how health care providers may use the predictive outcomes and in which part of their treatment, such as who is making the critical aspects of the care planning decisions or carrying out the care responsibilities if AI is used, would be important.[25]

As AI-powered technologies are intrinsically data-driven platforms that in turn amass a vast amount of heterogeneous forms of user data, respect for individual autonomy under the liberal conception includes providing transparent and understandable information about what types of data are being collected by the proposed AI health monitoring platform, how the data may be utilized in the predictive analytical process to facilitate health care management and delivery, who may have access to the collected data and for what purposes (e.g., family and professional caregivers, insurance companies, employers, other third parties), whether collected data will be anonymized, and how/whether one may be able to withdraw consent to the use of these technologies and data sharing at a later time. Given that much of AI health monitoring is still in research, developmental, or proof-of-concept stages, and that available algorithms are accompanied by varying levels of risks, limitations, and errors, promotion of self-determination requires that people have the freedom to discern and weigh the uncertain or unknown risks and benefits of AI health monitoring in the context of their other life goals or priorities. This is especially important given that the public may presume that any tools and interventions used in the highly regulated realm of medicine would have already been proven to be safe and effective. Moreover, misuse of people's personal and health data in the context of big data may have a magnified discriminatory impact or impose other devastating psychological, economic, and social harms, compromising people's ability to create and pursue their own pathways. We can imagine insurance companies wanting to use data collected through direct-to-consumer (DTC) health monitoring devices or AI home health monitoring to train other learning algorithms to predict prospective customers' future functional status and thereby determine long-term care or life insurance premiums. And since predictive algorithms may have biases and other limitations—ones that may be difficult to identify or isolate in the deep neural networks—the use of such algorithms will require transparent processes regarding how disputes about algorithmic decisions may be handled if we are to protect patients' capacities for self-determination. Recalling the example of the high-risk care management algorithm from the Introduction, patients should be informed regarding the role of the algorithm in their care management, and whether/how they can appeal their risk scores if they perceive that their illness severity is higher or lower than indicated by the algorithm.[26]

One important aspect of the liberal discussions and practices around respecting patient autonomy is that they generally assess autonomy in an individualistic manner, by looking at one person and one health care decision at a time; each decisional context is considered separate from one another rather than a part of a broader social or cultural practice.[27] A decision is deemed autonomous if a self-governing patient, construed as a "normal chooser," has and understands the relevant information about the available health monitoring options and makes an intentional choice according to their values and preferences, without coercion from others. The focus here is on ensuring that external parties, such as a patient's health care providers or family members, are not unduly influencing the patient's capacity to make that particular decision in ways that compromise the person's decisional process.[28]

Certainly, an individualistic focus on each person's capacity, authenticity, and decision-making process provides some level of autonomy protection, given that different individuals in diverse societies have varying practical identities and considerations as they discern whether or how AI health monitoring may promote their goals compared to other modalities. Nonetheless, I contend that an individualist focus is too narrow and is thus ultimately insufficient in addressing all the relevant normative and practical concerns surrounding prospective AI health monitoring users' motivational structure.[29] Individualist frameworks miss the significance of other external powers, which are not simply or always tied to individual actions (e.g., a health care provider directly exerts pressure on a patient to accept a particular AI home health monitoring platform).[30] Though blatantly paternalistic practices are now commonly criticized as compromising people's autonomy, power hierarchies—which are generally not key considerations under the individualist conception of autonomy—continue to structure medical encounters and health care recommendations in subtle but forceful ways, albeit masked as voluntary choices based on individual consent.

At the same time, not all curtailment of freedom hinders people's ability to reflectively form and exercise their practical identities. For example, some people may decline any form of data participation on a whim even when it is purely anonymous, requires no effort on their part, cannot be traced back to the person, and has no impact on their lives or interests. There are situations where some limits to individual freedom may be necessary to achieve important public health goals that are not otherwise attainable, as highlighted during the COVID-19 pandemic and in the ongoing American discourses around gun regulations. We thus cannot fully assess autonomy without critically evaluating how or whether the interconnected social, political, and structural frameworks may affect the availability of meaningful opportunities or how individuals approach their situations.[31]

2. Autonomy in AI Health Monitoring: The Need for a Relational Lens

In other words, promotion of autonomy involves more than having a process to obtain voluntary and informed consent for specific technologies or health outcomes. Social domination, oppressive or exploitative environments, deprivation, and other forms of injustice can thwart people's ability to fully develop and live according to their reflective self-concepts in the first place. In the context of AI health monitoring, various external and environmental factors can affect how our society decides to invest in certain health monitoring resources over others, thereby predetermining patients' resource and service eligibilities, including what types or levels of health monitoring they can receive. As health systems and commercial developers show increasing interest in integrating digital and remote health monitoring tools into people's everyday lives, promoting them as more accurate and efficient methods of care, these technological processes also exert new forms of power over people's own embodied experiences and predetermine their available choices, regardless of their practical identity or values as part of their self-concepts. An adequate conception of autonomy must therefore address how people's decisions around AI health monitoring are embedded within a complex set of social relations, professional practices, societal norms/expectations, and policies/regulations—they structure an individual's selfhood and can significantly affect their ability to exercise autonomy with respect to their choices.[32] A commitment to autonomy thus requires a relational lens, one that highlights not only individual but also structural conditions that may compromise or facilitate people's ability to develop their self-conception and navigate health monitoring decisions according to their practical identity.

In the United States, changing demographics, digitization of health care information and processes, involvement of technologists and entrepreneurs in health sectors, lax regulations for wellness technologies, as well as insurance coverage and reimbursements for health monitoring and diagnostic tests may affect how health promotion and acceptable risk tolerance are defined and managed at a system level.[33] As AI health monitoring technologies are increasingly proposed in response to these evolving social factors, health systems' rapid deployment or embrace of these technologies may drastically impact people's available options and ability to decide reflectively how they would like to manage their health according to their practical identities. The liberal individualist focus neglects how quickly evolving socio-technological practices and expectations may leave people who are uncomfortable with automated predictive technologies with no reasonable alternatives but to accept AI health monitoring. Some health systems have been sharing patients' de-identified electronic health record (EHR) data for AI development or using various forms of AI without seeking consent or explaining why such technology is believed to be more effective.[34] For example, without notifying patients about algorithmic involvement, a large health system in Minnesota has been utilizing an AI algorithm to help make discharge planning decisions, and other prominent health systems have been using a life-expectancy prediction algorithm to prompt physicians to have end-of-life care discussions with patients who are expected to die within a year.[35] Even if these may be "operational" decisions that do not generally require patient consent, as the utilization of these algorithms may affect how physicians approach their patients' care management (e.g., whether to begin end-of-life care planning with the patient during a particular hospital stay), failure to inform people about these practices and their rationales precludes opportunities to learn more about them, thus perpetuating technological illiteracy and potential distrust.

Given the effects of wider socio-contextual factors on people's freedom and opportunity to define their own good, it is important to consider whether a given individual would choose automated and continuous AI health monitoring if other care alternatives and living environments were available or accessible. To account for these factors, I adopt Catriona Mackenzie's relational theorization of autonomy as comprising three distinct but causally interdependent axes (self-governance, self-determination, and self-authorization), which attend to broader external and structural considerations of people's decisional contexts.[36] I argue that a normatively adequate framework of autonomy for AI health monitoring needs to go beyond determining whether an individual has the decisional authority to adopt a particular health monitoring technology. Such considerations are necessary but insufficient for fully establishing what would constitute meaningful conditions for people to exercise their autonomy. As we will see in subsequent chapters, these technologies are promoted as tools not only to improve health but also to democratize health information and facilitate people's desired living and care arrangements. Potential users' ability to make health care monitoring decisions based on their practical identity must thus be understood in the intersecting context of competing social, normative, and pragmatic considerations, given the technological requirements and functionality of AI outside of the clinics and hospitals. This relational approach draws attention to how various social and systemic forces that impose or predefine notions of healthy or independent living can impair people's autonomy, particularly for older adults and those with certain disabilities or mental conditions, whose ability to form their self-conception and whose power to act accordingly may be further constrained due to stigmatized identities. If we accept that AI health monitoring is a generally worthwhile social strategy, then we must also determine how to achieve what Rosamond Rhodes calls "collaborative necessity," as widescale participation and data sharing may be necessary to ensure algorithmic accuracy and equitable benefits for all populations,[37] but willingness to participate may require the public's trust in the integrity and governance of these activities. This raises intersecting questions of how to structure health monitoring and related data and care delivery practices in ways that will still promote people's ability to lead self-determining lives, their capacity for self-governance, and their confidence in being self-authorizing agents as they discern whether continuous algorithmic monitoring fits with their life and health priorities.

In the remainder of this chapter, I present a constitutively relational approach to autonomy that will serve as a conceptual foundation for analyzing the complex ethical implications and decisional considerations for AI health monitoring. This conception emphasizes that, because humans are embodied and socially constituted, the development of our practical identities and the competencies required for governing and expressing the self are intricately tied to the extensive interpersonal, social, and institutional structures that either support or deprive the development and exercise of autonomy. Such a conception asks how the social system ought to be organized to ensure that people have genuinely meaningful opportunities to form and critically reflect upon their priorities about health monitoring, understand how their data may be handled and shared in the new era of big data, and make health maintenance decisions that will realize their practical identities accordingly. This relational lens highlights the fact that utilization of AI in health monitoring is not simply a computational or technological endeavor to improve people's health and functioning.[38] Individuals' desire and ability to utilize these technologies (vs. other health monitoring modalities) partly depend on the social conditions within which the evolution and adoption of these platforms reflect and simultaneously reinforce various social and health care norms and expectations, thereby reframing people's available options and thus their decisional processes, regardless of their true desires. The objectives behind the development and promotion of AI health monitoring are fundamentally socio-relational, with deep moral meanings, and may affect people's ability to be the normative and practical authors of their own personal and health pursuits. This may in turn impact their self-conception and autonomy.

A relational approach to autonomy takes vulnerability, dependency, and socio-relational needs, whether temporary or permanent, as starting points. It recognizes the necessity of building a trustworthy governance system that acknowledges that humans desire and require different forms and extents of assistance throughout their life cycles, and critically informs evaluations of emerging AI health monitoring practices within a socio-relational context. In particular, it focuses on how structural privileges and oppressions manifest in health care and technological practices.[39] Attending to patterns of hierarchically structured social relations, it calls for the correction of professional, institutional, and systemic practices that may exert or reinforce social domination and compromise people's ability to self-govern.[40] In subsequent chapters, a relational analysis of various AI health monitoring use cases will illustrate how the experiences and concerns of agents navigating social deprivation, oppression, stigmatization, and injustice, which arise out of potentially and/or inherently unequal care and social relationships, can be exacerbated by continuous and automated monitoring. This relational lens will also help to explore potential solutions to these oppressive forces.

2.1 Self-Governance: Capacities in Navigating Evolving Health Monitoring Technologies

As we saw earlier, the liberal conception of autonomy often begins with ascertaining that a person has the skills and capacities necessary to make decisions about specific situations based on one's reflectively constituted practical identity. This includes having the requisite ability to understand the relevant technical information of how AI health monitoring works and how it may affect one's data and personal privacy, health maintenance, access to professional care, and health outcomes, so that one can make informed decisions about such care management possibilities.

Nonetheless, rational agents' ability to develop these capacities and skills, or self-governance, is not simply a matter of an individual's internal cognitive faculties operating in a cultural vacuum. It depends on socially shaped skills, self-identities, and self-evaluations regarding one's health goals as they intersect with other priorities and concerns. It also depends on externally structured opportunities that determine how the health system and health care providers promote patient education and information exchange, what health monitoring alternatives are available and affordable, and how our health care, social, and regulatory systems govern data practices in the increasingly overlapping commercial and public domains.[41] This last point is particularly important, as many AI algorithms require large amounts of data to enhance robustness and accuracy, such that successful AI development and iterative improvement requires people's willingness to continuously participate and share data in their regular clinical care settings and other digital activities, which may depend on users' understanding of these technological processes and their trust in the various entities developing, promoting, implementing, and regulating these practices.

Take health and digital literacy as examples. Health literacy is the degree to which people can obtain, process, and understand the basic health information and services necessary to make appropriate care decisions.[42] In the United States, over one-third of adults have only basic or below basic health literacy.[43] This raises social justice and health equity concerns, as layers of social disadvantage, shaped by both current and historical misdistributions of money, power, and resources, can unfairly affect a person's health literacy level and compromise their ability to process health information.[44] Low health literacy is associated with more advanced illness, poorer health outcomes, and higher care costs.[45] Moreover, in an era of increasingly complex technological processes, like AI health monitoring, these challenges may be compounded by low levels of digital literacy: In the United States, 16 percent of adults are not digitally literate.[46] Even as electronic and monitoring technologies have become more ubiquitous, and as diverse types of data from these technologies are increasingly merged with real-time data to build consumer and patient profiles for predictive analysis, most people have very limited awareness or understanding of how AI is involved in their everyday life, including in health monitoring.[47] It is important to note that the social determinants of health literacy and digital literacy are quite similar, such that maldistribution of opportunity and resources can affect people's access to both appropriate health information and digital technologies.[48] In the United States, people who are digitally illiterate tend to be less educated and older, and are more likely to be Black, Hispanic, or foreign-born compared to digitally literate adults.[49] Given the rapidly changing domain of AI development and the lack of education on these technologies, members of the lay public, especially those in socioeconomically disadvantaged groups, may be unable to foresee the impact or implications of new data collection and data sharing practices that often accompany AI-powered technologies.

Certainly, traditional research informed consent processes and health care consultations may help to build understanding for patients who are participating in the research development of, or are prescribed, specific monitoring technologies. Nonetheless, some of these requirements are absent outside of the federally funded research realms. Moreover, explaining these new and highly technical platforms and addressing prospective users' concerns in clinical encounters can be challenging, especially since the implications of data collection, data analysis, and data sharing for AI development and implementation often go beyond the particular technology being proposed or implemented.[50] Prospective users of these technologies need to have adequate health and technical literacy to understand how AI health monitoring operates, such as its basic functionality compared to in-person or non-AI remote monitoring to reach a particular goal (e.g., using traditional CCTV vs. computer vision to prevent falls), and the implication of these differences for one's practical identity and care pathways.

For example, as AI algorithms merge and process different types of historical and real-time user data computationally to make automated predictions or suggestions without explicit programming by humans, patients may need to know whether the predictive analytics serve as an assistive clinical decision support tool, or whether they are making automated decisions without human (clinician) involvement. As we will see in subsequent chapters, since AI health monitoring is increasingly promoted as a set of tools that can maintain and enhance people's health, self-governance also means having the capacity to consider how these technologies will affect patients' own roles and ability in managing their own health. Given that AI development relies on big data, people also need to understand how the collected data may be aggregated and shared for machine learning (ML) development and refinement, and the implications on data privacy and data ownership.

Building people's capacity to understand data collection and data sharing in the age of big data requires a considerable time investment from both the health care provider and the patient. For example, when algorithms make predictions from the data using inferential statistics and/or ML techniques, such as the chance of a skin lesion being cancerous, that knowledge remains inevitably uncertain.[51] Thus, it is important for physicians to clarify that even significant correlations do not necessarily imply a causal connection and explain to patients what this epistemic limitation implies, especially if the algorithm may only process users' narrow individual factors without considering the full scope of the user experience and/or various levels of socio-relational determinants of behavior and choice. Unfortunately, these capacity-promoting conditions are lacking in the current health care delivery structure, where physicians face pressure to get through information quickly during limited consultation sessions. Even though the shift from fee-for-service, or volume-based payment, to value-based payment in the United States has allowed clinicians more time with their patients, the average consultation time with a primary care physician is still only approximately 20 minutes.[52] Many topics compete for limited time, especially for patients with complex comorbidities or multiple concerns, such that further discussions on highly technical aspects of AI in these consultations may overwhelm patients rather than build their understanding or decisional capacity.[53]

Exacerbating such problems, doctors often use jargon-filled language in describing or explaining various health matters without confirming patients' understanding. This is significant from a relational self-governance perspective, as inadequate health and technology literacy accentuates the epistemic and power hierarchy between health care providers and patients, which may further affect patients' ability and willingness to ask questions and engage in shared decision-making.[54] Simply providing more technical information in fast-paced and sometimes anxiety-provoking care encounters may diminish rather than enhance understanding or decisional capacity, particularly given the inherent power imbalance in therapeutic relationships.[55] This is especially concerning for patients with declining or low cognitive understanding or mental illnesses, who may be subjected to monitoring based on their presumed health risks but have limited capacity to comprehend the complex algorithmic operations and implications of continuous AI health monitoring.

A related systemic or structural barrier to building people's capacity to understand AI health monitoring is that most medical and professional programs lack curricular requirements or training opportunities in new technologies and bioinformatics or ML/DL (deep learning), such that even physicians may have minimal understanding of how AI health monitoring works, rendering them ill-equipped to guide patients on these technologies. In addition, as we will see in subsequent chapters, AI health monitoring technologies are often developed by non-clinicians, and some are directly marketed to consumers as recreational devices, thus bypassing physician consultation, traditional requirements of informed consent, and other regulatory oversight. Marketing schemes for these "user-friendly" platforms often conflate automated and AI functions or oversimplify the analytical process of algorithms, confusing potential users and compromising their ability to fully understand what is involved in AI health monitoring. It is also noteworthy that black box or non-explainable algorithms, if not compensated by more transparent business and implementation practices, may further prevent potential users from advancing their understanding of how AI health monitoring would fit with their identities and health goals.

An adequate analysis of self-governance must acknowledge the extensive interpersonal, social, and institutional structures necessary for people to develop the cognitive skills and capacities required to navigate various forms of health monitoring decisions. A commitment to self-governance requires that we correct those conditions that may counter capacity development, and promote others that can facilitate it. Recognizing how socio-structural conditions affect people's capacity to understand AI health monitoring, a relational approach to self-governance highlights the need to reconstruct social, professional, educational, and regulatory practices to promote explainable AI and digital literacy. This may include regulations and guidelines for developing explainable AI health technologies and governing how predictive analytics would (not) be used in care delivery, as well as expanded general science and computer education to enhance people's confidence in engaging in AI health monitoring decision-making with their care providers. Moreover, an increased emphasis on knowledge management and communication in medical education may help physicians understand the fundamentals of AI work,[56] evaluate AI applications,[57] determine when to incorporate AI analytics into patient care, and guide patients regarding these technologies.[58] Curricula that instruct journalists and science writers on how to use plain language may also help to promote the public's skills in understanding the basic functions and possibilities of these technologies.

Given the limitations of traditional clinical encounters in facilitating understanding around AI health monitoring, as we will see in Chapter 5, we need a systems approach to restructure these encounters and/or supplement them with broader opportunity-enhancing efforts that promote agents' capacity to deliberate on the use of these technologies for their care. For example, having accessible education portals and technology navigators may enhance prospective users' capacity to understand and reflect on the risks and benefits of these monitoring technologies.

2.2 Self-Determination: AI Health Monitoring as the Best Option or the Only Feasible Option?

As we saw earlier, the liberal conception of autonomy emphasizes the basic freedom conditions that either compromise or facilitate rational agents' ability to make decisions according to their priorities, including their health management goals. However, while there is likely agreement among bioethicists that freedom from all forms of coercion, manipulation, and exploitation would be a precondition for self-determination in AI health monitoring decisions that have direct impact on the user, the liberal conception of self-determination focuses mostly on freedom conditions, such as whether a person has the final authority to consent to or decline proposed research or care options according to their values, perspectives, and priorities. Under this individualist framework, in the absence of direct imposition from external others or internal constraints (e.g., depression), self-determination is considered upheld by virtue of one's explicit or implicit consent to AI health monitoring practices, lending support to a non-interventionist view.[59] As we will see later in the case of DTC AI health monitoring, self-determination is also associated with the rhetoric of consumer sovereignty and self-regulating markets.[60]

While protection or promotion of freedom is important, I argue that a disproportionate focus on liberty conditions may compromise people's meaningful autonomy regarding AI health monitoring in various ways. On the one hand, a narrow emphasis on freedom neglects or masks important structural factors—including aforementioned social determinants of health and digital literacy—that may limit people's ability to determine what health maintenance goals are most important to them and carry out their health monitoring priorities accordingly. On the other hand, questions remain whether it may be legitimate to limit certain types or levels of freedom that are not crucial to people's practical identity and well-being. For example, we may ask whether anonymized EHR data that were already collected for clinical purposes can be routinely utilized by health systems to train, build, and test algorithms as part of the aforementioned "collaborative necessity,"[61] if these practices are responsibly governed to protect users' privacy and are crucial to promote important social good, such as algorithmic accuracy and equitable scientific benefits.

There are at least four reasons why the liberal focus on liberty or freedom conditions in the context of AI health monitoring are inadequate in addressing prospective users' autonomy. First, promotion of liberty requires that people have the requisite information and opportunities to make AI health monitoring decisions according to their broader values and goals. However, despite promises by AI enthusiasts, the utility or clinical value of continuous data collection and the specifics of its future applications are frequently unknown due to a paucity of high-quality prospective clinical trials and thus a lack of clear evidence.[62] In the era of big data, it is also often unclear how everyday personal and health data collected by health systems, clinical researchers, or corporations are used for AI development, and whether or how data that are collected from AI platforms may be used outside of the person's direct monitoring or care purposes. Moreover, the power to determine what and how much information to provide research participants and patients regarding the development and utilization of AI remains with researchers, health care providers, health systems, and, increasingly, for-profit enterprises that are developing these platforms. These entities may have other incentives beyond improving patient wellness when considering whether to recommend or implement AI health monitoring. For example, a health plan or primary care clinic may want to implement AI home health monitoring partly to reduce the cost of clinic space and administrative staff. These are legitimate goals, especially if the shift to AI health monitoring does not compromise patient outcomes and can promote value-based care. Nonetheless, without transparency to allow prospective users to understand and critically evaluate various implications and public investments that facilitate access and successful adoption for patients, such a technological shift can reinforce power asymmetry and contribute to patient distrust, even if monitored users' liberty is not directly violated.

Second, the individual liberty focus, which looks at one decision and technology at a time, is inadequate in handling the new technological reality of big data for AI health monitoring.[63] The use of algorithmic decision support is not new: Clinicians and health systems have long utilized expert systems and other algorithms to help diagnose various conditions and detect cancer in medical images. What is new, however, is partly the scale of information digitization, data linkage, and longitudinal sharing activities, which are intrinsic to Internet of Things (IoT) and AI development and functionality. The increasingly complex data types have raised concerns that even well-resourced companies and health systems have failed to fully control their massive datasets or understand how to secure various datapoints as per user agreements.[64] Depending on how or where the data are collected, shared, and merged with other datasets, these activities do not always fall neatly under a traditional research or clinical care category, accompanied by consent provisions that promote liberty. And while federally funded research involving human participants is subject to the Common Rule and associated institutional review board (IRB) reviews, corporations developing and testing AI health monitoring algorithms using only private funds are not subject to similar review requirements. As we saw in the Introduction, AI algorithms learn from large integrated datasets consisting of heterogenous forms of historical data. This may include not only de-identified data produced by the health care system, but also a growing variety of data from consumer wellness industries, socio-demographic sources, and people's digital activities.[65] For example, companies and organizations are increasingly exploring the physical and mental health aspects of consumers' social media posts, internet search histories, purchasing behaviors, location data, and movement habits. AI-powered technologies then continuously collect and analyze new real-time input data to produce user-tailored predictive output, further contributing to the expanding dataset. Liberty conditions for self-determination generally demand that individual consent be sought for collecting and sharing people's personal and health data for explicit research or care delivery purposes. However, as the ongoing COVID-19 pandemic has revealed, continuous analyses of collected health data, including for secondary research protocols beyond those for which the data were originally intended, may be necessary or helpful for timely health system responses to emerging population-level health needs. Moreover, as clinics, hospitals, and health systems increasingly partner with commercial entities to develop patient portals and health monitoring systems that may aggregate health information from multiple sources, there are logistical barriers to providing opt-out choices while retaining the public and social benefits of data collection. Traditional consent models, which are the main tools used to protect self-determination in research settings, do not adequately address complex issues of whether health systems may legitimately collect, utilize, or share people's heterogenous data for iterative AI system development and improvement without seeking explicit consent.[66]

Third, the liberty focus by itself does not delineate between important and trivial forms of liberty, rendering it inadequate to determine how to set the threshold of whether or when certain restrictions on freedom are justifiable to fulfill important social utility and scientific integrity goals. The collection and use of heterogeneous data from people of diverse backgrounds are essential to foster an equitable learning health system, defined by the National Academy of Medicine as one where the care of patients is integrated with medical research so that the health care practices offered in the system are continuously studied, updated, and improved during the care process.[67] Clinical data from health care encounters are aggregated and analyzed on an ongoing basis, creating a feedback loop whereby the new knowledge is iteratively incorporated into the improvement of future care. With regard to AI health monitoring more specifically, the inclusion of data from as many people of diverse backgrounds as possible is necessary to ensure representative training and testing datasets for ML algorithms and to promote scientific accuracy and equitable benefits. Relying on a liberty-focused model of separate informed consent processes, where individuals either opt in or opt out of data collection and sharing for AI development and testing purposes, may lead to missing data points and data biases, which can result in inaccurate systems. For example, if underserved population groups are more prone to declining data collection and data sharing because of health and digital literacy concerns or distrust in the system, then an emphasis on liberty conditions via individual consent without correcting root causes of declination may exacerbate inequity and distrust rather than enhance self-determination.[68] While respect for individual liberty remains important, it does not sufficiently address all the ways we design and conduct research in the name of transforming health services.[69] Ultimately, a recalibration of the tensions between the promotion of liberty and the evolving context and paradigm of AI research may be necessary to ensure accurate algorithms and equitable implementation.

Fourth, the increasing utilization of digital practices and IoT at a broader societal and health system level may expand certain technological options but reduce access to other currently available health monitoring alternatives, potentially leaving people who have lower digital literacy or a lower comfort level with technologies with no real opportunity to access appropriate health monitoring that is congruent with their broader context. While AI health monitoring is increasingly hailed as a way to promote patient empowerment, engagement, and autonomy, adopting predictive health monitoring and management platforms without addressing the social and care environment within which such monitoring is promoted and implemented may compromise people's ability to make goal-concordant decisions regarding how to track their health over time (e.g., having in-person vs. automated and continuous monitoring). Offering AI health monitoring as one of the methods or additional resources to track health progression can promote self-determination for patients who are interested in and appropriately resourced to utilize these tools. However, requiring or expecting patients to adopt AI health monitoring and related practices, or defunding in-person appointments and care management in favor of AI monitoring, regardless of the person's own preferences and technological literacy, counters self-determination for people who may already have been deprived of other social resources. Even without direct coercion, heavy promotion and widescale implementation of AI health monitoring technologies at the system level may exert undue power on patients by changing the motivational structure of their decisions. For people who may not be financially or technologically prepared or equipped to accept these complex digital processes, widescale implementation may not only impose the power of these technologies on them but may also remove opportunities to receive appropriate monitoring, and potentially lead to poorer health outcomes.

A relational approach to self-determination may provide guidance on building governance models that address broader socio-systemic considerations, going beyond isolated consent decisions about each technology or each type of information being collected. Such an approach highlights the importance of *both* liberty and opportunity conditions. Opportunity conditions are the types of opportunities or resources that are necessary in institutional and social environments for agents to make decisions according to their goals, values, and priorities. Under a relational lens, opportunity conditions may sometimes be prioritized over freedom conditions, as which freedom conditions are important may be determined by conditions that can promote equal opportunities. Opportunity conditions offer insight into which professional, institutional, and social practices may hinder people's meaningful opportunities to fulfill their health monitoring goals, and which may enhance patients' understanding and care goals. Patient navigator services that guide underserved or immigrant patients through hospital registration, help schedule patients' tests, take patients to appointments, and explain every step in patients' native language and culture are one example.[70] In the context of AI health monitoring, providing self-governing individuals the opportunity to receive and consider relevant information in their native language or in an appropriate format (e.g., infographics) may help them understand and make decisions based on what would best fit their identity and values. As some smaller or more remote communities may lack home care support or physician services, providing AI health monitoring may also allow patients expanded opportunities to determine what monitoring practices may best meet their ongoing care needs.

Opportunity conditions may also include ensuring affordable access to internet services and AI technologies, so that people who are open to adopting these technologies have real opportunities to reflect on and decide how they would like health monitoring to take place, as well as adequate and appropriate health monitoring alternatives for those who are less open to AI. For example, subsidized and expanded internet and technological access may reduce the digital divide or barriers to access and boost people's realistic health monitoring options, which in turn can enhance their self-determination. Attention to opportunity conditions may also guide concerted efforts to empower and enable people to have the appropriate information and resources to consider whether or how these emerging health monitoring technologies fit their health and life goals. Continuing efforts to ensure access to in-person monitoring for people who have a low comfort level with digital technologies, which may include providing incentives and supports for formal and informal caregivers, as well as broader consideration of whether or how one can challenge data use and the platform's recommendations, may also enhance self-determination. Providing prospective users free or affordable access to the proposed technology and help desk support for at least a trial period while they still have in-person monitoring may also help them to have direct comparison about the benefits and become more informed and comfortable with the technology, if they decide or need to transition to AI health monitoring.

2.3 Self-Authorization and Epistemic Injustice

We have seen how self-determining adults in liberal societies generally consider themselves as having the epistemic and moral privilege to determine their own good. Echoing John Stuart Mill's notion of individualism, even if we may disagree with rational agents' self-regarding decisions or believe they are taking excessive risks or making mistakes, whether in health care or other situations, they are presumably the ones best equipped to discern how they can promote their own values, priorities, and well-being. As health care can affect physical, emotional, relational, and socioeconomic aspects of one's life, it is difficult for anyone other than the patient to know which of the expanding number of treatment alternatives will be most compatible with their values and priorities. If we suspect that the agents have incorrectly calculated what strategies will best achieve their goals, we can advise or persuade them to re-evaluate their situation, and provide more accurate or relevant information so that they are better equipped to reconsider their decisions.[71] Nonetheless, we are limited in our knowledge of other people and their worldview, and thus cannot coercively override the agents' own reasons for action or their self-regarding decisions based on their practical commitments. Moreover, allowing people to make their own decisions—even if they may make non-ideal decisions—helps them to constitute themselves as full, active agents, rather than mere passive recipients of choices that others make for them.

Self-authorization, the third dimension of autonomy, involves people having confidence in their normative power to exercise practical control over matters of fundamental importance to them.[72] It emphasizes the role of self-evaluative attitudes such as self-trust in various decisional domains, including health care.[73] Self-authorization is particularly important as AI gradually moves outside of clinics and hospitals and into people's homes and everyday activities, which may substantially affect whether people have the sovereign authority to define their own health care priorities, determine their own risk tolerance, make their own tradeoffs between privacy and other multifaceted health and life goals, and pursue their desired living arrangements or care relationships accordingly. As we will see in the use case of AI home health and DTC health monitoring, questions abound whether predictive analytics from AI monitoring platforms may replace people's evaluation of their own haptic senses, or override their judgment around what types of assistance they might need.

It is noteworthy that self-authorization is inherently relational. Self-authorizing agents see themselves as the rightful authors of their destiny. They own their convictions, emotional responses, and judgments, but are also socially prepared to answer others who may have questions about these beliefs and values. Moreover, self-authorizing agents are open to revising their preferences in light of this questioning, engaging in dialogic and collaborative knowledge creation and decision-making. In the context of AI health monitoring, this may include a willingness to explain why one does not want to adopt these technologies or participate in data-sharing practices, or engagement in dialogic communication that may bring further information to light. Simultaneously, self-authorization requires that one's normative authority and credibility to be self-determining and self-governing be taken seriously by *others* as part of social, institutional, and regulatory practices.[74] This does not necessitate others agreeing with our commitments, reasons, or decisions to reject various recommendations.[75] Rather, it involves trusting oneself and being accountable to others, while simultaneously being trusted by them. For example, we can imagine a Black patient resisting the opportunity to use an AI algorithm to monitor their skin lesion growth because of their preference for in-person assessment with a physician and concerns that some of these algorithms have mostly been trained on lighter skin.[76] This self-authorizing agent recognizes the legitimacy of their doubts about algorithmic accuracy, but would be willing to reconsider if they were provided with accessible and transparent information about validation methods to assuage their worries, or if they could still rely on their clinicians to provide "checks and balances" or a second opinion on algorithmic recommendations.[77] At the same time, when a physician or health system recognizes the patient's self-authorization, they take the patient's concerns seriously, giving them due consideration, accommodating them when feasible, and adjusting funding and access accordingly as part of dialogic inquiry among stakeholders. In other words, self-authorization is relational because it is fundamentally a form of social recognition; the ability to hold and exercise self-evaluative attitudes depends on intersubjective social and professional relations, which can either facilitate or thwart people's capacity to trust and implement reflexive self-interpretations and evaluations of their commitments.

The socio-relational dimension of self-trust highlights how some individuals or social groups may face barriers to self-authorization due to epistemic injustice, which is particularly concerning as health care monitoring becomes increasingly high tech. In brief, epistemic injustice is both a moral and distinctly epistemic concept, whereby relations of power can deprive our functioning as rational agents and hinder self-authorization. It consists in a wrong done to someone specifically in their capacity as a knower, and occurs when people's ability to contribute to and benefit from knowledge creation is unfairly rejected by others.[78]

As Miranda Fricker explains, there are at least two forms of epistemic injustice, hermeneutical injustice and testimonial injustice, both of which result from the operation of socio-political power in epistemic interactions.[79] First, epistemic injustice can assume the form of hermeneutical injustice, which happens when a gap in collective interpretive resources of a particular phenomenon puts someone at an unfair disadvantage in their effort to make sense of their experiences. A health care example may be medical paternalism in a hospital culture that still lacks or dismisses that critical concept. Patients may face hermeneutical interference of dominant background narratives that are misguided and inappropriately resistant to counter-evidence.[80] Hermeneutical injustice can also happen when some people do not have adequate resources and prospects to acquire knowledge or reach a correct assessment of their experiences (e.g., due to a lack of societal investment), robbing them of equal opportunities to engage in dialogic exchanges about these experiences and affecting their social identity. Hermeneutical injustice is particularly concerning in highly technical and specialized domains such as AI health monitoring, as technology developers, clinicians, and health system administrators have increasing power and social authority to conceptualize what or who is unsafe and thus in need of continuous monitoring and analysis, determine how various forms of data are labeled or interpreted according to such conceptualization, and set threshold standards for algorithmic alerts and follow-up actions, thereby structuring collective understandings of and agendas for these new technological practices.[81] Moreover, as mentioned earlier, disparities in health and digital literacy abound. Patients of lower socioeconomic status may lack access to the conceptual and technical resources to understand important aspects of predictive analytics, articulate their concerns or experience in dialogic communication, or address those concerns systematically.

Second, epistemic injustice can happen in the form of testimonial injustice, when some people's testimonies or narratives are prematurely dismissed as having less credible normative and epistemic authority due to their stigmatized identity or presumed inherent inadequacies. In health care, there is generally a presumed methodological hierarchy, whereby scientific methods of inquiry and technologically enhanced care are categorically recognized to be superior to other methods or sources of knowledge. Health care providers, particularly physicians, presumably have superior cognitive abilities to apply the privileged scientific methods, medical knowledge, and diagnostic and procedural skills compared to lay patients, and are thus conferred the designated professional authority to determine how conditions and symptoms should be clinically managed.[82] Even though clinicians have expert domain in their specialized clinical areas but not patients' situated and global experiences, patients' own narratives and experiential knowledge are nonetheless often dismissed as less trustworthy than professional and clinical determination of best interests. With medical and digital advances, the increasingly vast asymmetry of informational and conceptual resources may exacerbate testimonial injustice, whereby lay patients' assertions or testimonies are not accepted because they are unfairly judged as lacking the requirements to be credible informants or collaborative decision-makers in their own care pathway.[83] This may prejudicially lead patients, especially those who do not have high medical or technical literacy, to undervalue their own experience or expertise relative to clinicians, compromising their ability or confidence to further advocate for themselves.[84] As we will see in subsequent chapters, older adults as well as people with disabilities or mental illnesses are in particular often *made* vulnerable by others due to prejudicial assumptions about their identity, their capacity to determine acceptable risk levels, and their veracity in reporting their health-related behaviors. Their sovereign authority to refuse continuous and predictive monitoring may be unfairly rejected as suspect in health care encounters.

A relational approach to self-authorization highlights how respect for autonomy demands attention to and elimination of epistemic injustice, which can distort what types of health data and testimonies are deemed relevant in guiding care pathways, impede people's ability to acquire appropriate care and health monitoring, and reinforce power domination in therapeutic relationships. Self-authorization is particularly important in the context of AI health monitoring because the ability to diagnose or predict health decline, even when enhanced by predictive algorithms, does not automatically answer the normative questions of how people form their health and overall goals and how they should balance health and privacy risks. Patients' priorities and health goals involve broader considerations of practical identity that often go beyond clinical considerations. As we will see in various use cases, in the context of AI health monitoring, popular notions of healthy aging, independent living, treatment compliance, and self-management may predefine acceptable ways for people to manage their health needs and usurp their authority to determine or negotiate how much risk they are allowed to take.

In the context of AI health monitoring, a relational interpretation of self-authorization helps to explain the importance of providing evidence to support AI implementation. Relational self-authorization recognizes the bidirectionality of accountability in dialogic exchange. To uphold patients' normative authority in deciding whether to accept AI health monitoring, *others*—including technologists, prescribing clinicians, and/or health systems that decide to implement these algorithms—also need to be answerable to their positions. For example, if prospective users who reject continuous health monitoring are subjected to critical questioning of their reasons, then the commercial developers and health systems that promote these technologies, or that intend to replace some of the existing health monitoring methods with AI technologies, must also be prepared to demonstrate the explainability and accuracy of these algorithmic tools. Otherwise, people's normative authority to reject these technologies may be compromised.

As AI health technologies are often uncritically promoted by enthusiasts as being more effective and efficient, even when there is minimal to no evidence of these claims,[85] they are increasingly utilized to resolve subjective and value-laden health care questions that are disguised as objective clinical decisions, overriding patients' own testimonies and desires due to the social power of technology. To illustrate these ideas more fully, we will turn to the use case of AI home health monitoring in the next chapter.

Notes

1. Stacy M. Carter et al., "The Ethical, Legal and Social Implications of Using Artificial Intelligence Systems in Breast Cancer Care," *The Breast* 49 (2020): 25–32, https://doi.org/10.1016/j.breast.2019.10.001.
2. Catriona Mackenzie, "Three Dimensions of Autonomy: A Relational Analysis," in *Autonomy, Oppression, and Gender*, ed. Andrea Veltman and Mark Piper (New York: Oxford University Press, 2014), 15–41.
3. Jennifer Nedelsky, *Law's Relations: A Relational Theory of Self, Autonomy, and Law* (New York: Oxford University Press, 2012).
4. Catriona Mackenzie, "Relational Autonomy, Normative Authority and Perfectionism," *Journal of Social Philosophy* 39, no. 4 (December 2008): 512–33, https://doi.org/10.1111/j.1467-9833.2008.00440.x.
5. Susan Sherwin, "A Relational Approach to Autonomy in Health Care," in *The Politics of Women's Health: Exploring Agency and Autonomy*, ed. Susan Sherwin (Philadelphia: Temple University Press, 1998), 19–47.
6. Stephen Scher and Kasia Kozlowska, "The Rise of Bioethics: A Historical Overview," in *Rethinking Health Care Ethics*, ed. Stephen Scher and Kasia Kozlowska (Singapore: Palgrave Pivot, 2018), 31–44, https://doi.org/10.1007/978-981-13-0830-7_3.
7. Sherwin, "A Relational Approach to Autonomy in Health Care."
8. Rahul K. Nayak and Steven D. Pearson, "The Ethics of 'Fail First': Guidelines and Practical Scenarios for Step Therapy Coverage Policies." *Health Affairs (Millwood)* 33, no. 10 (October 2014): 1779–85. doi: 10.1377/hlthaff.2014.0516. PMID: 25288422.

9. Sherwin, "A Relational Approach to Autonomy in Health Care."
10. Mark Siegler, "The Progression of Medicine: From Physician Paternalism to Patient Autonomy to Bureaucratic Parsimony," *Archives of Internal Medicine* 145, no. 4 (1985): 713–15, https://doi.org/10.1001/archinte.1985.00360040147031.
11. See Jonathan Moreno, Ulf Schmidt, and Steve Joffe, "The Nuremberg Code 70 Years Later," *Journal of the American Medical Association* 318, no. 9 (2017): 795–96, https://doi:10.1001/jama.2017.10265.
12. Scher and Kozlowska, "The Rise of Bioethics: A Historical Overview."
13. Scher and Kozlowska, "The Rise of Bioethics: A Historical Overview."
14. Christine Korsgaard, *The Sources of Normativity* (Cambridge: Cambridge University Press, 1996); Christine Korsgaard, *Self-Constitution: Agency, Identity, and Integrity* (Oxford: Oxford University Press, 2009).
15. Matthew Silverstein, "Agency and Normative Self-Governance," *Australasian Journal of Philosophy* 95, no. 3 (2017): 517–28, https://doi.org/10.1080/00048402.2016.1254263.
16. Immanuel Kant, *Foundations of the Metaphysics of Morals*, trans. Lewis White Beck (Indianapolis: Bobbs-Merrill, 1959).
17. Matti Häyry, "The Tension between Self Governance and Absolute Inner Worth in Kant's Moral Philosophy," *Journal of Medical Ethics* 31, no. 11 (2005): 645–47, https://doi.org/10.1136/jme.2004.010058. It is worth noting that Kant was mostly interested in moral agents' rational capacity to act in accordance with moral laws and the moral respect that is owed to autonomous agents, rather than the actual empirical decisions they make.
18. Mackenzie, "Three Dimensions of Autonomy."
19. Jesper Ahlin Marceta, "A Non-ideal Authenticity-Based Conceptualization of Personal Autonomy," *Medicine, Health Care and Philosophy* 22 (2019): 387–395, https://doi.org/10.1007/s11019-018-9879-1
20. Mackenzie, "Three Dimensions of Autonomy."
21. Robert M. Nelson et al., "The Concept of Voluntary Consent," *American Journal of Bioethics* 11, no. 8 (2011): 6–16, https://doi.org/10.1080/15265161.2011.583318.
22. However, it is important to note that confidentiality protection in and of itself does not necessarily prevent discrimination within a therapeutic relationship, especially when some patients may have already been marginalized due to their stigmatized identities—an issue that will be further discussed in various use cases.
23. Tom Beauchamp and James Childress, *Principles of Biomedical Ethics*, 7th ed. (New York: Oxford University Press, 2012).

24. Rebecca Robbins and Erin Brodwin, "An Invisible Hand: Patients Aren't Being Told about the AI Systems Advising Their Care," STAT, July 15, 2020, https://www.statnews.com/2020/07/15/artificial-intelligence-patient-consent-hospitals/.
25. I. Glenn Cohen, "Informed Consent and Medical Artificial Intelligence: What to Tell the Patient?" *Georgetown Law Journal* 108 (2020): 1425–69, https://doi.org/10.2139/ssrn.3529576.Mackenzie, "Three Dimensions of Autonomy."
26. Ziad Obermeyer et al., "Dissecting Racial Bias in an Algorithm Used to Manage the Health of Populations," *Science* 366, no. 6464 (October 2019): 447–53, https://doi.org/10.1126/science.aax2342.
27. Anita Ho, "The Individualist Model of Autonomy and the Challenge of Disability," *Bioethical Inquiry* 5 (2008): 193–207, https://doi.org/10.1007/s11673-007-9075-0.
28. Ho, "Individualist Model of Autonomy."
29. Ho, "Individualist Model of Autonomy."
30. I. M. Young, *Justice and the Politics of Difference* (Princeton, NJ: Princeton University Press, 1990).
31. Catriona Mackenzie and Natalie Stoljar, eds., *Relational Autonomy: Feminist Perspectives on Autonomy, Agency, and the Social Self* (New York: Oxford University Press, 2000).
32. Susan Sherwin, "A Relational Approach to Autonomy in Health Care."
33. Marilyn Friedman, *Autonomy, Gender, and Politics* (New York: Oxford University Press, 2003).
34. I. Glenn Cohen, "Informed Consent and Medical Artificial Intelligence: What to Tell the Patient?" *Georgetown Law Journal* 108 (2020): 1425–69, https://doi.org/10.2139/ssrn.3529576.
35. Rebecca Robbins, "An Experiment in End-of-Life Care: Tapping AI's Cold Calculus to Nudge the Most Human of Conversations," STAT, July 1, 2020, https://www.statnews.com/2020/07/01/end-of-life-artificial-intelligence/.
36. Mackenzie, "Three Dimensions of Autonomy."
37. Rosamond Rhodes, "When Is Participation in Research a Moral Duty?" *Journal of Law, Medicine & Ethics* 45, no. 3 (2017): 318–26, https://doi.org/10.1177/1073110517737529.
38. Carter et al., "The Ethical, Legal and Social Implications."
39. Hilde Lindemann Nelson, "Feminist Bioethics: Where We've Been, Where We're Going," *Metaphilosophy* 31, no. 5 (2000): 492–508, https://doi.org/10.1111/1467-9973.00165.
40. Mackenzie, "Three Dimensions of Autonomy."

41. S. M. Carter, V. A. Entwistle, and M. Little, "Relational Conceptions of Paternalism: A Way to Rebut Nanny-State Accusations and Evaluate Public Health Interventions," *Public Health* 129, no. 8 (August 2015): 1021–29, https://doi.org/10.1016/j.puhe.2015.03.007.
42. Lynn Nielsen-Bohlman, Allison M. Panzer, and David A. Kindig, eds., *Health Literacy: A Prescription to End Confusion* (Washington, DC: National Academies Press, 2004), https://doi.org/10.17226/10883.
43. Steven S. Coughlin et al., "Health Literacy and Patient Web Portals," *International Journal of Medical Informatics* 113 (2018): 43–48, https://doi.org/10.1016/j.ijmedinf.2018.02.009.
44. Dean Schillinger, "The Intersections between Social Determinants of Health, Health Literacy, and Health Disparities," *Studies in Health Technology and Informatics* 269 (June 2020): 22–41, https://doi.org/10.3233/SHTI200020.
45. Steven S. Coughlin et al., "Health Literacy, Social Determinants of Health, and Disease Prevention and Control," *Journal of Environment and Health Sciences* 6, no. 1 (2020), https://www.ncbi.nlm.nih.gov/pmc/articles/PMC7889072/.
46. Saida Mamedova and Emily Pawlowski, "A Description of U.S. Adults Who Are Not Digitally Literate," American Institutes for Research, May 1, 2018, https://www.air.org/resource/brief/description-us-adults-who-are-not-digitally-literate.
47. Robbins and Brodwin, "An Invisible Hand."
48. Don Nutbeam and Jane E. Lloyd, "Understanding and Responding to Health Literacy as a Social Determinant of Health," *Annual Review of Public Health* 42 (April 2021): 159–73, https://doi.org/10.1146/annurev-publhealth-090419-102529; Louis Rice and Rachel Sara, "Updating the Determinants of Health Model in the Information Age," *Health Promotion International* 34, no. 6 (December 2019): 1241–49, https://doi.org/10.1093/heapro/day064.
49. Mamedova and Pawlowski, "A Description of U.S. Adults."
50. If there is no consent required for the implementation of a particular AI technology, clinicians may also be reluctant to spend precious consultation time on discussing the technological process.
51. Brent Daniel Mittelstadt et al., "The Ethics of Algorithms: Mapping the Debate," *Big Data & Society* 3, no. 2 (December 2016), https://doi.org/10.1177/2053951716679679.
52. Greg Irving et al., "International Variations in Primary Care Physician Consultation Time: A Systematic Review of 67 Countries," *BMJ Open* 7, no. 10 (2017): e017902, https://doi.org/10.1136/bmjopen-2017-017902.

53. Ming Tai-Seale, Thomas G. McGuire, and Weimin Zhang, "Time Allocation in Primary Care Office Visits," *Health Services Research* 42, no. 5 (October 2007): 1871–94, https://doi.org/10.1111/j.1475-6773.2006.00689.x.
54. Michael K. Paasche-Orlow and Michael S. Wolf, "The Causal Pathways Linking Health Literacy to Health Outcomes," *American Journal of Health Behavior* 31, Suppl. 1 (October 2007): S19–S26, https://doi.org/10.5555/ajhb.2007.31.supp.S19.
55. Natalie Joseph-Williams, Glyn Elwyn, and Adrian Edwards, "Knowledge Is Not Power for Patients: A Systematic Review and Thematic Synthesis of Patient-Reported Barriers and Facilitators to Shared Decision Making," *Patient Education and Counseling* 94, no. 3 (March 2014): 291–309, https://doi.org/10.1016/j.pec.2013.10.031.
56. Lawrence Carin, "On Artificial Intelligence and Deep Learning Within Medical Education," *Academic Medicine* 95, no. 11S (2020): S10–S11, https://doi.org/10.1097/ACM.0000000000003630.
57. Thomas Robert Savage, "Artificial Intelligence in Medical Education," *Academic Medicine* 96, no. 9 (2021): 1229–30, https://doi.org/10.1097/ACM.0000000000004183.
58. Steven A. Wartman and C. Donald Combs, "Medical Education Must Move From the Information Age to the Age of Artificial Intelligence," *Academic Medicine: Journal of the Association of American Medical Colleges* 93, no. 8 (August 2018): 1107–9, https://doi.org/10.1097/ACM.0000000000002044.
59. Anita Ho, "Relational Autonomy or Undue Pressure? Family's Role in Medical Decision-Making," *Scandinavian Journal of Caring Sciences* 22, no. 1 (March 2008): 128–35, https://doi.org/10.1111/j.1471-6712.2007.00561.x.
60. Catriona Mackenzie, "Feminist Innovation in Philosophy: Relational Autonomy and Social Justice," *Women's Studies International Forum* 72 (2019): 144–51, https://doi.org/10.1016/j.wsif.2018.05.003.
61. Rhodes, "When Is Participation in Research a Moral Duty?"
62. Konstantin Genin and Thomas Grote. "Randomized Controlled Trials in Medical AI: A Methodological Critique," *Philosophy of Medicine* 2, no. 1 (2021), https://doi.org/10.5195/philmed.2021.27.
63. Celia B. Fisher and Deborah M. Layman, "Genomics, Big Data, and Broad Consent: A New Ethics Frontier for Prevention Science," *Prevention Science: The Official Journal of the Society for Prevention Research* 19, no. 7 (October 2018): 871–79, https://doi.org/10.1007/s11121-018-0944-z.

64. Sophie Putka, "Meta, Hospitals Sued for Sharing Private Medical Info," Medpage Today, August 3, 2022, https://www.medpagetoday.com/special-reports/features/100050.
65. Deven McGraw and Kenneth D. Mandl, "Privacy Protections to Encourage Use of Health-Relevant Digital Data in a Learning Health System," *npj Digital Medicine* 4, no. 1 (2021), https://doi.org/10.1038/s41746-020-00362-8.
66. Stephanie A. Kraft et al., "Beyond Consent: Building Trusting Relationships with Diverse Populations in Precision Medicine Research," *American Journal of Bioethics* 18, no. 4 (2018): 3–20, https://doi.org/10.1080/15265161.2018.1431322.
67. Nancy E. Kass et al., "The Research–Treatment Distinction: A Problematic Approach for Determining Which Activities Should Have Ethical Oversight," *Hastings Center Report* 43, no. 1 (2013): S4–S15, https://doi.org/10.1002/hast.133; Ruth R. Faden et al., "An Ethics Framework for a Learning Health Care System: A Departure from Traditional Research Ethics and Clinical Ethics," *Hastings Center Report* 43, no. 1 (2013): S16–S27, https://doi.org/10.1002/hast.134; Nancy E. Kass and Ruth R. Faden, "Ethics and Learning Health Care: The Essential Roles of Engagement, Transparency, and Accountability," *Learning Health Systems* 2, no. 4 (2018): e10066, https://doi.org/10.1002/lrh2.10066.
68. Stephanie R. Morain, Nancy E. Kass, and Ruth R. Faden, "Learning Is Not Enough: Earning Institutional Trustworthiness through Knowledge Translation," *American Journal of Bioethics* 18, no. 4 (2018): 31–34, https://doi.org/10.1080/15265161.2018.1431708.
69. Kayte Spector-Bagdady and Jonathan Beever, "Rethinking the Importance of the Individual within a Community of Data," *Hastings Center Report* 50, no. 4 (July 2020): 9–11, https://doi.org/10.1002/hast.1112.
70. Ruben Castaneda, "Creative Ways Hospitals Reach Diverse Populations," *US News & World Report*, January 23, 2017, https://health.usnews.com/wellness/slideshows/creative-ways-hospitals-reach-diverse-populations.
71. John Stuart Mill, *On Liberty* (Peterborough, Ontario: Broadview, 1999).
72. Mackenzie, "Three Dimensions of Autonomy."
73. Carolyn McLeod, *Self-Trust and Reproductive Autonomy* (Cambridge, MA: MIT Press, 2002).
74. Joel Anderson and Axel Honneth, "Autonomy, Vulnerability, Recognition, and Justice," in *Autonomy and the Challenges to Liberalism: New Essays*, ed. John Christman and Joel Anderson (Cambridge: Cambridge University Press, 2005), 127–49.
75. Mackenzie, "Three Dimensions of Autonomy."

76. Adewole S. Adamson and Avery Smith, "Machine Learning and Health Care Disparities in Dermatology," *JAMA Dermatology* 154, no. 11 (November 2018): 1247–48, https://doi.org/10.1001/jamadermatol.2018.2348.
77. Jordan P. Richardson et al., "Patient Apprehensions about the Use of Artificial Intelligence in Healthcare," *npj Digital Medicine* 4, no. 1 (September 2021): 140, https://doi.org/10.1038/s41746-021-00509-1.
78. Miranda Fricker, *Epistemic Injustice: Power and the Ethics of Knowing* (Oxford: Oxford University Press, 2007).
79. Anita Ho, "Epistemic Injustice," in *Encyclopedia of Bioethics*, ed. Bruce Jennings, 4th ed. (Belmont, CA: Wadsworth Publishing, 2014).
80. H. Hänel, "Hermeneutical Injustice, (Self-)Recognition, and Academia," *Hypatia* 35, no. 2 (2000): 336–54, doi:10.1017/hyp.2020.3.
81. Ho, "Epistemic Injustice."
82. Ho, "Epistemic Injustice."
83. Fricker, *Epistemic Injustice.*
84. Joseph-Williams et al., "Knowledge Is Not Power."
85. Michael Roberts et al., "Common Pitfalls and Recommendations for Using Machine Learning to Detect and Prognosticate for COVID-19 Using Chest Radiographs and CT Scans," *Nature Machine Intelligence* 3, no. 3 (2021): 199–217, https://doi.org/10.1038/s42256-021-00307-0.

2

Independent Living With(out) Privacy

Artificial Intelligence Home Health Monitoring

As we saw in the last chapter, the focus on individual autonomy in bioethics has led to increased professional and policy attention on how to empower patients (and healthy individuals) to make health-related decisions according to their values and priorities. As the global population continues to age, and as chronic conditions and disabilities become more prevalent, promotion of individual autonomy intersects with public discourses and campaigns that emphasize helping older adults avoid disease and disability, maintain physical and mental functioning, and actively engage in community and civic life.[1]

With the continuing advancement of medical and consumer technologies, self-care practices of body monitoring and improvement with the aid of technology, including artificial intelligence (AI) health monitoring, are now touted as a strategy to empower older adults to prevent or delay potential health problems associated with aging, as well as minimize dependency on others.[2] It is widely recognized that people prefer to live at home, which can allow freer self-expression and stave off unwanted interference from others. However, for some older adults and people with chronic conditions and various impairments regardless of their age, higher functional support needs and the risk of unwitnessed health decline or adverse events (e.g., falls) are potential barriers to living safely in the community. Continuous and automated health monitoring technologies are thus increasingly promoted as tools to enhance proactive, ongoing health management, with proponents assuming a receptive audience and downplaying potential resistance to unwanted surveillance. A few small studies have indicated that community-dwelling older adults experience a greater sense of safety using automated home monitoring systems,[3] suggesting that these technologies may be acceptable alternatives or enhancements to in-person monitoring in support of independent living.[4] Nonetheless, there is a dearth of large-scale empirical studies on older adults' perceived benefits of AI health monitoring,[5] as well as limited supporting clinical evidence indicating that home health monitoring technologies can indeed translate to fewer hospitalizations or emergency room visits.[6]

In this chapter, I explain how the common individualist autonomy-based argument for promoting AI home health monitoring fails to capture the complex factors that affect people's capacity and opportunity to reflect on and make decisions about home health monitoring. Using a relational framework of autonomy introduced in the last chapter, I highlight various socio-contextual factors that frame people's practical identity around aging and "independent living," their available options for health monitoring, and their decisional motivations regarding the use of AI home health monitoring. Section 1 details the perceived need for alternatives to traditional in-person home health monitoring. Section 2 investigates the common claim that AI home health monitoring can promote users' autonomy and well-being, looking at various technologies that have been proposed, developed, or implemented to monitor people's functioning and health status at home. Section 3 utilizes a relational lens to explain how the individualist approach to autonomy neglects important contextual and structural issues that may affect people's ability to make health monitoring decisions that truly respect their autonomy. Contextualizing the discussion against the backdrop of an aging population, changing family patterns, and inadequate social or system support, this section examines how AI health monitoring may affect older adults' self-governance, self-determination, and self-authorization. It cautions that uncritical promotion of AI health monitoring without systemic improvement in the care environment may paradoxically exacerbate caregiver burden and isolation of those being remotely monitored.

1. Healthy Aging and Independent Living: An Artificial Dream?

Internationally, life expectancy continues to rise, climbing from an average of forty-seven years in 1900 to almost seventy-nine years in 2017, although there is notable regional variation due to different socioeconomic realities, levels of political stability, and prevalence of various health conditions.[7] In 2009, there were 39.6 million Americans over age sixty-five, and this number is projected to reach 94.7 million by 2060.[8] This aging demographic shift increases health challenges, both in terms of older adults' health and functional status as well as having adequate resources and support to meet population health needs. Old age itself is not a disease, and people at all ages may have different levels or forms of physical and cognitive impairment. Various socioeconomic determinants of health, such as education, employment, income, familial-social support, and community safety, have contributed to variability in health outcomes among different population groups.[9] Nonetheless, increasing longevity often means the development of multiple chronic diseases, including cardiovascular disease, stroke, cancer, osteoarthritis, and dementia later in life,[10] potentially affecting older adults' ability to perform daily activities or ambulate without assistance.[11] Moreover, the likelihood of having a disability increases with age, with those seventy-five years and older being five times as likely to have a disability as adults under twenty-four years old.[12] In the United States, more than half of older adults (58.5 percent) between ages eighty-five and eighty-nine receive a family caregiver's help due to health problems or functional limitations.[13] From age ninety onward, only a minority of individuals (24 percent) do *not* need active assistance from others.[14]

Most older adults and people with disabilities, including those who have extended health and functional needs, prefer to live and age in place.[15] In other words, they want to reside in their own home or community with appropriate support rather than in residential care facilities,[16] many of which are chronically crowded and understaffed, as revealed and exacerbated by the COVID-19 pandemic.[17] Given that hospitals, assisted living facilities, and residential care facilities have also implemented various types and levels of visitation restrictions throughout the pandemic, many older adults and/or their families have been seeking support services or assistive technologies that may allow the older adults to leave long-term care and live in the community. Studies have shown that aging in place is positively perceived by older adults in terms of security, familiarity, and sense of identity.[18]

In addition to recognizing that home is the preferred site of care for many older adults and disabled individuals, health systems around the country have been shifting ongoing care and monitoring out of institutions and into people's homes to lower costs for the system.[19] This is particularly the case for chronic illnesses and other long-term impairments, which require ongoing management that may last throughout the patient's life. Long-entrenched acute care–focused treatment and reimbursement paradigms are gradually making way for new models of care coordination and disease management that are further redistributing various care responsibilities from the state, medical institutions, and formal caregivers to informal caregivers, such as voluntary organizations and the family.[20] In the United States, health systems such as the Mayo Clinic and Kaiser Permanente have adopted remote patient monitoring platforms to shift certain advanced medical care to patients' homes, under the direction of system physicians and providers.[21]

Unfortunately, the availability of in-person care to support older adults living in their own home is dwindling due to demographic changes and corresponding human resource shortages. First, mirroring the general demographic trend, the health workforce is also aging. Replacing retired clinicians and recruiting new care workers to keep up with demand remains a challenge. In the United States, demand for geriatricians is projected to exceed supply, resulting in a forecasted national shortage of almost 27,000 full-time equivalencies (FTEs) by 2025.[22] As the new generation of medical professionals seeks to limit working hours to achieve better work–life balance, further workforce shortages are anticipated.[23] There are also inadequate direct care workers, such as home health aides, 90 percent of whom are women, and nearly two-thirds of whom are people of color.[24] Low salaries and benefits for these positions may partly explain the labor shortage in this field,[25] with personal care aides making only $14.27 an hour in 2021.[26] While the Biden administration sought in 2021 $400 billion in new spending for Medicaid home and community care, there were inadequate Senate votes even after the House pared it down to $150 million.[27] In states with fewer immigrants, who are disproportionately represented in many low-wage home health occupations,[28] the workforce availability for publicly funded or subsidized programs to fulfill long-term home care needs is particularly low. Disabled adults often have higher levels of medical debt and food insecurity and lower incomes than nondisabled adults, and many older adults live on restricted pension incomes,[29] such that they generally cannot afford private in-person home care, the median annual cost of which was $54,912 in 2020 for a forty-four-hour week.[30] Individuals can only qualify for a Medicaid subsidy if they have less than $2,000 in assets, and due to insufficient funding, the waiting list for the 800,000 low-income Americans who do qualify for home- and community-based services is around thirty-nine months.[31] In other words, systemic or structural issues around how home care is financed and organized are directly affecting people's ability to receive in-person care, particularly for those who have lower incomes—but not low enough to qualify for subsidies.

Second, at a time when health systems are trying to shift more caregiving and health monitoring duties to family members and other social support persons to reduce costs, there are signs that the availability of informal caregivers to meet increasing demands is also constrained. As a result of the changing nature of family relationships, decreasing family size, and women's growing participation in the workforce, the elderly support ratio around the world is expected to continue to drop sharply.[32] In the United States, it is estimated that between 2010 and 2050, the number of potential family caregivers available to provide long-term support for every older adult over the age of eighty with substantial care needs will decrease from more than seven to fewer than three.[33] Without other forms of financial or respite support for caregivers, this shortage will likely intensify the unmet care needs for older and disabled adults as well as the pressure on available or potential family caregivers. Moreover, despite ongoing calls for greater gender equality in liberal societies, familial caregiving duties continue to fall mostly on women (61 percent in the United States),[34] regardless of whether they are employed outside of the home and/or also take care of their children. Caring for disabled or older adult family members at home, attending to their functional and health needs if they live elsewhere, and taking them to medical appointments imposes substantial responsibilities and time commitments, which can significantly affect women's professional and personal lives as well as physical, mental, and financial well-being, thereby exacerbating gender inequity. According to a 2020 report from the AARP (formerly known as the American Association of Retired Persons),[35] an organization that aims to empower people to choose how they live as they age, 18 percent of family caregivers reported high financial strain due to caregiving, with 28 percent having stopped saving and 23 percent taking on more debt.

The growing imbalance between the number of older adults and the available formal and informal caregivers in an aging population highlights the need for alternative and affordable ways to support those in need of home health monitoring and their prospective caregivers.[36] While health monitoring is only one component of care management, automated monitoring technologies with remote communication features that allow users to contact or share information with loved ones or care providers are increasingly proposed as complementary or even replacement tools to enhance health management and active engagement at home. Advocates also promise that these technologies can reduce or delay the disabling effects of various conditions.[37]

The use of technologies to support home health monitoring is not a new phenomenon. Medical alert systems have for decades provided some support, but often only after injuries or adverse events have already occurred. Some older models also require users to activate the help button themselves. Other non-AI remote monitoring technologies, such as those that use CCTV cameras and ambient sensors to observe people's activities at home, can alert observers of adverse events or physiological decline. However, these technologies rely on human operators or family caregivers to watch video feeds or monitor other signals continuously in real time and respond accordingly. They are labor intensive and thus share some of the same human resource limitations as in-person monitoring, especially since these methods are also prone to human distractions and errors.[38] Without training, informal caregivers and rotating care aides may be unable to detect subtle changes in a person's behavior or motor/cognitive skills that indicate potential health concerns. Thus, the preventive potential of these technologies for effective ongoing health monitoring is limited, as the observer may only be able to alert a professional caregiver or assist after the monitored person has already suffered harm or has exhibited explicitly risky behavior, such as after an older adult with mobility challenges has been seen walking without a cane or has already fallen. These monitoring technologies do not analyze stored data and are also unhelpful when the observer is away from the monitor.

Observed users and their caregivers may also consider certain types of non-AI remote monitoring intrusive. For example, video monitoring in bedrooms or bathrooms to track users' mobility getting in and out of bed or entering and exiting the shower subjects the monitored individual to the direct gaze of others. It may invade the person's privacy or intimate space in their own home. Some studies have shown that even when older adults recognize that activity and fall detection may help keep them safer at home, they are reluctant to adopt camera monitoring for privacy reasons.[39] CCTV also captures and records the activities of other people appearing in the frame and may therefore be considered intrusive by those who provide direct care but do not themselves benefit from being monitored.

2. AI to the Rescue: The Artificial Dream Comes True

As information and assistive technologies continue to advance, AI health monitoring has been touted as a more effective tool for promoting older adults' autonomy and well-being while also reducing family care burden and health workforce pressure. Even though many technologies are still in research or developmental stages, and more evidence-based platforms that have undergone end user evaluation are needed to evaluate AI's potential to adequately support these populations, there is great optimism among technologists and health systems that these technologies can not only counteract growing institutional failures to provide high-quality human care,[40] but also can increase people's control over their living environment. They promise that these platforms can allow users to extend the duration of time they can live safely, independently, and comfortably in their own private dwellings, thereby promoting their quality of life and overall autonomy. AI enthusiasts believe that algorithmic devices that are trained on high-quality big datasets can provide ongoing monitoring, accurate detection of different behaviors, and effective predictive analysis of the monitored person's disease progression or health status, all while preserving users' personal privacy better than other monitoring technologies. These devices may be particularly beneficial for people with degenerative conditions, as ongoing monitoring of physiological and cognitive changes may inform care management and improve health outcomes.

Take Parkinson's disease (PD) and Alzheimer's disease (AD) as examples, both of which are progressive neurological disorders that have a higher prevalence among older adults and are garnering increasing attention from AI developers.[41] PD is characterized by cardinal motor signs, such as slowness, rigidity, tremor, loss of balance, and freezing of gait, whereas AD is characterized by a continuous decline in cognition as well as in behavioral and social skills. There is currently no known cure for either condition, and neurologists generally rely on clinical assessment of patients' mobility, cognitive function, memory, and the presence of psychological comorbidities to inform decisions on drug regimens for symptom management. Neuropsychiatric symptoms such as apathy and depression are common in AD but are often underreported by patients and family caregivers, who may not notice subtle changes over time.[42] Moreover, screenings have limited utility when a patient's ability to articulate their emotions and thoughts declines.[43] Assessment of nonverbal communication changes, such as involuntary facial expressions, may be helpful, but due to logistical limitations and funding constraints, these clinical evaluations are sparsely performed. Patients' gradual changes between professional consultations are also generally not actively monitored by professionals, except via patients' or family members' reports. As health care providers may not have a complete picture of a patient's status over time, people with PD and AD often endure a lengthy, exhausting journey of visiting their physicians, experimenting with various therapies, and reactively adjusting medications to manage symptoms as the disease progresses.

Machine learning (ML) algorithms that can continuously measure, analyze, and predict disease and functional status based on the observed person's data may complement infrequent clinical assessments and serve as clinical decision support to enhance ongoing and timely care. Some promising use cases of AI home health monitoring for people with PD and AD include AI-enabled sensors or computer vision systems, which aim to provide continuous and real-time observation of users' health-related activities, altered behavior patterns, disease progression, and adverse events such as falls.[44] Sophisticated deep learning (DL) computer vision analytics trained on big data on various forms and durations of motor functioning can classify different activities, such as standing or walking, from raw image data, and then iteratively learn the expected movements or behaviors for a particular user. Data on the effort and amount of time a person spends getting out of bed, for example, may help to predict the progression of an older adult's functional decline and the anticipated need for assistance. Information for other extrinsic risk factors such as poor lighting or inappropriate footwear may also help determine the most appropriate interventions.

Some of these platforms use ML or DL algorithms within the local monitoring system to process the input data, without human involvement in interacting with the raw data. For example, advanced computer vision programs can automatically convert video footage into stick figures, heat maps, and quantified information within the unit to detect the monitored user's posture and gait, track the person's movement within a spatial environment, and describe the types and durations of various activities in that environment to help predict the person's health status.[45] As no humans directly view the images and videos of identified users, these AI systems can provide more privacy protection than the aforementioned CCTV recordings. If the machine is capable of distinguishing the designated user from others who may be within the monitoring range, it may also protect the anonymity and privacy of caregivers, visitors, and other bystanders. Such protection is particularly important in the context of Internet of Things (IoT) and big data, where collected data may be shared across platforms and merged with other heterogeneous types of data for further analysis.

AI-powered ambient sensors installed in a person's home and other microsensors in smart devices (e.g., smartphones, tablets) have also been developed to track monitored individuals' total daily activity, time spent outside of the home and in different areas within the home, walking speed, etc.[46] These devices may help to detect that an observed person is gradually taking longer to gain balance while trying to stand up or slowly exhibiting more sporadic tremors—something that a busy family caregiver who is simultaneously looking after young children or working from home may miss. With advances in computational and architectural technologies, there is also an expanding availability of voice-activated smart devices and AI home technologies that can learn from users' routines over time and anticipate their needs to control lighting, room temperature, and household appliances, thereby enhancing people's ability to live at home safely and conveniently. Analyzing historical datasets as well as the user's own comprehensive longitudinal and real-time data points from these technologies may help to identify the individual's types, sequences, patterns, and durations of activities within various physical surroundings and at different times of day. There is great hope that these heterogeneous data can produce a more personalized assessment of the user's changing functional status and future progression,[47] provide timely alerts, and inform users of what types of architectural features or behavioral and environmental adjustments may enhance or compromise their ability to move around freely and safely in their own home.

In other AI advancements, natural language processing (NLP) algorithms, which use speech-to-text processing to detect changing or unusual speech patterns, have been developed to predict cognitive decline for older adults, including those with AD.[48] In recent years, there has also been increasing enthusiasm for, and commercial development of, conversational virtual intelligent assistants (e.g., chatbots). These devices combine physical and cognitive health monitoring with conversational functions to monitor users' functional changes and nudge them to adopt lifestyle adjustments that aim to promote healthy aging. Some of these devices use NLP to remind people to take their medication, recommend diets and activities based on the user's responses and other functional data, as well as engage in tailored conversations with the user based on previously stored and processed data. The ML algorithms utilize monitored users' longitudinal responses to various questions to detect the length of time users take to search for words, patterns in their vocabulary use and sentence structures, and tones of voice in order to identify or forecast cognitive, emotional, and functional changes. Advocates argue that, by integrating health and "social" functions, these technologies, including commercial robotic "pets," can act as both predictive and interventional devices to promote active engagement and ease isolation or loneliness—issues of particular concern during the COVID-19 pandemic. Some of these AI-enabled technologies use voice commands, which may give older adults and those with limited movement more control over their environment, allowing them to play music, get medication reminders, or call for help.[49]

As AI health monitoring continues to develop, many are hopeful that data from these platforms can facilitate more effective and efficient care delivery at both the individual and health system levels. First, at the individual level, instead of relying solely on a limited set of markers observed during a short clinical visit in a controlled environment, or on patients' and families' self-reports, multimodal data from AI health monitoring may provide valuable information on a wider array of relevant markers that evolve over time under identifiable and real-life circumstances.[50] If data from these technologies can be seamlessly integrated and analyzed with an older adult's electronic health record (EHR), AI home health monitoring may enable a better understanding of the dynamic nature of a person's degenerative condition and associated environmental factors. It has the real-world potential of further enhancing therapeutic interactions by offering health care providers more comprehensive and context-specific data, and may be particularly helpful to support people who live alone and/or have difficulty remembering or articulating their symptoms, needs, and concerns,[51] especially when there is a significant time lapse between noticing the symptoms and consulting a physician.[52] In providing ongoing predictive analysis of a user's health status, AI-powered home health monitoring technologies may help to assure monitored users and their caregivers when they are doing well, and facilitate timely assistance and safe care tailored to the users' longitudinal data when AI-indicated.

Second, at the health system delivery level, continuous and real-time data may also help clinicians to prioritize patients who require more comprehensive or urgent consultations and provide remote support to others who can be managed safely at home. If fully integrated into the health care infrastructure, these technologies may help to enhance system capacity by preserving and allocating health care resources responsibly and responsively. AI-powered platforms may also promote more equitable access to health information and corresponding management options for people living in remote areas. As traveling to clinics for check-ups can be burdensome for older adults, people with disabilities, and the family caregivers of these individuals, uninterrupted and automated collection, analysis, and sharing of key health data with family or professional caregivers by algorithmic monitoring platforms may facilitate proactive and continuing interventional assistance, thus easing caregiver burden while also promoting safety at home.[53] These technologies can potentially facilitate earlier and broader care management to prevent acute deteriorations or serious injuries, thereby preserving people's well-being and delaying or avoiding the use of costly institutional care.[54]

The COVID-19 pandemic has highlighted both the need for and convenience of remote patient monitoring for people with chronic and non-acute conditions. Home health monitoring and virtual care allow people to receive medical attention without fear of viral exposure or transportation inconveniences. They are accelerating the shift towards a future where patients can self-manage their conditions with the assistance of remote and automated technologies to the greatest extent feasible and without compromising their health outcomes. In light of the intersecting concerns of an aging population, a declining formal/informal caregiver ratio, overstretched health systems, and an uncertain pandemic outlook, AI home health monitoring reflects and contributes to changes in how care work is conceptualized and organized. If successfully and equitably implemented, this can be helpful not only for older or disabled individuals with mobility challenges, but also for patients who face other barriers to in-person consultation for routine or chronic conditions due to work and other personal responsibilities.

The increasing interest among health care providers and health systems in adopting or expanding AI health monitoring is significant not only from a service access and health outcome perspective—it is also ethically significant. Messages around the adoption of AI home health monitoring are increasingly moralized, touting these technologies as a means of promoting individual autonomy by enhancing people's engagement in and management of their own health, as well as their ability to live at home independently.[55] Optimism abounds that these tools will facilitate individuals' self-governance, self-determination, and self-authorization, which are essential to individual autonomy.

First, AI health monitoring technologies that provide continuous data collection and predictive analysis may promote people's self-governance by enhancing their capacity to recognize and understand potential health changes and remedies to prevent further deterioration. As seen in the PD and AD examples, instead of patients having to wait for professional consultations to gain access to their health information and insight around their disease progression, ongoing monitoring and data collection, display, and analysis may help monitored users recognize and respond to their physiological changes as per algorithmic advice. For adults whose cognitive and functional capacities may decline over time, automated home health monitoring that allows them to participate in AI-guided routines, facilitated by predictive reminders and health alerts such as fall prevention warning signals, may help to maintain people's self-governance by optimizing their ability to safely navigate their familiar environment. As the ability to live in one's home allows people more control over architectural design, furniture arrangement, and display items that reflect their identity and will, AI home health monitoring may also help to preserve people's competencies and authenticity, which are crucial to self-governance. This may in turn help delay or prevent the need for moving to an unfamiliar institutional environment and interacting with rotating caregivers, which can exacerbate confusion and further compromise individuals' ability to comprehend their situations.

Second, if AI home health monitoring can enable people with otherwise high health risks and care needs to live at home, these technologies may promote self-determination by contributing to de-institutionalization. De-institutionalization refers to the idea that people with disabilities, whatever their age, should have the same rights as anyone to live free and independent lives and participate in the community to whatever extent they desire. They should not be subjected to unwanted custodial care or segregated institutional living, which is often accompanied by paternalistic attitudes and numerous environmental and operational restrictions. Such restrictions are generally not under the residents' control and can significantly limit their mobility and social interaction with family, friends, or even other residents and staff, all based on the facility's operational capacity rather than the desire or functional capability of the particular resident. Early lockdowns and continuing worries about viral spread at the 15,000+ nursing homes in the United States during the COVID-19 pandemic compounded the impact of institutional restrictions and further decreased in-person care and monitoring for older adults in residential care facilities, exacerbating an estimated 1.3 million residents' social isolation and health risks.[56] Living at home with AI health monitoring support may promote self-determination by allowing users who can afford, navigate, and consent to these platforms to move freely and have more control over their spatial arrangement, meal times, food choices, or other daily and social activities.

Third, AI home health monitoring has the potential to enhance observed users' self-authorization, particularly for people who experience functional or cognitive limitations and whose testimony about their ability to live at home safely may be questioned by family members and health care professionals. It may also help to de-medicalize one's functional changes. De-medicalization involves shifting away from the power-based medical model that pathologizes different physical characteristics and disabilities as inevitable results of natural inferiority that can only be resolved or addressed by medical or clinical strategies, as determined by professionals. Just as a driver's ability to get from one location to another can now be augmented by AI-enabled interactive routing systems, an older or disabled adult's ability to move around safely in their own home may also be enhanced by predictive technologies that can adjust lighting, warn them of physical barriers and fall risks, or remind them to rest between steps. Ongoing feedback loops and predictive analytics from AI health monitoring may allow all stakeholders to recognize that a particular individual's ability to live safely at home is not static. In addition to suggesting architectural and other environmental adjustments, assistive technologies can enhance a person's functional capability and safety by providing clinically relevant alerts, reminders, and recommendations based on user environment and responses. For people with memory or cognitive challenges, AI health monitoring devices can act as extended minds, helping users to remember various safety protocols, medications, appointments, etc. so that they can be more confident about their ability to exercise practical control over their lives. In addition, monitoring platforms that can share information, alerts, and predictive outputs with formal and informal caregivers may boost individuals' authority and testimonial credibility about their proclaimed ability to live safely at home or their expressed need for follow-up care and other services.

3. The Promise of Independent Living and Autonomy Reassessed

As emerging AI health monitoring technologies bring forth new tools to potentially enhance older and/or disabled adults' ability to live safely at home, there are lingering questions as to whether these technologies may inadvertently compromise people's self-governance, self-determination, and self-authorization in ways that cannot be remedied through traditional models of informed consent. While consent requirements are helpful for preventing explicitly coercive acts in dyadic power relationships, they are insufficient for addressing whether the shift to automated and predictive health monitoring technologies may exacerbate hierarchically structured social relations and institutional practices that affect people's ability to live according to their practical identity. As evolving technological developments intersect with social norms around healthy aging and independent living, institutional and system promotions of AI health monitoring may affect monitored people's normative and practical authority to determine how they want to live and be cared for. Moreover, the individualist conception of autonomy neglects important socio-relational questions of how to reconcile the freedoms and opportunities of monitored users with those who are providing care in this new technological environment. Since people's ability to live at home with AI health monitoring depends on others' willingness and ability to facilitate and support such arrangements, these technologies can affect caregivers' own freedom and well-being and/or exacerbate power imbalances.

In what follows, I utilize a relational autonomy lens to explore how AI home health monitoring may reinforce hierarchical care relations and power-based practices, impose new expectations or responsibilities for self-management, and constrain targeted populations' ability to make home health monitoring decisions that would best support their practical identities and life plans. AI health monitoring is not a neutral technological process; it takes place within—and can therefore affect—human relationships and power dynamics, raising questions of whether or how people can truly choose how they want to monitor their health in accordance with their self-conception and reflective values in this broader techno-cultural and socio-relational context. In particular, I focus on how AI home health monitoring may compromise people's self-governance, self-determination, and self-authorization by (1) stigmatizing older and disabled adults as well as dependency conditions, (2) framing independent living as an individual civic responsibility while neglecting social determinants of health, (3) medicalizing people's homes and restructuring their motivations and expectations at home, (4) reorganizing care work and care relationships in ways that reinforce but disguise power relations, and (5) foreclosing other reasonable health monitoring options.

3.1 Re-stigmatization of Dependency

As we have seen, AI health monitoring is increasingly touted as a panacea that can fill home care gaps and support people's ability to live at home. These technologies promise to enhance the autonomy of older and disabled people, whose risks of suffering from unobserved health decline and injuries may compromise their ability to live in the privacy and safety of their own home. In the public discourse, it is often presumed that these population groups are (potentially) vulnerable and would welcome continuous and automated monitoring and alerts in their homestead as part of rational self-interest. As healthy aging and independent living movements focus on maintaining function and preventing debilitating conditions (or minimizing their effects), AI health monitoring technologies are increasingly interpreted as care practices that promote older and disabled adults' interests and preferences for de-medicalization and de-institutionalization.[57] When Diane (see Preface) experienced declining cognition and suspected surreptitious visitors, for example, her physician quickly suggested continuous monitoring. The physician viewed it as a benevolent act that would undoubtedly be accepted by—or could be legitimately imposed on—her patient, even though Diane was already wary of uninvited guests.

The idea that older adults and people with disabilities require or can benefit from special protection through continuous monitoring is not new. According to longstanding stereotypes, older and disabled people are less capable of acting autonomously, and others can therefore decide what they would be willing to accept based on their presumed vulnerability.[58] However, while AI health monitoring technologies purport to provide benevolent support and restore the autonomy of monitored individuals, they may in fact further stigmatize older and disabled people, as well as the notion of dependency itself, thereby compromising their self-governance, self-determination, and self-authorization.

First, while advocates of AI home health monitoring promise to promote individuals' autonomy by helping them to retain independence at a time when they may be experiencing increasing frailty, dependency, and engagement with medical services, continuous and automated technological monitoring extends sick roles to those targeted for such monitoring, potentially reinforcing negative stereotypes regarding their capabilities. Despite the diverse range of cognitive and functional capabilities among older and disabled adults, the underlying message around AI health monitoring technologies is that old age and disability entail such unique levels of risk and vulnerability that those so categorized constitute a separate class, requiring, or at least legitimizing, ongoing surveillance for their own protection. This message is especially troubling given that many targeted individuals only require help with certain daily activities, such as getting dressed, bathing, preparing meals, or managing medication, rather than continuous observation algorithms in search of "repetitive eating motions."[59] In liberal societies, proposals for ongoing surveillance would generally raise concerns of privacy violation of moral agents. Nonetheless, proposals by health systems, professionals, and family members to continuously monitor older adults and people with disabilities based on their theoretical risks appear to play out somewhat differently.[60] They generally frame continuous surveillance, assessment, and nudging as medical and social responsibilities grounded in paternalistic benevolence. Indeed, continuous surveillance of older and/or disabled adults is often construed as part of a collective or public duty to care for these individuals, whereby looking *at* them is equated to looking *out for* them as a caring practice.[61] People with disability and older adults who are subjected to such dominant narratives about inherent weaknesses or vulnerabilities may also internalize these oppressive viewpoints and adapt their preferences according to these circumstances.[62] For people with cognitive decline or impairments, who may lack adequate capacity to decide on or articulate their preferences around these technologies, there is also a presumption that these individuals would welcome continuous monitoring if they were able to understand their risks, or that they would be willing to forfeit personal privacy from ongoing data collection in exchange for a higher sense of physical safety.

Second, as the rhetoric around AI health monitoring focuses on how these technologies, particularly ambient monitoring technologies, can reduce or bypass the need for in-person assistance or caregiving *itself*,[63] it may reinforce the stigmatizing ideology that dependency on other human beings for health monitoring, reminders, and assistance in daily activities negates self-determination and autonomy. Technology developers and policymakers often frame dependence on in-person monitoring and assistance as a lack of self-sufficiency, yet they conceptualize similar reliance on technological health monitoring as a form of self-regulation and self-improvement that empowers and enhances independent living and healthy aging at home.[64]

Certainly, empirical data suggest that most people, regardless of age and functional ability, prefer the privacy and comfort of living at home, where they have resources to preserve their practical identity, rather than in crowded institutional care facilities that impose various disempowering policies and practices on residents.[65] And people with (and without) disabilities have long used assistive technologies to enhance their ability to live healthy and productive lives. There is also evidence that self-governing and self-determining agents shun lopsided in-person care relationships. Nonetheless, there is a paucity of research indicating that older adults prefer automated technological tools to positive and empowering care relationships and/or nontechnical solutions that can preserve privacy. For example, individuals from diverse nondominant cultural groups that value personal interdependence may prefer other socio-relational strategies that enhance their capacity to live at home safely, such as providing subsidies for in-person care or respite for family caregivers.[66] For many, constructive care relationships that can foster their capacities and promote their well-being are more important than independence in promoting their autonomy as they navigate their living environment and health needs.[67] There can be important relational and moral goods internal to such practice of caregiving, teaching us the moral meaning and importance of reciprocity and fostering empathy.[68]

It is worth noting that "independent living" as a civil rights movement focuses on the removal of physical, structural, social, and systemic barriers that compromise people's ability to exercise their self-governance and self-determination regarding where and how they want to live. Autonomy within this framework is about having the socially recognized self-authority to make decisions about one's goals, pursuits, and daily life, rather than maintaining physical independence or self-sufficiency.[69] It is perfectly possible to rely on others for functional and health needs and simultaneously experience high levels of autonomy if one is in interdependent and/or positive relationships that enhance self-esteem, self-determination, purpose in life, personal growth, and continuity of the self.[70] Self-authorizing agents can accept help and still have ample opportunities for self-expression if their normative power to direct their lives and make decisions accordingly is respected by others.[71]

In other words, autonomy is about people's ability to participate, cohabitate, and interact with family and others in ways they see fit, rather than a rejection of personal assistance by others or a desire to achieve one's goals in isolation.[72] The quest for autonomy in this context is a denunciation of overreach by professionals, public officials, and others in deciding how aging, disability, or embodied experience are defined, what levels and types of monitoring and support services people may need, and how these needs will be met or supported. Moreover, independence is not a fixed concept or experience.[73] Instead, it is socio-relational and multidimensional, based on an individual's sense of choice and control over personal support and self-conception.[74] It is also the authority to determine what kinds of health monitoring and follow-up practices one would like to pursue without fear of prejudicial attitudes about aging and disability, which can subtly but profoundly impact people's motivational structure and ability to uphold their practical identity. The promotion of AI health monitoring as a tool for people to minimize their functional reliance on others and reclaim their physical independence misses how the ideology and practices around these technological solutions may perpetuate such stigmas of dependency.

As Alasdair MacIntyre has noted, humans flourish and discover their own "goods" by acknowledging the virtue of independent practical reasoning in and through social relationships and the achievement of common goods.[75] Given that we are embodied beings who are inevitably dependent on others for care in at least some stages of life,[76] interdependence and positive care relationships are essential not only for survival but also for autonomy.[77] Accepting interdependency as a universal condition and recognizing the inevitability or even the virtue of dependency, autonomy is about building a socio-relational environment whereby people can request and obtain communal assistance in the manner they see fit without fear of stigma and discrimination. AI can enhance some of these efforts to provide additional support, but replacing human monitoring with AI technologies to enhance self-sufficiency without correcting stigmatizing stereotypes about aging and disability may ironically compromise people's practical self-identity and emotional well-being. This is particularly concerning, since the shift from in-person to AI monitoring for people who live alone and "independently" may result in less frequent family visits or in-person professional consultations, if AI is presumed to be adequate or superior in replacing such needs. During the COVID-19 pandemic, social isolation has been found to correlate with worsening mental health, especially for individuals living in limited physical space.[78] Even though online contacts provide some protection, prolonged replacement of in-person interaction with online modalities may contribute to other forms of mental health degradation.[79] Questions abound as to whether an increasing reliance on AI home health monitoring may ironically compromise users' cognitive capacity and opportunities to flourish; for example, reduced social contact may lower cognitive engagement, stimulation, or other forms of daily and civic activities.[80]

3.2 Self-Monitoring as Individual Responsibility

Intersecting with concerns of stigmatizing dependency are the moral tensions between individual empowerment and individual responsibility. In many democratic societies that emphasize the importance of individual autonomy, the ideal of healthy aging, or *successful* aging, is promoted as both an intrinsic goal and a means to maintain independence, especially the ability to live in one's own home. Framing healthy aging as something that empowered individuals can decide and act on, public health campaigns across many countries encourage older adults to engage in healthy eating, physical activities, and other positive lifestyle "choices."[81] For example, Health Canada identifies healthy eating and physical activity as "determinants" that play key roles in healthy aging; it advises older adults to "keep [themselves] healthy" and reduce the risk of chronic disease by making these "positive" lifestyle "choices."[82] In the United Kingdom, the 2010 *Healthy Lives, Healthy People* policy paper names the "promotion of active ageing" as a central public health strategy, while the National Health Services web portal promotes "exercises for older people" and "eat[ing] well over 60" as key ways to "help you stay healthy, energetic and independent as you get older."[83] In the United States, the Department of Health and Human Services promotes healthy aging as a "national priority" and "encourages all Americans to lead a healthy and active life" by "adopting healthy habits and behaviors, staying involved in [their] community, using preventive services, managing health conditions, and understanding all [their] medications."[84]

Granted, there is evidence that certain lifestyles (e.g., avoiding tobacco, alcohol, and substance misuse; engaging in moderate to vigorous physical activity) are associated with a longer life expectancy free of major chronic diseases.[85] And health promotion programs do not generally coerce people into following certain recommendations, at least not explicitly. Nevertheless, the obligation to take responsibility for one's own health remains integral to what it means to be a rational and responsible citizen within Western neoliberal contexts.[86] Despite advances made in public health research on how various social determinants of health, institutional policies, and socio-environmental factors can affect people's ability to adopt or sustain various health-promoting activities, the civic-moral imperative to actively engage in proactive and preventive risk management of one's own aging process is increasingly pronounced for older citizens, who are exhorted to stave off the effects of aging and emerging health problems to maintain a "productive and meaningful life" through self-care practices of body monitoring and improvement, risk management, and an active lifestyle.[87]

Within this discourse, acceptance of AI health monitoring technologies to enhance one's ability to stay in one's own home is increasingly couched in normative or moralized terms.[88] Older adults are urged to accept the free choice of fulfilling the idealized notion of independent living to liberate themselves from medical paternalism, but also to spare individual, familial, and societal costs of institutional care.[89] Such emphasis on self-empowerment through disciplining technologies implies that people who require a higher level of in-person care may be blamed for not staying active, productive, or independent.[90] However, this individualist focus on self-management and successful aging treats degenerative conditions and the aging process as something mostly or wholly under individual control, without addressing structural-political-economic dimensions of healthy living. Such rhetoric effectively places blame on those who were predisposed to various conditions and cannot gain control over their lifestyle and health to maintain self-sufficiency—even when that may not have been a realistic or desired goal based on the person's context and competing priorities, or when health care and social policies and practices have not supported people's abilities to pursue their health goals.[91] As we recall from the last chapter, social determinants of health and digital literacy can have substantial impact on people's ability to understand health information and act accordingly. The uncritically accepted directive of independent living paradoxically perpetuates ageism and ableism, distorts the meaning of good quality of life by neglecting the relational and communal dimension of healthy living and aging, and further marginalizes people who have higher care needs or require long-term dependency care. As Holstein and Minkler caution, the new paradigm of "healthy aging," which idealizes the positive features of aging and promotes conventional notions of autonomy as empowering, may be counterproductive or even oppressive, unwittingly imposing unrealistic and overbearing standards that can negatively affect the identity and self-worth of people who fail to live up to these normative ideals.[92] It is worth noting that, even if people accept the self-obligation to be digitally engaged, metrics that measure disability and functioning show that only 27.2 percent of older adults are able to achieve "successful aging."[93] If learning algorithms and associated health promotion programs use these metrics to forecast and enhance people's ability to achieve "healthy aging" and "independent living," despite users' own priorities or subjective self-conceptions,[94] they may marginalize people who do not conform to such narrow notions of independence and lead to further restrictions.

3.3 Hospital at (Artificial) Home

As health systems increasingly shift health monitoring from clinics and hospitals to patients' homes—using AI technologies, such as various hospital-at-home programs, for self-management—they are restructuring monitored users' living environments and redefining the meaning of a home. Even though these technologies can be valuable resources for short-term post-acute or post-discharge transition for patients returning home from hospitals, long-term continuous AI health monitoring may restructure people's practical identities and motivations. While these monitoring technologies are generally promoted as ways to de-institutionalize and de-medicalize care by enhancing people's ability to receive ongoing attention in the comfort and safety of their familiar home environment, they may paradoxically extend medicalized and asymmetrical power relations into people's homes in ways that curb users' self-governance or capacity for self-expression.

Traditionally, clinics, laboratories, hospitals, and other medical spaces operate under specific regulatory and licensing guidelines that structure the parameters within which various health monitoring practices formally take place. They designate and authorize health care providers with predefined roles, responsibilities, and accountabilities, guiding how all stakeholders must behave and interact with each other during the scheduled consultation appointments and within professional spaces. In the United States, the Health Insurance Portability and Accountability Act (HIPAA) also regulates how identifiable patient information and data collected in these HIPAA-covered entities will be handled to ensure data privacy or confidentiality. Feminist bioethicists have raised legitimate concerns regarding various institutional and systemic practices that reinforce professional hierarchies and power relations, which can compromise patients' self-governance, self-determination, and self-authorization. Ultimately, boundaries to professional reach play an important role in preventing abuse of power and violation of personal privacy in health care delivery.

In contrast to these formally structured environments and highly regulated encounters, liberal democratic societies typically define the home (for people who reside in stable housing) as a private space where individuals are free to express themselves according to their evolving practical identities, preferences, and priorities, without the constant gaze or interference of uninvited others. Homes are often full of personal memories, relationships, and possessions that turn material spaces or physical structures into places with symbolic meanings that elicit a sense of belonging and attachment.[95] For people who have been subjected to various unjust institutions and practices, home can be a vehicle for developing resistance to oppression and other forms of intrusion, where one can have control over the space.[96] Patients who return home after prolonged hospitalizations, where they have been under the constant scrutiny of machines and care professionals, often find comfort in transitioning out of their illness-defined experience and identity and returning to "normal" life.[97] The freedom and opportunity for self-determination in one's own space is precisely why many people consider their homestead as the best environment to facilitate independent living.

As medicalized technological objects or functions are increasingly proposed for people's living quarters, however, there is a paradox in conceptualizing the unobserved home—one that is supposed to provide privacy and comfort—as a potentially unsafe physical space that legitimates ongoing surveillance in the name of protecting the targeted occupant from harm. This intersects with increasing adoption of smart doorbells in higher-income populations, where these technologies are promoted not only as necessary protections against potential intrusion from unknown others, but also as portals to simply watch and track what happens in their home or around the neighborhood.[98] As the watchful eyes of technologies move into the health care arena, the line between one's private home and a clinical care space under professional norms and surveillance becomes blurry. This is especially the case if AI home monitoring is recommended or ordered by a patient's clinical care provider, who will receive continuous data and algorithmic outputs from the monitoring system. Home is not a neutral physical space,[99] and the implementation of AI health monitoring in one's home is not a value-free technological endeavor to simply promote health outcomes. By indefinitely collecting heterogeneous data in the name of comprehensive and personalized predictive analysis, AI-powered technologies transform one's home into an ongoing medical observation unit, converting personal and intimate home experiences into medical information awaiting further analysis and recommendations.

Moreover, AI home health monitoring, especially ambient technologies that automatically collect and transfer various types of data to care teams and device companies, perpetually places monitored individuals under the watchful eyes of not only the machines but also anonymous others who receive the data and/or algorithmic outputs. Even though some technologies such as computer vision may convert raw footage to a de-personalized data format, these technologies can still alter and disrupt the nature, structure, ambience, and symbolic meanings of the physical environment, including the resident's relationship with the place and with any cohabitants. As ongoing monitoring allows observation even when there is no danger, such practices can change expectations of what information health care professionals and others may legitimately collect, access, and share with third parties in the name of risk management and health protection. In the era of IoT and big data, where different sources and types of data are merged for ML and algorithmic analysis, patients and users of AI health monitoring often do not know in advance how their data may be handled or shared with other parties, and whether the use of multiple datapoints to promote personalized care may increase the identifiability of technology users. Paradoxically, health monitoring platforms that are touted as enhancing personal privacy by facilitating living at home may in fact introduce more avenues for data access by (unknown) others, even when the targeted user is at theoretical rather than actual risk, and thus monitoring would not provide much clinical value. While small units or ambient sensors that are not highly visible may seem unobtrusive, just being aware that one is subjected to continuous and one-way observation and analysis by others based on one's presumed vulnerability and lower capability can feel belittling and damage people's self-trust and practical identity.[100] It can also affect one's relationship with those who are recommending such monitoring or receiving data from these technologies.

Michel Foucault's concept of disciplining acts is helpful here. It highlights additional concerns that AI home health monitoring may alter people's self-identity and compromise their relational autonomy in subtle ways that are nonetheless difficult to resist.[101] Disciplining (and self-disciplining) acts are acts of power relations solidified by social and cultural discourses, practices, and institutions. This is particularly true for biomedicine, where emerging technologies such as AI home health monitoring serve as new engines for medicalizing and redefining human embodied experiences. Expert systems and other supervised learning algorithms predetermine thresholds and teach machines to categorize various labeled physiological and behavioral patterns as problems, and govern how these predicted troubles should be communicated and managed in people's homes.[102] Many monitored users or even their caregivers may not understand or agree with the predictive analytical outputs produced by these opaque systems, but they are expected to follow the prescriptive recommendations by virtue of using these devices. Users who do not comply will be continuously nudged by the automated system, which never gets tired or frustrated. Promises of user-tailored outputs notwithstanding, these devices are not generally set up for users to question the algorithmic recommendations or negotiate a mutually acceptable response, except for allowing the user to turn off monitoring and possibly some of the alert or notification functions. Unless the algorithm is learning continuously and is capable of self-adjusting various threshold levels for alerts or algorithmic recommendations based on the users' own desires or evolving baselines, monitored individuals whose subjective embodied experience differs from the outputs indicated by the predictive algorithms may doubt themselves or worry that they may not be trusted by others. As we will see in Chapter 5, most AI systems are "locked" algorithms that do not adapt over time on their own based on new data.[103] Thus, what is touted as an empowering technology for enhancing independent living can function more akin to a disciplinary tool that forces monitored users to abide by various healthy aging goals, predetermined by professionals, health systems, and technology developers without consideration for users' dynamic priorities and risk tolerance that may evolve over time.[104]

3.4 Whose Care Work Is It Anyway?

The shift from in-person care to automated home health monitoring not only medicalizes one's home but also imposes and reorganizes care work and care relationships, highlighting the inadequacy of considering autonomy only at the individual level of the monitored person. These emerging technological practices may reinforce existing power asymmetries and introduce new power relations that can compromise the autonomy of not only the people being monitored, but also their family or informal caregivers (who are predominantly women), raising ethical questions of how to reconcile conflicting priorities and concerns.[105]

As social and health care institutions increasingly redistribute care from the state and formal caregivers to informal caregivers and individuals themselves,[106] the significant involvement of family in supporting older adults and disabled people as they seek to live "independently" at home highlights the complexity of navigating a physical and moral space where individual and familial interests intertwine and diverge. For family caregivers who live with the monitored person, AI health monitoring technologies also impose significant restrictions on caregivers' practical and relational identities, transforming their caregiver's living space into a continuous health data collection site as well as their role and relations in that space. The implementation of these automated monitoring platforms reconfigures how care work is conceptualized, recognized, delegated, and carried out.[107] It may counter how these caregivers identify themselves, their care roles and responsibilities, and their relationship to those whom they are caring for. These technological practices redefine various expectations that family members may have of each other, including the timing and frequency of providing care based on algorithmic recommendations rather than the family caregivers' capacity and the monitored person's desires. They reflect and potentially reinforce power imbalances that may affect different stakeholders' autonomy and well-being in various ways.[108]

First, while the home usually serves as a place of social relations and personal life,[109] the adoption of AI health monitoring, which turns the home into a site of care, can change feelings of privacy, control, and power relations for *all* residents, not just the monitored individual. Despite the rhetoric of promoting independent living via technology, older and disabled people who are continuously observed and analyzed due to their presumed inability to determine their own risk levels may face disempowerment in their care relationships. On the one hand, family caregiving is deeply symbolic,[110] especially in cultures where filial interdependency is highly valued, and many family caregivers accept such care responsibilities willingly in order to uphold what they perceive to be their loved one's values and/or best interests. Some caregivers fully accept and embrace their capacity to care well as part of their and their loved ones' flourishing.[111] On the other hand, because people with higher care needs often depend on family caregivers to live at home, caregiving is also inherently fraught with power asymmetry that can compromise monitored adults' ability to determine their practical identity and priorities. As family caregivers work with and against dependency,[112] the connectivity between these stakeholders' well-being raises questions regarding how much control family caregivers may have over loved ones under their care. This includes whether they can impose or withhold AI health monitoring in their shared living space, how much health information family caregivers should be able to access through the AI system, and who should have control over the algorithmic settings (e.g., frequency or types of alerts), especially if the stakeholders may have different levels of risk tolerance.[113] In one study with Meals on Wheels clients and their adult children regarding their perceptions of in-home health monitoring technologies, researchers found that the children preferred these technologies more than their elderly parents.[114] Other studies show that older adults desire control over what information AI systems may share with family and caregivers and when they should be monitored.[115] For example, an older adult may want to be able to turn the monitoring system on and off based on their perceived needs or well-being rather than allow others to indirectly monitor them at all times. They may want the AI system to alert others when they have fallen and are injured, but not when they have fallen but are uninjured and able to get up unassisted, or when they are unstable on their feet but manage to not fall. Moreover, prescriptive outputs from AI analytics that are trained on predefined thresholds through supervised learning, such as behavioral change recommendations, may counter an older adult's desires or their own risk assessments (e.g., getting out of bed without assistance).

While disagreements with family caregivers or medical professionals are not new, algorithms are often promoted as being fairer or more objective than humans, such that older adults may face additional scrutiny if they decline AI monitoring or reject the algorithm's safety recommendations. This thinly veiled power and control may deny the person self-authorization in the name of benevolence and AI superiority,[116] restricting rather than expanding the decisional domains of those being monitored.[117] If monitoring technologies have the power to impose "objective" recommendations, regardless of older adults' own priorities and concerns in their own home, users may simply abandon the technology altogether in order to retain or regain certain levels of control, or may try to manipulate the data (e.g., find various means to trick the system).[118]

Second, and relatedly, AI home health monitoring may have a significant impact on potential family caregivers, whose interests and concerns are generally neglected in the liberal bioethics discussion of individual autonomy, wherein patients' priorities often take precedence over those of others. The value placed on filial interdependency notwithstanding, we need to be cautious of idealizing caregiving at home, which has been socially constructed as a predominantly female activity and responsibility. Women have been historically and/or socially expected to take on caregiving work regardless of their resources, capacities, or priorities. Gender oppression continues to shape many women's practical identities and motivational structures around caregiving, and how much personal privacy they can expect. According to the aforementioned AARP report, in 2020, 55 percent of women who provided care felt that they had no choice but to take on their caregiving role (compared to 50 percent in 2015).[119] Compounding the burden on these (predominantly female) family caregivers, their work is often devalued and uncompensated, despite the fact that many of these individuals must give up other employment opportunities to provide at-home care.[120] Given that AI technologies are often touted as innovative tools that can help reduce caregiver workload and support people to live safely and "independently" at home, family members who are ambivalent about their ability to manage these technologies and carry out care duties may nonetheless feel obliged to accept such monitoring platforms and associated care work, regardless of their own comfort level. These new technological practices may further shape or predetermine potential family caregivers' views of who they are and what roles they can accept or reject, as these technologies may send the message that there are fewer "excuses" for family members to refuse care responsibilities for their loved ones or ask for additional help, as the predictive algorithmic outputs purportedly take on the bulk of the monitoring work and guide caregivers to attend to the monitored individuals.

The hyperbolic promises of what AI home health monitoring can do on its own reflect and exacerbate the disproportionate prestige and confidence afforded to high-tech medicine, compared to the low social status, recognition, and compensation for both paid and informal caregivers who provide ongoing health monitoring and personal care.

Continuous automated monitoring and predictive analytics still require humans to verify output accuracy and respond accordingly for safe and successful implementation. Despite AI enthusiasts' optimism that automated health monitoring can decrease hospital readmissions and prevent medical emergencies, many studies on these technologies have poor reference standards and no explicit critical appraisal. One systematic review reports that only 6 percent of surveyed studies achieved Level 1 evidence or good reference standards,[121] even as the objectivity, accuracy, and efficacy of AI algorithms continue to be hyped in the public discourse. Given the lower technological literacy among older adults, family caregivers will likely have to perform quality assurance tasks and provide other forms of technology support to the monitored users, in addition to personal care work. Demonstrating the Foucauldian concept of disciplining acts, AI alerts trigger and impose behaviors not only on the monitored person but also on their caregivers.[122] They impress upon caregivers the need to intervene according to algorithmic outputs, and may continue to issue alerts until caregiver compliance is achieved, thereby simultaneously disciplining them. We can imagine family or professional caregivers rushing to the monitored person's side when an alert indicates that the person is walking unsteadily, even if that may be the person's baseline. Depending on the sensitivity and specificity of the algorithm, and how well the algorithm can adjust according to the user's environment (e.g., if there are railings) and adaptation to their own changing functional status, frequent triggers and false alarms may intensify caregivers' worries and workload rather than reduce their burden. Reactive caregiving based on algorithmic alerts also raises questions of whether the expanding use of AI health monitoring technologies may lead to more detached and medicalized caregiving experiences, turning relational caregiving into care work.[123]

Because caregivers' responses to alerts are also recorded and analyzed as part of an AI system,[124] caregivers are subjected to indirect surveillance. Although the privacy of monitored users has received much attention in the literature, there is a paucity of practice or policy discussions on how to minimize potential intrusion and burden on caregivers, and whether they have moral and legal claims to data privacy. Further shifting health monitoring and related care responsibilities to informal caregivers, while also downplaying the resources, technological skills, labor, and privacy sacrifices required to implement these platforms successfully, reinforces gendered social and familial relationships, further renders care work invisible, and marginalizes women, who predominantly provide the care required to uphold monitored users' autonomy. In 2020, 57 percent of women caregivers (compared to 50 percent in 2015) reported acting as an advocate when interacting with care providers, community services, or government agencies in addition to monitoring and providing care to their loved ones.[125]

3.5 You Can't Have This. And You Can't Have That.

While accurate AI health monitoring can be a useful supplement to care that may otherwise be unavailable, a relational lens of autonomy that attends to power relations and socio-structural contexts of people's choices helps to reveal the ways in which the expanding practice of shifting home health monitoring to AI technologies may compromise people's ability to live autonomously. On the one hand, questions abound as to whether these technologies are truly accessible to people who may desire or benefit from ongoing monitoring. On the other hand, there are concerns that the wider promotion of these products may gradually restrict other opportunities for desired health monitoring alternatives.

First, relational self-determination considers both liberty and opportunity conditions that either enhance or hinder people's ability to carry out their desired choices, with special attention on ensuring that people have equal access to personal, social, and political opportunities for achieving self-determination.[126] As technologists and policymakers continue to tout the benefits of AI health monitoring, there are questions of whether these platforms may be prohibitively expensive and too technologically complex, rendering them accessible only to those of higher socioeconomic status and digital skills. The effectiveness of these technologies in promoting people's ability to live at home safely relies on the monitored users' and/or caregivers' ability to navigate these platforms and respond according to algorithmic recommendations. From a relational perspective, an empowering paradigm that supports older adults or people with disabilities would require taking into account their own agendas, technical capacities, and material and social circumstances.[127] In order for individuals to truly have the opportunity to exercise self-determination in fully evaluating and adopting AI home health monitoring, institutional and infrastructure support is needed to ensure that these options are genuinely accessible to all populations, particularly members of marginalized, disadvantaged, or historically oppressed groups. Populations that lack the financial means to hire in-person care or do not have family support may also have limited resources to utilize AI home health monitoring. For example, Nobi, an AI-powered ceiling-mounted smart lamp for one's home that touts its ability to detect falls, prevent user dehydration by encouraging them to drink enough water, recognize the monitored user's activity patterns, detect smoke/fire, and other functions, costs $2,499 plus a monthly subscription fee (although cheaper platforms are increasingly available).[128] It is postulated that shifting health monitoring to people's homes may save health systems the high costs of institutional care. Those savings could be funneled into financial subsidies for monitoring devices, infrastructure for reliable internet access, and technology training and support, which would help provide the necessary and fair opportunity conditions to ensure that people from different socioeconomic backgrounds and geographical locations (e.g., rural or isolated areas) have equitable means to consider utilizing appropriate AI to support their health monitoring.

Second, we need to consider how the expanding use of AI home health monitoring may gradually affect the array of health monitoring opportunities or options available to people. As health systems increasingly turn to AI health monitoring technologies as a cost-effective way to replace or reduce rather than enhance in-person monitoring, these institutional practices may predetermine the options available to people with varying levels of functional and health needs, as well as how much risk they are allowed to take in their own home. Studies have shown that health care providers' trust in older adults' ability to self-manage relates significantly to their own perception of the person's capacity, but not to the person's self-rated ability.[129]

Interestingly, people who would have been able to live at home prior to AI health monitoring may now be subjected to more restrictions and privacy intrusion due to our ability to continuously monitor their behavior. Moreover, just as economically disadvantaged or historically oppressed individuals are more likely to have trouble accessing AI health monitoring technologies, even if they are eager to adopt them, these same individuals are at a higher risk of being pressured to accept technologies they are not comfortable with, especially as health care funding decisions by insurance and other health coverage payment plans are increasingly tied to the adoption of electronic and digital practices.[130] As hospitals may refuse to discharge patients based on care providers' risk perception and institutional risk management, some older adults and people with disabilities may resign themselves to these tools due to funding constraints or heavy nudging from family and clinicians, such that resistance may be unrealistic or futile.

4. Conclusion

As we can see, AI home health monitoring technologies are redefining the problem of inadequate in-person health monitoring, how the problem should be addressed, and which values should be prioritized, reconstructing the normative, relational, and practical goals of independent, at-home living in the process. Systemic concerns about human resource shortages for in-person monitoring and care have been reframed as opportunities to use AI health monitoring to empower otherwise dependent people to become independent. As these technologies are increasingly promoted and implemented, we must carefully weigh the proposed benefits for older adults and people with disabilities against the potential risks for both users and their caregivers. While these technologies may promote faster and more convenient monitoring, the ability to delay or prevent deterioration and institutional care, greater accuracy in tracking functional changes, and reduction in family care burden and health workforce pressure, they may also stigmatize dependency, medicalize the home, reduce in-person monitoring and care, distort care relationships, exacerbate social isolation, and invade privacy. Moreover, if paternalistic recommendations from algorithms do not align with users' desires or goals, or if these technologies are not affordable to all, they may also reinforce hierarchical care relations and inequitable access.

As home health monitoring becomes increasingly commercialized and integrated with other consumer technologies to track and predict both specific medical conditions and general wellness, bioethical questions regarding whether continuous monitoring compromises people's privacy and autonomy also gradually take on new directions. If targeting older and disabled people might stigmatize aging, disability, and dependency care, would broadening AI health monitoring to healthy "consumers" help to reduce such stigma and simultaneously democratize health information to promote users' autonomy? To explore this and other related issues, I will now turn to the area of direct-to-consumer AI health monitoring.

Notes

1. Toni Calasanti and Neal King, "Successful Aging, Ageism, and the Maintenance of Age and Gender Relations," in *Successful Aging as a Contemporary Obsession: Global Perspectives*, ed. Sarah Lamb (New Brunswick, NJ: Rutgers University Press, 2017), 27–40.
2. Stephen Katz, "Growing Older without Aging? Positive Aging, Anti-Ageism, and Anti-Aging," *Generations* 25 (2001/2002): 27–32.
3. Margriet Pol et al., "Older People's Perspectives Regarding the Use of Sensor Monitoring in Their Home," *Gerontologist* 56, no. 3 (2016): 485–93, https://doi.org/10.1093/geront/gnu104; J. van Hoof et al., "Ageing-in-Place with the Use of Ambient Intelligence Technology: Perspectives of Older Users," *International Journal of Medical Informatics* 80, no. 5 (2011): 310–31, http://doi.org/10.1016/j.ijmedinf.2011.02.010; Vimal Sriram, Crispin Jenkinson, and Michele Peters, "Informal Carers' Experience of Assistive Technology Use in Dementia Care at Home: A Systematic Review," *BMC Geriatrics* 19, no. 1 (2019): 160, https://doi.org/10.1186/s12877-019-1169-0.
4. Helen Hawley-Hague et al., "Older Adults' Perceptions of Technologies Aimed at Falls Prevention, Detection or Monitoring: A Systematic Review," *International Journal of Medical Informatics* 83, no. 6 (2014): 416–26, https://doi.org/10.1016/j.ijmedinf.2014.03.002.

5. Jui-Chen Huang, "Remote Health Monitoring Adoption Model Based on Artificial Neural Networks," *Expert Systems with Applications* 37, no. 1 (2010): 307–14, https://doi.org/10.1016/j.eswa.2009.05.063.
6. Riyad Al-Shaqi, Monjur Mourshed, and Yacine Rezgui, "Progress in Ambient Assisted Systems for Independent Living by the Elderly," *SpringerPlus* 5 (2016): 624, https://doi.org/10.1186/s40064-016-2272-8.
7. Elizabeth Arias and Jiaquan Xu, "United States Life Tables, 2017," *National Vital Statistics Reports* 68, no. 7 (2019): 1–66.
8. "2020 Profile of Older Americans," Administration for Community Living, U.S. Department of Health and Human Services, last modified November 24, 2021, https://acl.gov/aging-and-disability-in-america/data-and-research/profile-older-americans.
9. Adam Karpati et al., "Variability and Vulnerability at the Ecological Level: Implications for Understanding the Social Determinants of Health," *American Journal of Public Health* 92, no. 11 (2002): 1768–72, https://doi.org/10.2105/ajph.92.11.1768.
10. Luigi Fontana et al., "Medical Research: Treat Ageing," *Nature* 511 (2014): 405–7, https://doi.org/10.1038/511405a.
11. "Chronic Conditions Charts: 2018," Centers for Medicare & Medicaid Services, last modified December 1, 2021, https://www.cms.gov/Research-Statistics-Data-and-Systems/Statistics-Trends-and-Reports/Chronic-Conditions/Chartbook_Charts.html; National Academies of Sciences, Engineering, and Medicine, *Families Caring for an Aging America* (Washington, DC: National Academies Press, 2016), https://www.ncbi.nlm.nih.gov/books/NBK396397/.
12. Danielle M. Taylor, "Americans with Disabilities: 2014," United States Census Bureau, November 29, 2018, https://www.census.gov/library/publications/2018/demo/p70-152.html.
13. Vicki Freedman and Brenda Spillman, "Disability and Care Needs among Older Americans," *Milbank Quarterly* 92, no. 3 (2014): 509–41, https://doi.org/10.1111/1468-0009.12076.
14. National Academies of Sciences, Engineering, and Medicine, *Families Caring for an Aging America*.
15. Damien Stones and Judith Gullifer, "'At Home It's Just So Much Easier to Be Yourself': Older Adults' Perceptions of Ageing in Place," *Ageing and Society* 36, no. 3 (2016): 449–81, https://doi.org/10.1017/S0144686X14001214.
16. Cara Bailey Fausset et al., "Challenges to Aging in Place: Understanding Home Maintenance Difficulties," *Journal of Housing for the Elderly* 25, no. 2 (2011): 125–41, https://www.doi.org/10.1080/02763893.2011.571105; J. Kevin Eckert, Leslie A. Morgan, and Namratha Swamy, "Preferences

for Receipt of Care among Community-Dwelling Adults," *Journal of Aging & Social Policy* 16, no. 2 (2004): 49–65, https://www.doi.org/10.1300/J031v16n02_04.

17. Michael Sainato, "US Workers Who Risked Their Lives to Care for Elderly Demand Change," *The Guardian*, April 19, 2021, https://www.theguardian.com/us-news/2021/apr/19/nursing-home-care-workers-coronavirus.
18. Janine L. Wiles et al., "The Meaning of 'Aging in Place' to Older People," *Gerontologist* 52 (2012): 357–66, https://doi.org/10.1093/geront/gnr098.
19. Christine Milligan, *There's No Place Like Home: Place and Care in an Ageing Society*, 1st ed. (London: Routledge, 2009).
20. Janice L. Clarke et al., "An Innovative Approach to Health Care Delivery for Patients with Chronic Conditions," *Population Health Management* 20, no. 1 (2017): 23–30, https://www.doi.org/10.1089/pop.2016.0076; Nelly Oudshoorn, "How Places Matter: Telecare Technologies and the Changing Spatial Dimensions of Healthcare," *Social Studies of Science* 42, no. 1 (2012): 121–42, https://www.doi.org/10.1177/0306312711431817.
21. Andrew Donlan, "Kaiser Permanente, Mayo Clinic, Johns Hopkins and Others Form 'Advanced Care at Home Coalition,'" Home Health Care News, October 14, 2021, https://homehealthcarenews.com/2021/10/kaiser-permanente-mayo-clinic-johns-hopkins-and-others-form-advanced-care-at-home-coalition/.
22. U.S. Department of Health and Human Services et al., *National and Regional Projections of Supply and Demand for Geriatricians: 2013–2025* (Rockville, MD, 2017), https://bhw.hrsa.gov/sites/default/files/bureau-health-workforce/data-research/geriatrics-report-51817.pdf.
23. Bertalan Meskó, Gergely Hetényi, and Zsuzsanna Győrffy, "Will Artificial Intelligence Solve the Human Resource Crisis in Healthcare?" *BMC Health Services Research* 18 (2018), https://doi.org/10.1186/s12913-018-3359-4.
24. California Future Health Workforce Commission, "Meeting the Demand for Health: Final Report of the Future Health Workforce Commission" (2019), https://futurehealthworkforce.org/wp-content/uploads/2019/03/MeetingDemandForHealthFinalReportCFHWC.pdf.
25. Jeff Stein, "'This Will Be Catastrophic': Maine Families Face Elder Boom, Worker Shortage in Preview of Nation's Future," *Washington Post*, August 14, 2019, https://www.washingtonpost.com/business/economy/this-will-be-catastrophic-maine-families-face-elder-boom-worker-shortage-in-preview-of-nations-future/2019/08/14/7cecafc6-bec1-11e9-b873-63ace636af08_story.html.

26. Christopher Roland, "Seniors Are Stuck Home Alone as Health Aides Flee for Higher-Paying Jobs," *Washington Post*, September 25, 2022, https://www.washingtonpost.com/business/2022/09/25/seniors-home-health-care/.
27. Roland, "Seniors Are Stuck Home Alone."
28. Sainato, "US Workers Who Risked Their Lives."
29. Pireh Pirzada et al., "Ethics and Acceptance of Smart Homes for Older Adults," *Informatics for Health and Social Care* (July 2021): 1–28, https://doi.org/10.1080/17538157.2021.1923500.
30. "Cost of Care: Trends and Insights," Genworth, accessed February 8, 2022, https://www.genworth.com/aging-and-you/finances/cost-of-care/cost-of-care-trends-and-insights.html.
31. Office of U.S. Senator Bob Casey, "Disability Digest," *Aging Newsletter* 1, no. 1 (May 2020), https://www.aging.senate.gov/imo/media/doc/CASEY%20Aging%20Newsletter%20Issue%201.1.pdf.
32. National Academies of Sciences, Engineering, and Medicine, *Families Caring for an Aging America*; Donald Redfoot, Lynn Feinberg, and Ari Houser, "The Aging of the Baby Boom and the Growing Care Gap: A Look at Future Declines in the Availability of Family Caregivers," AARP Public Policy Institute, August 2013, https://www.aarp.org/home-family/caregiving/info-08-2013/the-aging-of-the-baby-boom-and-the-growing-care-gap AARP-ppi-ltc.html.
33. Redfoot et al., "Aging of the Baby Boom."
34. AARP and National Alliance for Caregiving, *Caregiving in the U.S. 2020* (Washington, DC: AARP, 2020), https://www.aarp.org/content/dam/aarp/ppi/2020/05/full-report-caregiving-in-the-united-states.doi.10.26419-2Fppi.00103.001.pdf.
35. AARP and National Alliance for Caregiving, *Caregiving in the U.S. 2020*.
36. Tijs Vandemeulebroucke, Bernadette Dierckx de Casterlé, and Chris Gastmans, "The Use of Care Robots in Aged Care: A Systematic Review of Argument-Based Ethics Literature," *Archives of Gerontology and Geriatrics* 74 (January 2018): 15–25, https://doi.org/10.1016/j.archger.2017.08.014.
37. Kaare Christensen et al., "Ageing Populations: The Challenges Ahead," *Lancet* 374, no. 9696 (October 2009): 1196–208, https://doi.org/10.1016/S0140-6736(09)61460-4.
38. Serena Yeung et al., "Bedside Computer Vision—Moving Artificial Intelligence from Driver Assistance to Patient Safety," *New England Journal of Medicine* 378, no. 14 (April 2018): 1271–73, https://doi.org/10.1056/NEJMp1716891.

39. Giles Birchley et al., "Smart Homes, Private Homes? An Empirical Study of Technology Researchers' Perceptions of Ethical Issues in Developing Smart-Home Health Technologies," *BMC Medical Ethics* 18, no. 1 (April 2017): 23, https://doi.org/10.1186/s12910-017-0183-z.
40. Shannon Vallor, *Technology and the Virtues: A Philosophical Guide to a Future Worth Wanting* (New York: Oxford University Press, 2016).
41. Ole-Bjørn Tysnes and Anette Storstein, "Epidemiology of Parkinson's Disease," *Journal of Neural Transmission* 124, no. 8 (August 2017): 901–5, https://doi.org/10.1007/s00702-017-1686-y; Alzheimer's Association, "2021 Alzheimer's Disease Facts and Figures," *Alzheimer's and Dementia* 17, no. 3 (March 2021): 327–406, https://doi.org/10.1002/alz.12328.
42. L. Teri and A. W. Wagner, "Assessment of Depression in Patients with Alzheimer's Disease: Concordance among Informants," *Psychology and Aging* 6, no. 2 (June 1991): 280–85, https://doi.org/10.1037//0882-7974.6.2.280.
43. E. M. Frank, "Effect of Alzheimer's Disease on Communication Function," *Journal of the South Carolina Medical Association* 90, no. 9 (September 1994): 417–23.
44. Yueng Santiago Delahoz and Miguel Angel Labrador, "Survey on Fall Detection and Fall Prevention Using Wearable and External Sensors," *Sensors* 14, no. 10 (October 2014): 19806–42, https://doi.org/10.3390/s141019806; Ramesh Rajagopalan, Irene Litvan, and Tzyy-Ping Jung, "Fall Prediction and Prevention Systems: Recent Trends, Challenges, and Future Research Directions," *Sensors* 17, no. 11 (November 2017), https://doi.org/10.3390/s17112509.
45. Zelun Luo et al., "Computer Vision-Based Descriptive Analytics of Seniors' Daily Activities for Long-Term Health Monitoring," *Proceedings of Machine Learning Research* 85 (2018): 1–18.
46. Ikram Asghar, Shuang Cang, and Hongnian Yu, "A Systematic Mapping Study on Assistive Technologies for People with Dementia," *9th International Conference on Software, Knowledge, Information Management and Applications (SKIMA)* (2015): 1–8, https://doi.org/10.1109/SKIMA.2015.7399989.
47. Nazia Gillani and Tughrul Arslan, "Intelligent Sensing Technologies for the Diagnosis, Monitoring and Therapy of Alzheimer's Disease: A Systematic Review," *Sensors* 21, no. 12 (June 2021): 4249, https://doi.org/10.3390/s21124249.
48. Sweta Karlekar, Tong Niu, and Mohit Bansal, "Detecting Linguistic Characteristics of Alzheimer's Dementia by Interpreting Neural Models," *Proceedings of the 2018 Conference of the North American Chapter of the*

Association for Computational Linguistics: Human Language Technologies, Volume 2 (Short Papers) (June 2018): 701–7, https://doi.org/10.18653/v1/N18-2110.

49. Deborah Vollmer Dahlke and Marcia G. Ory, "Emerging Opportunities and Challenges in Optimal Aging with Virtual Personal Assistants," *Public Policy & Aging Report* 27, no. 2 (May 2017): 68–73, https://doi.org/10.1093/ppar/prx004.
50. Hyun Gu Kang et al., "In Situ Monitoring of Health in Older Adults: Technologies and Issues," *Journal of the American Geriatrics Society* 58, no. 8 (August 2010): 1579–86, https://doi.org/10.1111/j.1532-5415.2010.02959.x.
51. Anita Ho, Stephen J. Pinney, and Kevin Bozic, "Ethical Concerns in Caring for Elderly Patients with Cognitive Limitations: A Capacity-Adjusted Shared Decision-Making Approach," *Journal of Bone and Joint Surgery* 97, no. 3 (2015): e16, https://doi.org/10.2106/JBJS.N.00762.
52. Roy P. C. Kessels, "Patients' Memory for Medical Information," *Journal of the Royal Society of Medicine* 96, no. 5 (May 2003): 219–22, https://doi.org/10.1258/jrsm.96.5.219.
53. Yeung et al., "Bedside Computer Vision."
54. Josephine McMurray et al., "The Importance of Trust in the Adoption and Use of Intelligent Assistive Technology by Older Adults to Support Aging in Place: Scoping Review Protocol," *JMIR Research Protocols* 6, no. 11 (November 2017): e218, https://doi.org/10.2196/resprot.8772; E. Ray Dorsey et al., "Moving Parkinson Care to the Home," *Movement Disorders* 31, no. 9 (September 2016): 1258–62, https://doi.org/10.1002/mds.26744.
55. A. Hasan Sapci and H. Aylin Sapci, "Innovative Assisted Living Tools, Remote Monitoring Technologies, Artificial Intelligence-Driven Solutions, and Robotic Systems for Aging Societies: Systematic Review," *JMIR Aging* 2, no. 2 (November 2019): e15429, https://doi.org/10.2196/15429.
56. Matt Sedensky and Bernard Condon, "Not Just COVID: Nursing Home Neglect Deaths Surge in Shadows," AP News, November 19, 2020, https://apnews.com/article/pandemics-us-news-coronavirus-pandemic-daac7f011bcf08747184bd851a1e1b8e.
57. Louis Neven, "By Any Means? Questioning the Link between Gerontechnological Innovation and Older People's Wish to Live at Home," *Technological Forecasting and Social Change* 93 (April 2015): 32–43, https://doi.org/10.1016/j.techfore.2014.04.016.

58. Laura Pritchard-Jones, "Ageism and Autonomy in Health Care: Explorations Through a Relational Lens," *Health Care Analysis* 25, no. 1 (March 2017): 72–89, https://doi.org/10.1007/s10728-014-0288-1.
59. Zoë Corbyn, "The Future of Elder Care Is Here—and It's Artificial Intelligence," *The Guardian*, June 3, 2021, https://www.theguardian.com/us-news/2021/jun/03/elder-care-artificial-intelligence-software.
60. Anita Ho, Anita Silvers, and Tim Stainton, "Continuous Surveillance of Persons with Disabilities: Conflicts and Compatibilities of Personal and Social Goods," *Journal of Social Philosophy* 45, no. 3 (2014): 348–68, https://doi.org/10.1111/josp.12067.
61. Ho et al., "Continuous Surveillance of Persons with Disabilities."
62. Catriona Mackenzie, "Three Dimensions of Autonomy: A Relational Analysis," in *Autonomy, Oppression, and Gender*, ed. Andrea Veltman and Mark Piper (New York: Oxford University Press, 2014), 15–41.
63. Vallor, *Technology and the Virtues*.
64. Giovanni Rubeis, "The Disruptive Power of Artificial Intelligence: Ethical Aspects of Gerontechnology in Elderly Care," *Archives of Gerontology and Geriatrics* 91 (November 2020): 104186, https://doi.org/10.1016/j.archger.2020.104186.
65. Neven, "By Any Means?"
66. Rob Ranzijn, "Active Ageing—Another Way to Oppress Marginalized and Disadvantaged Elders? Aboriginal Elders as a Case Study," *Journal of Health Psychology* 15, no. 5 (July 2010): 716–23, https://doi.org/10.1177/1359105310368181.
67. Jennifer Nedelsky, *Law's Relations: A Relational Theory of Self, Autonomy, and Law* (New York: Oxford University Press, 2012).
68. Vallor, *Technology and the Virtues*.
69. Solveig Magnus Reindal, "Independence, Dependence, Interdependence: Some Reflections on the Subject and Personal Autonomy," *Disability & Society* 14, no. 3 (1999), 353–67.
70. Jenny Secker et al., "Promoting Independence: But Promoting What and How?" *Ageing and Society* 23, no. 3 (2003): 375–91, https://doi.org/10.1017/S0144686X03001193.
71. Sarah Hillcoat-Nallétamby, "The Meaning of 'Independence' for Older People in Different Residential Settings," *Journals of Gerontology: Series B* 69, no. 3 (May 2014): 419–30, https://doi.org/10.1093/geronb/gbu008; Pritchard-Jones, "Ageism and Autonomy in Health Care."
72. Anita Ho, "Are We Ready for Artificial Intelligence Health Monitoring in Elder Care?" *BMC Geriatrics* 20, no. 1 (September 2020): 358, https://doi.org/10.1186/s12877-020-01764-9.

73. Parvaneh Rabiee, "Exploring the Relationships between Choice and Independence: Experiences of Disabled and Older People," *British Journal of Social Work* 43, no. 5 (July 1, 2013): 872–88, https://doi.org/10.1093/bjsw/bcs022.
74. Pritchard-Jones, "Ageism and Autonomy in Health Care."
75. Alasdair MacIntyre, *Dependent Rational Animals* (London: Duckworth, 1999).
76. Martha Fineman, *The Autonomy Myth: A Theory of Dependency* (New York: The New Press, 2004).
77. Pritchard-Jones, "Ageism and Autonomy in Health Care."
78. Luca Pancani et al., "Forced Social Isolation and Mental Health: A Study on 1,006 Italians under COVID-19 Lockdown," *Frontiers in Psychology* 12 (2021): 663799, https://doi.org/10.3389/fpsyg.2021.663799.
79. Maya E. Rao and Dhananjai M. Rao, "The Mental Health of High School Students during the COVID-19 Pandemic," *Frontiers in Education* 6 (2021): 275, https://doi.org/10.3389/feduc.2021.719539.
80. Vimal Sriram, Crispin Jenkinson, and Michele Peters, "Informal Carers' Experience of Assistive Technology Use in Dementia Care at Home: A Systematic Review," *BMC Geriatrics* 19, no. 1 (June 2019): 160, https://doi.org/10.1186/s12877-019-1169-0.
81. Philippa Spoel, Roma Harris, and Flis Henwood, "The Moralization of Healthy Living: Burke's Rhetoric of Rebirth and Older Adults' Accounts of Healthy Eating," *Health* 16, no. 6 (April 2012): 619–35, https://doi.org/10.1177/1363459312441009.
82. "Seniors," Healthy Living, Health Canada, last modified November 5, 2014, https://www.canada.ca/en/health-canada/services/healthy-living/seniors.html.
83. Spoel et al., "Moralization of Healthy Living."
84. "Healthy Aging," U.S. Department of Health and Human Services, last modified May 2, 2022, https://www.hhs.gov/aging/healthy-aging/index.html; "Healthy Aging," Office of Disease Prevention and Health Promotion, U.S. Department of Health and Human Services, last modified September 24, 2021, https://health.gov/our-work/national-health-initiatives/healthy-aging.
85. Yanping Li, Josje Schoufour, Dong D. Wang, et al., "Healthy Lifestyle and Life Expectancy Free of Cancer, Cardiovascular Disease, and Type 2 Diabetes: Prospective Cohort Study. *BMJ* 368 (2020), 16669, doi:10.1136/bmj.16669.
86. Sara Henderson and Alan Petersen, eds., *Consuming Health: The Commodification of Health Care* (London: Routledge, 2002).

87. Debbie Laliberte Rudman, "Shaping the Active, Autonomous and Responsible Modern Retiree: An Analysis of Discursive Technologies and Their Links with Neo-Liberal Political Rationality," *Ageing and Society* 26 (March 2006): 181–201, https://doi.org/10.1017/S0144686X05004253; "Healthy Aging," Office of Disease Prevention and Health Promotion, U.S. Department of Health and Human Services.
88. Spoel et al., "Moralization of Healthy Living."
89. Bettina Schmietow and Georg Marckmann, "Mobile Health Ethics and the Expanding Role of Autonomy," *Medicine, Health Care, and Philosophy* 22, no. 4 (December 2019): 623–30, https://doi.org/10.1007/s11019-019-09900-y.
90. Ranzijn, "Active Ageing."
91. Philippa Spoel, Roma Harris, and Flis Henwood, "Rhetorics of Health Citizenship: Exploring Vernacular Critiques of Government's Role in Supporting Healthy Living," *Journal of Medical Humanities* 35, no. 2 (June 2014): 131–47, https://doi.org/10.1007/s10912-014-9276-6.
92. Martha B. Holstein and Meredith Minkler, "Critical Gerontology: Reflections for the 21st Century," in *Critical Perspectives on Ageing Societies*, ed. Miriam Bernard and Thomas Scharf (Bristol: Policy Press, 2007), 13–26.
93. Colin A. Depp and Dilip V. Jeste, "Definitions and Predictors of Successful Aging: A Comprehensive Review of Larger Quantitative Studies," *American Journal of Geriatric Psychiatry* 14, no. 1 (January 2006): 6–20, https://doi.org/10.1097/01.JGP.0000192501.03069.bc.
94. Paul Stenner, Tara McFarquhar, and Ann Bowling, "Older People and 'Active Ageing': Subjective Aspects of Ageing Actively," *Journal of Health Psychology* 16, no. 3 (April 2011): 467–77, https://doi.org/10.1177/1359105310384298.
95. Liliane Rioux, "The Well-Being of Aging People Living in Their Own Homes," *Journal of Environmental Psychology* 25, no. 2 (June 2005): 231–43, https://doi.org/10.1016/j.jenvp.2005.05.001.
96. bell hooks, "Homeplace: A Site of Resistance," in *Undoing Place? A Geographical Reader*, ed. Linda McDowell (London: Routledge, 1997), 33–38.
97. Carol H. Cain et al., "Patient Experiences of Transitioning from Hospital to Home: An Ethnographic Quality Improvement Project," *Journal of Hospital Medicine* 7, no. 5 (June 2012): 382–87, https://doi.org/10.1002/jhm.1918.
98. Drew Harwell, "Ring and Nest Helped Normalize American Surveillance and Turned Us into a Nation of Voyeurs," *Washington Post*, February 18,

2020, https://www.washingtonpost.com/technology/2020/02/18/ring-nest-surveillance-doorbell-camera/.
99. Oudshoorn, "How Places Matter."
100. J. J. Rolison, Y. Hanoch, and A. M. Freund, "Perception of Risk for Older Adults: Differences in Evaluations for Self versus Others and across Risk Domains," *Gerontology* 65, no. 5 (2019): 547–59, https://doi.org/10.1159/000494352.
101. Black Hawk Hancock, "Michel Foucault and the Problematics of Power: Theorizing DTCA and Medicalized Subjectivity," *Journal of Medicine and Philosophy: A Forum for Bioethics and Philosophy of Medicine* 43, no. 4 (August 2018): 439–68, https://doi.org/10.1093/jmp/jhy010; Michel Foucault, *Discipline and Punish: The Birth of the Prison*, trans. Alan Sheridan (New York: Pantheon Books, 1977).
102. Peter Conrad, "The Shifting Engines of Medicalization," *Journal of Health and Social Behavior* 46, no. 1 (March 2005): 3–14, https://doi.org/10.1177%2F002214650504600102.
103. Sara Gerke et al., "The Need for a System View to Regulate Artificial Intelligence/Machine Learning-Based Software as Medical Device," *npj Digital Medicine* 3, no. 1 (April 2020): 53, https://doi.org/10.1038/s41746-020-0262-2.
104. Rubeis, "Disruptive Power of Artificial Intelligence."
105. Oudshoorn, "How Places Matter."
106. Milligan, *There's No Place Like Home*.
107. Oudshoorn, "How Places Matter."
108. Milligan, *There's No Place Like Home*.
109. Milligan, *There's No Place Like Home*.
110. Pamela Wisniewski et al., "We Have Built It, But They Have Not Come: Examining the Adoption and Use of Assistive Technologies for Informal Family Caregivers," in *Advances in Usability, User Experience and Assistive Technology*, ed. Tareq Z. Ahram and Christianne Falcão (Cham: Springer International Publishing, 2019), 824–36; Clara Berridge and Terrie Fox Wetle, "Why Older Adults and Their Children Disagree about In-Home Surveillance Technology, Sensors, and Tracking," *Gerontologist* 60, no. 5 (July 2020): 926–34, https://doi.org/10.1093/geront/gnz068.
111. Vallor, *Technology and the Virtues*.
112. Simon van der Weele et al., "What Is the Problem of Dependency? Dependency Work Reconsidered," *Nursing Philosophy* 22, no. 2 (April 2021): e12327, https://doi.org/10.1111/nup.12327.
113. Rolison et al., "Perception of Risk."

114. Berridge and Wetle, "Why Older Adults."
115. Colleen Galambos et al., "Living With Intelligent Sensors: Older Adult and Family Member Perceptions," *CIN: Computers, Informatics, Nursing* 37, no. 12 (2019), https://journals.lww.com/cinjournal/Fulltext/2019/12000/Living_With_Intelligent_Sensors__Older_Adult_and.3.aspx; Clara Berridge, "Breathing Room in Monitored Space: The Impact of Passive Monitoring Technology on Privacy in Independent Living," *Gerontologist* 56, no. 5 (October 2016): 807–16, https://doi.org/10.1093/geront/gnv034.
116. W. Ben Mortenson, Andrew Sixsmith, and Robert Beringer, "No Place Like Home? Surveillance and What Home Means in Old Age," *Canadian Journal on Aging* 35, no. 1 (March 2016): 103–14, https://doi.org/10.1017/S0714980815000549; Danton S. Char, Nigam H. Shah, and David Magnus, "Implementing Machine Learning in Health Care—Addressing Ethical Challenges," *New England Journal of Medicine* 378, no. 11 (March 2018): 981–83, https://doi.org/10.1056/NEJMp1714229.
117. Alison Marie Kenner, "Securing the Elderly Body: Dementia, Surveillance, and the Politics of 'Aging in Place,'" *Surveillance & Society* 5, no. 3 (2008), https://doi.org/10.24908/ss.v5i3.3423.
118. "Uninvited Guests," short film by SuperFlux Lab, uploaded May 26, 2015, https://vimeo.com/128873380.
119. AARP and National Alliance for Caregiving, *Caregiving in the U.S. 2020.*
120. Evelyn Nakano Glenn, *Forced to Care: Coercion and Caregiving in America* (Cambridge, MA: Harvard University Press, 2012). Glenn points out that even paid home health care workers in the United States are often excluded from critical rights such as minimum wage, retirement benefits, and workers' compensation.
121. Sapci and Sapci, "Innovative Assisted Living Tools."
122. Pascale Lehoux, Jocelyne Saint-Arnaud, and Lucie Richard, "The Use of Technology at Home: What Patient Manuals Say and Sell vs. What Patients Face and Fear," *Sociology of Health & Illness* 26, no. 5 (July 2004): 617–44, https://doi.org/10.1111/j.0141-9889.2004.00408.x.
123. John Vines et al., "Making Family Care Work: Dependence, Privacy and Remote Home Monitoring Telecare Systems," *Proceedings of the 2013 ACM International Joint Conference on Pervasive and Ubiquitous Computing* (September 2013), 607–16, https://doi.org/10.1145/2493432.2493469.
124. Berridge, "Breathing Room."
125. AARP and National Alliance for Caregiving, *Caregiving in the U.S. 2020.*
126. Mackenzie, "Three Dimensions of Autonomy."

127. Vikki A. Entwistle et al., "Involving Patients in Their Care," *Current Breast Cancer Reports* 6, no. 3 (September 2014): 211–18, https://doi.org/10.1007/s12609-014-0151-2.

128. Andrew Gebhart, "Nobi Will Watch over Your Grandparents, Literally, from a Ceiling Mounted Smart Lamp," CNET, January 12, 2021, https://www.cnet.com/home/smart-home/nobi-will-watch-over-your-grandparents-literally-from-a-ceiling-mounted-smart-lamp.

129. Kirti D. Doekhie et al., "Trust in Older Persons: A Quantitative Analysis of Alignment in Triads of Older Persons, Informal Carers and Home Care Nurses," *Health & Social Care in the Community* 27, no. 6 (November 2019): 1490–1506, https://doi.org/10.1111/hsc.12820.

130. "National Nurses United Condemns Industry Plans to Maximize Profit by Sending Patients Home All Alone, Replacing 24/7 Hands-on Nursing Care with Technology," National Nurses United, November 4, 2021, https://www.nationalnursesunited.org/press/nnu-condemns-industry-plans-to-maximize-profit-by-sending-patients-home-alone.

3

Artificial Doctoring

The Case of Direct-to-Consumer Health Monitoring

As we saw in the last chapter, the health care industry has been working to move more services out of the hospital or clinic and into people's homes.[1] One industry study from 2019 of 100 clinical informatics and health information technology (IT) thought leaders found that 88 percent of surveyed providers were already investing in or exploring investment in remote monitoring for high-risk chronically ill patients to help provide early symptom management and reduce the rate of hospital admission.[2] This trend has accelerated during the COVID-19 pandemic. In the United States, as part of the federal government's pandemic response, the Centers for Medicare and Medicaid Services is now allowing not only primary care providers to prescribe Medicare beneficiaries remote health services in the home, but also home health care providers to use remote health monitoring technology to adjust the frequency and types of in-person visits with patients.[3] With more health care providers using telehealth and remote patient monitoring, technologists and health systems claim that these technologies will improve access and outcomes. Nonetheless, the health system and health care providers generally retain control over which virtual technologies are utilized in care delivery and how.

As the pandemic persists and continues to delay consultations and services for non-urgent health concerns, which can nonetheless worsen health outcomes and psychological anguish, people are increasingly turning to direct-to-consumer (DTC) health technologies. These technologies promise to help patients and consumers monitor non-acute health concerns and ongoing health trends on their own or supplement professional consultation with artificial intelligence (AI)-guided self-management, thereby minimizing dependency on or even bypassing traditional health care facilities and providers. While many home health monitoring platforms we saw in the last chapter focus on older adults and people with higher physical and cognitive limitations, there is a rapidly growing market of heterogeneous DTC AI health monitoring products using various forms of predictive analytics that target a much broader population, including not only those with chronic conditions but also young, healthy, and asymptomatic populations. While there have been very few scenarios where published evidence suggests that DTC AI health technologies *may* improve health outcomes,[4] developers and enthusiasts insist that these products will promote voluntary self-tracking and personalized outputs, thus enhancing self-management and preventive care. One industry report from 2021 estimates that there are over 350,000 health applications available worldwide, with more than 90,000 new ones introduced in 2020.[5] Some commentators acknowledge that most of these apps have not yet been prospectively tested, but nonetheless argue that this area "deserves aggressive pursuit," as it *could* reduce health care costs without sacrificing patient convenience and comfort.[6]

DTC AI health monitoring platforms collect and generate a broad spectrum of health and activity data. Some types of software act as medical devices, collecting and analyzing physiological health data such as blood pressure and heart rate. Others focus on wellness data, including physical activity, diet, and passive physiological data—although the line between these two categories is increasingly blurry. The fact that non-medical devices often collect similar types of data as medical devices and aggressively market themselves as health promotion tools further blurs the line between medical and commercial data and products. As these technologies monitor, record, and graph users' various bodily functions and habits, they promise to facilitate a proactive, informed, tech-enabled, interactive, and individualized approach to self-management.

This chapter explores how the expanding availability and marketing of DTC AI health applications affect potential users' autonomy. Section 1 introduces the common claim that these products can democratize health information and promote users' autonomy. Section 2 provides a brief overview of the different purposes and categories of DTC AI health applications, illustrated with examples of platforms currently on the market. Utilizing the concept of relational autonomy, Section 3 explores how these technologies affect (prospective) users' self-governance, self-determination, and self-authorization. It examines how the broader social phenomenon of self-quantification via indefinite tracking changes our practical identities and may ironically reinforce medical dominance that can further reduce (prospective) patients' power. Drawing on lessons learned from other DTC health products such as genetic tests, this section warns of the possibility that DTC AI health monitoring may alienate and marginalize people's embodied experience in ways that compromise their self-identity rather than promoting self-knowledge.

1. Democratization of Health Information?

The idea of using technology to track one's bodily processes and emotional states, with the goal of managing and improving one's health, is not new, even though advancing mobile technologies and the expanding commercialization of health services are accelerating its adoption. Most households have a thermometer to check body temperature as needed, and home pregnancy tests have been available in the United States since the 1970s. In other wellness areas, healthy individuals have long used scales to monitor their weight and adjust their diet and exercise regimens accordingly.[7]

People with various chronic conditions have also used DTC health products to facilitate self-monitoring and disease management. For example, individuals with diabetes routinely carry out finger strip tests for blood glucose monitoring between laboratory visits, and patients with hypertension can purchase inflatable cuffs for blood pressure monitoring at home. In the lingering COVID-19 pandemic, many patients with chronic cardiac and lung diseases are relying on DTC pulse oximeters to help determine oxygen saturation and monitor for potential "silent hypoxia," as even people who are not experiencing severe shortness of breath may nonetheless have dangerously low oxygen levels that require medical attention.

The advancement of AI/machine learning (ML) and the wider availability of clinical and personal data are further propelling the development and capabilities of DTC health monitoring devices. Conventional DTC health monitoring products, even when digitized, are generally active monitoring technologies, which collect and display exact measurements for a particular physiological characteristic or health condition (e.g., heart rate) when initiated by the user at specific times. They do not analyze the data or provide recommendations to users. Most of these devices store the data locally without intersecting or integrating with other systems or data, although some newer Internet of Things (IoT) devices allow users to upload their data to related websites, social media platforms, or physician portals.

DTC AI health monitoring is taking physiological and activity tracking to the next level by going beyond simply recording discrete events at various times. Many of these applications are passive technologies. Once activated, they continuously operate in the background and are automated to collect, store, and analyze different forms of data simultaneously, without the user's active prompt or involvement. Various fitness devices that track users' steps, heart rate, and duration of activities are some examples. DTC AI health monitoring platforms use a variety of predictive analytical techniques to identify, classify, or diagnose various health outcomes or concerns. However, many companies are opaque about the specific techniques utilized by their platforms and do not share any data on evidence of how well their products perform. Most of these devices currently on the market apply a fixed predictive function such as a decision tree or a complex classifier to a given set of inputs, and performance validation and improvement would require manual processes. Nonetheless, most developers do not provide information on whether or how often the platform will be updated if new evidence arises.[8] These platforms collect and analyze longitudinal user-generated data to produce probabilistic outputs about the person's current and future health status.[9] Many AI DTC health technologies also interact with users, such as through natural language processing (NLP) conversations or text messages, to gather additional self-reported information and progressively learn more about the users. Examples include chatbots that engage in conversation with users about their symptoms, personal information, medicines, and previous diagnoses, and provide real-time suggestions. In delivering personalized recommendations, some devices also nudge users to change their behavior by sending notifications and tracking progress accordingly. Some companies offer human consultation support for an additional fee, but most shift the cost of follow-up consultations and care management back to the health system by prompting concerned users to contact their primary care doctor or urgent care center for help.[10]

Enthusiasts of DTC AI health monitoring promise that these emerging technologies can revolutionize health care management by democratizing health information in ways that will truly promote patient and consumer autonomy. In the traditional and formal health care monitoring models in the United States, insurance companies and licensed health care providers are the gatekeepers of resources and information. Even in countries that have tax-funded systems and provide universal coverage for all its citizens and residents (e.g., Canada), health systems generally determine what services are covered and their frequency, often based partly on practice guidelines, physician recommendations, and/or resource availability. As we saw in previous chapters, the professionalization of (and presumed epistemic hierarchy in) modern medicine has given physicians the socially designated authority and responsibility to define health and determine how various constellations of symptoms or concerns should be understood and managed.[11] Funding models that dictate what types of consultation and referral services are covered by publicly or privately funded health insurance impose further parameters on health care delivery. Operating within this structure, physicians have the power and responsibility to determine who can receive screening and diagnostic services, what patient-specific information will be collected and analyzed, when and how frequently that may occur, and the settings through which such services and information may be delivered. Patients generally have minimal control over how consultations and data collection will take place.

Under this conventional health care delivery model, even symptomatic patients must take multiple sequential steps and rely exclusively on their physicians or other designated licensed professionals for assessment and interpretation of their health concerns, or for other direct information regarding their health. For non-emergency conditions, patients may have to endure long wait times for an appointment, a phenomenon that has been exacerbated in the COVID-19 pandemic. They then must arrange transportation, secure childcare, or take time off work and other socio-familial responsibilities to attend appointments during business hours. Further inconvenience and delay of information ensues if laboratory tests or scans have to be scheduled at specific times and locations. Patients in countries such as the United Kingdom often have to take the initiative to obtain their results,[12] whereas many American physicians adopt the "no news is good news" approach and only contact patients for follow-up appointments if there are concerning laboratory results.[13] Sometimes reports are missed and patients who require follow-up investigations or treatments are not notified,[14] potentially delaying necessary care and compromising health outcomes.

Electronic health records (EHRs) have closed some of the data access gap by allowing digitally enabled patients more convenient access to their laboratory results, although patients with flagged indicators often still need to wait for an appointment with their physician to interpret the findings and discuss follow-up and treatment options. Moreover, as patients' physiological responses (e.g., heart rate) may fluctuate depending on various circumstances (e.g., work stress, sleep deprivation, time since last meal), sparsely collected and time-specific clinical data may not provide a complete picture of the patient's disease progression. However, repeated screenings or diagnostic tests and follow-up consultations may add financial and logistical burdens to both patients and health systems, especially during the COVID-19 pandemic, when many clinics and laboratories have been overwhelmed with conducting and processing COVID tests in addition to their other regular screening and diagnostic tests.

Enthusiasts of AI DTC health technologies claim that DTC AI health monitoring platforms introduce new and flexible ways for ordinary people to directly manage their own health by producing and utilizing their own data, thereby promoting users' well-being, preventing sickness, and addressing unmet patient needs. They believe that wider access to one's health information and the associated predictive analytics provided by these new platforms can enhance people's agency and improve their overall health. As we will see shortly, these applications' mobility and capacity to be used continuously across diverse spatial and temporal settings, often synced on different mobile devices, brings health management to consumers wherever they are and allows them to produce and access physiological data on demand.

If these technologies can enhance users' autonomy, as promised, then they would promote self-governance, self-determination, and self-authorization as well. First, there is great hope that these participatory platforms can augment ordinary people's self-knowledge and expertise in monitoring their bodies, thereby enhancing their self-governance. As these technologies often prompt users to enter self-evaluative information (e.g., mood, food intake) in addition to collecting passive sensor data, they may help train users' "inner sensitivity" to their own body, such as how a person with diabetes feels when they are at various blood sugar levels.[15] This enriched understanding may guide active, deliberate, and informed agents to manage and improve their own health. Second, by enhancing users' sense of control over their data and behavior, these platforms promise to promote self-determination. Finally, there is optimism among technologists and consumer advocates that self-generated information using low-cost applications may promote a more mutual therapeutic relationship and enhance self-authorization: If patients can become more in tune with their own experiences while also presenting longitudinal data and predictive outputs from their DTC platforms as complementary information to validate their testimonial credibility, this in turn could result in patients feeling more confident in seeking care and advocating for themselves. This can presumably lead to more appropriate preventive care, more accurate diagnoses, timelier treatments, and better health outcomes.

Expanded and continued access to one's own health data, accompanied by tailored advice, may become part of personalized preventive health maintenance that can be particularly helpful in building the self-management capacity of the growing number of people with chronic illnesses, potentially allowing them to shift care away from institutions and reduce unnecessary or non-urgent encounters with health care professionals. In the United States, top chronic illnesses such as heart disease, cancer, and diabetes are the leading causes of death and disability.[16] Prior to the COVID-19 pandemic, these conditions incurred 90 percent of the nation's $3.8

trillion in annual health care expenditures and surpassed infectious diseases in premature death and morbidity.[17] Six in ten adults in the United States have at least one chronic condition, and four in ten have two or more comorbidities. Chronic disease management can be challenging for patients, since it often requires long-term adherence to dietary or other lifestyle changes that may impose significant inconvenience and unpleasant restrictions. These complex conditions typically involve multiple intersecting features and contributors, such as genetics, lifestyle, and environmental factors. Changes in one area without tackling other contributing factors often lead to suboptimal health improvement. Managing chronic conditions has thus traditionally required intensive in-person patient engagement, regular and time-consuming clinic check-ups, ongoing health and behavioral coaching, and longitudinal symptom monitoring to address problems at incremental intervals and prevent serious complications. Gaps in information and disease management can easily occur, especially when costs and other practical limitations curtail the frequency or duration of care encounters.

Instead of waiting to receive clinician advice or instructions at an in-person consultation, many hope that DTC AI health monitoring platforms can facilitate information gathering and sharing that will empower self-management.[18] As users continue to generate data, they can receive not only ongoing assessment but also personalized alerts and interactions to remind and encourage them to eat healthier, get more exercise, take medication as instructed, or seek professional or institutional help (only) when indicated. When users who change their behavior according to algorithmic recommendations witness a direct response in subsequent health indicators, they may feel more confident in their ability to adjust their behavior and improve their health. The continuous analytical feedback loops may fulfill people's desire for control and a sense of accomplishment in ways that can enhance their autonomy.[19]

Proponents of AI DTC health monitoring also believe that these technologies can democratize information for people who are healthy but may have predispositions to various conditions, such as diabetes or heart disease. As we will see shortly, there is a burgeoning industry of DTC AI health technologies that target younger and healthier populations who are not (yet) patients and are thus not routinely monitored by health care providers. Proliferating AI-powered self-tracking devices, wearable sensors, and mobile applications allow users to collect, measure, and display data concerning virtually any form of bodily function or behavioral activity.[20] They are thus providing people with unprecedented access to their basic physiological and health data. Healthy individuals are often unaware of their own susceptibility to various conditions and have to wait until they are symptomatic before receiving medical attention or advice. By continuously generating and reviewing physiological and activity data, DTC AI health monitoring may enhance risk management and analysis of potential illness as part of ordinary everyday life.[21] These technologies may empower users to proactively address personalized root causes of illness, adjust their lifestyle, and consult professionals for follow-up care as indicated, instead of only managing sickness after disease onset or a specific health event (e.g., heart attack, stroke). They may also help users gain access to health data that would otherwise be unavailable as well as facilitate participatory health management and personalized preventive care.[22]

2. Leaving Patients to Their Own Devices

As development of and demand for DTC AI health monitoring devices continue to grow, questions abound as to whether or how we can ensure that the wider adoption of this diverse category of technologies as well as the comprehensive and routinized data collection will truly promote patient autonomy and better health management. In the United States, there are currently no established best practices or specific AI regulatory pathway for evaluating DTC AI health algorithms to ensure reliability and safety. However, the Food and Drug Administration (FDA) seeks to effectively regulate the quality and safety of AI/ML health devices, including physical hardware/devices and software as medical devices (SaMD),[23] without impeding the rapid, innovative characteristic of the industry.[24] Guided by the FDA Modernization Act of 1997, the agency uses the "least burdensome means" or the "minimum amount of information necessary" to evaluate medical devices.[25] The agency's stand was reaffirmed by the 21st Century Cures Act of 2016, which was designed in large part to accelerate device approval.[26]

There are at least two broad categories of DTC AI health platforms, although their respective marketing claims and implicit messages often blur the distinction between them. First, DTC AI health platforms that use medically oriented AI/ML-based algorithms can seek approval as a medical device under Section 201(h) of the Federal Food, Drug, and Cosmetic Act (FDCA) based on (1) the intended use of the device and (2) the device's indications for use.[27] The intended use denotes the general purpose or objective of the algorithms, and the indications for use describe the diseases or conditions that the algorithms claim to diagnose, treat, or prevent, as well as the target populations. The FDA makes approval and compliance enforcement decisions by considering the degree of potential risk that the commercially marketed AI medical device would pose to individual users if it were not to function as intended.[28] These technologies can be granted a de novo pathway clearance, a 510(k) clearance, or premarket approval (PMA). A de novo pathway classification is for novel devices and algorithms that do not yet have legally marketed counterparts and that offer sufficient safety and effectiveness with general controls according to a risk-based assessment.[29] A 510(k) clearance, which requires less stringent review, is granted when an algorithm is shown to be at least as safe and effective as a similar, legally marketed algorithm,[30] even though it is conceivable that an adaptive algorithm will gradually diverge from the original device. Finally, PMA approval, which involves the most rigorous review, is reserved for medical devices that may have a higher risk or larger impact on human health.[31]

An online database shows that, as of the end of 2021, there were at least seventy-nine FDA-cleared AI-based algorithms as medical devices.[32] Amongst AI/ML-based software approved as a medical device, only 12.5 percent received de novo pathway clearance, compared to 85.9 percent that obtained the 510(k) clearance.[33] It is worth noting that not all "medical" devices are designed to manage disease, an issue that will be further considered later in the chapter. For example, the first FDA-cleared AI DTC birth control application, Natural Cycles, received de novo clearance in 2018 as a fertility awareness device that is "unlike others on the market."[34] The company boasts that the app can help patients become more knowledgeable about their menstrual cycle, fertility, and general body. The device collects a woman's basal body temperature readings, menstrual cycle data, heart rate variability, self-reported mood changes, and other sex data (e.g., the days the user had unprotected sex) to predict the user's ovulation cycle or fertile window.[35] According to a study co-authored by the company's CEO, the app is more accurate than calendar-based methods, such as the rhythm method and standard days method, which rely solely on the date of menstruation.[36] The study reported a 99 percent effectiveness with perfect use and 93 percent with "typical" use.[37]

Another DTC digital contraceptive algorithm, Clue, was not considered novel, as the FDA had already established the category of software application for fertility awareness based on the Natural Cycles clearance. In this case, the device received 510(k) clearance in 2021 based on being "substantially equivalent" to the first device. The equivalence is more of a conceptual or categorical similarity: Both are fertility awareness algorithm-based systems that utilize users' menstrual cycles to predict fertility window, though Clue does not collect or utilize temperature data in its algorithmic predictions.[38] Despite different methodologies, both applications are promoted by their respective companies as personalized and low-risk tools to help women take control of their reproductive health so they can make informed and autonomous decisions to prevent or plan pregnancy.[39] Both fertility algorithms describe their products as alternatives to hormonal birth control and were considered low to medium risk to individual users if they were not to function as intended. In making this determination, the FDA likely focused solely on the physiological risk of pregnancy in the general population rather than broader or additional socioeconomic, emotional, and relational risks of undesired pregnancy, even though many consumers use this product primarily to *avoid* becoming pregnant. The U.S. Supreme Court's overturn of *Roe v. Wade* in June 2022 may further heighten concerns of the accuracy of AI fertility awareness/prediction apps. As the ruling has triggered a growing number of states to limit or ban access to abortion,[40] consumers who utilize fertility monitoring apps for birth control purposes may face tremendous physical, psychological, legal, and financial burdens if the devices deliver inaccurate predictions.

The approval category that requires the most thorough safety and efficacy review for marketing approval is the PMA, which is issued to algorithms for Class III medical devices that may have a higher risk or larger impact on human health.[41] Applications are generally accompanied by at least one prospective trial to demonstrate reasonable assurance of safety and effectiveness. A 2020 review of the FDA database showed that only 1.2 percent of approved AI/ML software medical devices fall into this category.[42] One such device, the Guardian Connect System, which received PMA in 2018, is designed to help users manage diabetes by offering continuous or periodic monitoring of glucose levels in the interstitial fluid under the skin.[43] The system is approved for adjunctive use, requiring at least two daily fingerstick calibrations to convert the raw measurements to glucose values and preserve sensor accuracy.[44] Another mobile diabetes management platform from WellDoc received 510(k) class II clearance for being substantially equivalent to an already marketed device. This patient coaching and clinical decision support system can analyze data entered by the patient (e.g., blood glucose level, dietary information, insulin data), compare past data trends, provide automated personalized guidance to the user, and create a summary of curated data analytics that patients can present to their health care team.[45]

For other chronic conditions, FDA-authorized DTC AI medical devices include smartwatch electrocardiogram (ECG) applications for people with heart disease, which continuously record electric impulses from a patient's heart to detect and warn users of potential atrial fibrillation (i.e., irregular heart rate).[46] These devices can record the user's heart rate at different times and during various activities, such as sleeping, resting, running errands, exercising, or going through stressful events, which may help provide a fuller picture of the person's baseline and overall cardiac health. Some of these devices are integrated into other smart technologies that people already use every day. An example includes Apple's ECG app, intended to be used with the Apple Watch, which received authorization by the FDA as a de novo Class II medical device in 2018.[47]

The second (and much larger) category of DTC AI health platforms includes wellness technologies that track users' mental and/or physical well-being but are not subjected to FDA regulatory scrutiny or approval. The agency does not regulate software functions "intended for maintaining or encouraging a healthy lifestyle that are unrelated to the diagnosis, cure, mitigation, prevention, or treatment of a disease or condition."[48] For AI wellness algorithms, this may include technologies that are (1) intended for general patient education and the facilitation of access to commonly used reference information, (2) intended as a means for individuals to log, record, track, evaluate, or make decisions related to general fitness, health, or wellness, or (3) intended to help patients with specific conditions or chronic diseases (e.g., diabetes, heart disease) to organize and record their health information.[49] Many of these platforms are developed by lay entrepreneurs with no to minimal health care professional involvement,[50] and there is currently no required process of scientific or peer review to ascertain the accuracy or validity of these proprietary algorithms. Any reviews of these products generally come in the form of a simple online anonymous user satisfaction rating scale.[51]

Among DTC AI wellness platforms, many target the same chronic conditions and health concerns as FDA-approved medical devices, further confusing users of their classification. These products aim to enhance users' ability to prevent, detect, and manage these conditions, which often require long-term management and active patient engagement. In the aforementioned area of diabetes care, numerous wellness applications allow users to record their glucometer readings and other information about medications, mood, exercise, weight, food intake, blood pressure, etc. One such mobile app company highlights that the process of glucose control and lifestyle adjustment is "tough and lonely," and patients often do not know how to communicate with their care provider.[52] The platform thus serves as a "partner" by encouraging users to input their information, make use of notes and photos to keep a complete record of their vitals, and track their history and trends through charts and tables. The app can then send personalized reminders and recommendations to help users make lifestyle adjustments that may enhance their ability to control their glucose levels. It can also share the information and records with family and care providers if the user so desires, although it is unclear whether health care providers would need to be first notified of such data sharing. Other subscription-based AI diabetes management services claim to harness the benefits of big data and use connected glucometer readings, genetic test results, diet and activity information, mood reports, and AI coaching to provide a "hyper-personalized" or "genetically matched" chronic care experience.[53]

In the area of mental health, concerns abound that many individuals with known mental conditions, such as anxiety and depression, do not seek professional help due to lack of access and/or ongoing stigmas and discrimination against people with these conditions. In addition, people without a diagnosis but who have struggled with various symptoms may not be aware of or eligible for associated services and resources. The mental health burden has been exacerbated by the COVID-19 pandemic, which has seen an increase in both demand and wait times for mental health services around the world.[54] The ongoing physical, economic, and social stressors associated with the prolonged pandemic are affecting people with pre-existing mental health concerns and others who did not have a formal diagnosis prior to the pandemic but are now experiencing symptoms of depression, insomnia, post-traumatic stress disorder, and anxiety. Some of these concerns are particularly prevalent among patients who have contracted COVID-19. One study following more than 230,000 survivors of COVID-19 found that 34 percent of these patients were diagnosed with neurological or psychiatric conditions in the six months after the infection, with 13 percent being diagnosed with such disorders for the first time.[55]

Advocates of DTC AI wellness applications are optimistic that these technologies will democratize mental health and offer support in an area that has seen significant service gaps.[56] Some existing AI mental health monitoring apps claim to track users' physical and emotional stress over time, then personalize mindfulness, counseling, and supported therapy techniques based on the user's needs to manage stress, anxiety, and depression. One AI DTC app, BioBase, combines real-time wearable passive physical data (e.g., sleep and activity data, heart rate variability) with user responses around mood and cognitive function to calculate a personalized well-being score.[57] Other AI chatbots, such as Wysa, profess to leverage evidence-based techniques to help users self-manage stressors and feel heard.[58]

Another popular category of DTC AI health wellness platforms is digital reproductive monitoring, which targets women's reproductive cycles and pregnancies. In addition to the aforementioned AI DTC fertility awareness applications that are often used for birth control purposes, many AI pregnancy applications combine physiological data, self-reported symptoms, and other behavioral information (e.g., diet, exercise) to predict and inform pregnant women who want to carry their pregnancy to term of potential health problems, monitor progress and fetal growth, offer behavioral or dietary suggestions, and advise women on which symptoms are common or expected and which ones may require medical attention.

In addition to targeting users with specific health conditions or concerns, there is also a proliferation of AI wellness smartphone applications and wearable mobile sensors that promise to inform and empower healthy and asymptomatic individuals who currently have no specific health concerns. These platforms automatically and continuously collect and analyze users' steps taken, food intake, calories burned, menstrual cycles, blood chemistry, sleep patterns, mood, and/or other physiological characteristics to inform personalized nutrition or exercise plans. With colorful displays and gamified reward incentives,[59] these platforms are often branded as fun, exploratory, interactive, accessible, and collaborative, pledging to inform people of their health status and promote healthier lifestyles. Some device companies also encourage users to turn self-tracking practices into a biosocial and communal activity by sharing information about their physical activities and physiological data and motivating one another in achieving their health goals on online forums.[60] To maximize appeal, many companies integrate mobile applications into products that people already use daily, such as smartphones and tablets.

DTC AI health platforms are intended for easy and frequent personal use, as ongoing interaction can provide further data and feedback loops for both the user and the algorithm. A study published in 2015 indicated that more than half of smartphone users in the United States had downloaded a health-related app, most using the app at least once a day for wellness tracking and advice.[61] As of 2020, 1 million out of an estimated 4.5 million apps available in the Google and Apple app stores pertained to health, fitness, nutrition, and general wellness, potentially expanding the offering of accessible low-cost options to assist people in managing clinical conditions.[62] With continual interactive data collection, users can adopt personalized lifestyle recommendations and improve their metrics and health accordingly, while developers can update and improve the performance of the algorithm.[63] Users who receive information that identifies potential clinical concerns (e.g., melanoma risks) or find out that they may have a predisposition to various conditions (e.g., prediabetes) can also contact their health care providers for further testing or professional monitoring, thereby promoting early intervention. Because wellness applications are not subject to FDA approval procedures, they are cheaper and quicker to produce, and can target a much broader and more diverse set of users than DTC AI medical devices.

3. Relational Autonomy and DTC AI Health Monitoring

In many ways, the discourse around using DTC AI health monitoring to enhance self-knowledge and control over one's health fits well with the liberal conception of self-governance. Under this framework, rational and self-interested agents seek opportunities to improve their skills, capacity, performance, behavior, and habits through individual responsibility and effort. Intersecting with the discourses and practices of digitized health promotion, health risks are increasingly individualized and viewed as controllable as long as people adopt the appropriate technologies for self-monitoring and self-care.[64] DTC AI health monitoring is increasingly targeting younger, healthier, and more affluent populations,[65] who generally have higher educational and socioeconomic assets, comfort levels with technologies, and expectations that a wide array of services, information, and recommendations can be delivered to them digitally and at their convenience.[66] For example, internet search engines, product and social recommendations (e.g., online shopping, friends, and dating suggestions), interactive travel route suggestions, and traffic and arrival time predictions have become routine parts of many people's lives. As we saw in the last chapter, smart doorbells and other home monitoring devices that can be controlled on one's mobile phone are also increasingly popular among those who can afford these IoTs, despite privacy experts' ongoing warnings that many of these devices have inadequate data security protection.[67] Many users seem willing to forgo some informational privacy for the sake of convenience, as evidenced by their increasing utilization of or even reliance on algorithms and virtual assistants to provide pertinent information and support their activities, including their efforts to monitor their health.

As health monitoring increasingly takes place outside of hospitals, clinics, and laboratories, user-friendly DTC AI health applications now allow ordinary people with varying levels of technological or health literacy to navigate these digital platforms with relative ease. In particular, health applications that are built into everyday consumer mobile devices often utilize familiar activities (e.g., text conversations, voice memos, or photo uploads) to collect data and convert otherwise heterogeneous and complex information into simple graphs and display charts. Through personalized prompts and alerts, these technologies encourage users to continuously log their data, review the updated predictive outputs or findings,[68] and join forums to share their data and experiences, which further facilitates the aggregation or crowdsourcing of data.[69] Many hope that these interactive designs can replace (or at least supplement) hierarchical consultations and medical jargon, democratize health information, enhance users' capacity to understand and track their health status, and help them make health-related decisions and lifestyle changes accordingly. If the algorithmic outputs are clinically relevant, accurate, understandable, and actionable, they may facilitate informational access and health literacy, which can in turn enhance self-governance. There is optimism that patient-generated health data can help patients ask their clinicians new or more relevant questions, seek second opinions, or reflect further about their care decisions.

However, promises aside, a relational perspective reminds us that narrow, individualist definitions of consumer autonomy miss the bigger picture of how the proliferation and integration of these devices into our everyday lives may negatively impact prospective users' autonomy in other ways. To capture these important considerations, we need to attend to how the broader social practice of shifting health monitoring from traditional and highly regulated therapeutic relationships and professional practices to low-cost and rapidly evolving commercial AI platforms may affect people's agency and autonomy as they seek to take charge of their health and well-being. A relational approach to autonomy, which looks beyond isolated technologies and people's specific decisions about a particular platform, can help to determine how these emerging technologies and accompanying social and data practices may create a power paradox by restructuring people's practical identities and motivations in health tracking. Given that many DTC AI health platforms intersect with a variety of applications and devices, and that user data may be shared with other vendors for marketing and technology development purposes, a relational approach explores the broader social practices surrounding these technologies and their impact on people's embodied experiences, as well as their ability to form their own values, preferences, and desires regarding health monitoring. While some of these platforms may facilitate more informed self-management, the overly simplistic and overwhelmingly positive attention that AI DTC health monitoring has received in the public discourse neglects other ways that these emerging practices may compromise people's self-governance, self-determination, and self-authorization. While users turn to AI health monitoring to increase self-empowerment, they may inadvertently surrender power due to a lack of data privacy and identity control.[70]

3.1 Quantified Self-Governance: The Numbers Don't Lie?

Recall from Chapter 1 that under a relational conception of autonomy, self-governance involves having the skills and capacities necessary to enact decisions that express or cohere with one's reflectively constituted or authentic practical identity. This section thus critically explores how DTC AI health technologies may affect users' capacity and skills to understand their health and make informed decisions. I discuss how these technologies, which turn complex embodied experiences into quantified data, may oversimplify health experiences and concerns in ways that affect people's practical identities.

Enthusiasts of DTC AI health monitoring promise that medical and wellness applications can help users know more about their bodies and overall health, and that the data generated can enhance behavioral changes and decision support. Nonetheless, a crucial question is whether these techno-cultural practices may inadvertently alienate people from their rich and complex embodied experiences, ironically compromising their understanding of their bodily functioning and overall well-being. "Datafication," or the Quantified Self movement, which has been growing in industrialized countries, encourages people to embrace measuring and analyzing the details of their daily habits and activities through digital devices, mobile apps, and online platforms.[71] DTC AI health monitoring is playing an integral role in this social phenomenon, converting aspects of life not previously quantified, such as mood and other behavioral experiences, into numbers.[72] With the motto of "self-knowledge through numbers," this expanding global movement claims that the use of commercial, wearable digital devices, sensing technologies, and virtual agents to record, monitor, analyze, and quantify one's biometric data and other qualitative aspects of everyday activities allows digitized humans to gain more accurate, objective, and granular insight into their own health.[73] Enthusiasts claim that these technologies can enhance people's agency by helping them acquire more detailed knowledge about themselves, which they can then use to actively control and improve their health.

While the appeal of such claims is undeniable, it is important to recognize that even continuous streams of digital biomarkers cannot tell a patient's full story if we do not understand the context within which patients acquire certain habits and/or develop various conditions. We need to consider whether the reduction of people's rich narratives and embodied experiences to quantifiable numbers in AI processes may redefine their relationship to their own health, bodies, and self-identities,[74] thereby subtly restructuring their motivations. Prioritization of algorithmic predictive processes in the digital era assumes that experiences that can be converted to arithmetic or quantifiable data are more precise, epistemically superior, or more relevant in the production of self-knowledge.[75] Yet ML/DL (deep learning) requires training data to be organized and sometimes labeled in ways that *computers* can understand, even when doing so transforms human experiences into data formats that *people* can no longer identify with or comprehend. For example, one study exploring AI-enabled chatbot symptom checker apps found that, despite promising various benefits such as support for medication information and triage decisions, these apps do not adequately consider users' basic personal and medical history, require rigid input by asking users to choose symptoms from a preset list, ask confusing or irrelevant questions, lack sufficient sophistication to support diverse diagnoses and user groups, and do not have adequate functions for follow-up actions,[76] raising questions of not only their clinical value but also the potential alienating effect on people's embodied experience.

I contend that uncritical reduction of our experiences into numbers neglects or downplays the embodied knowledge that comes from people's complex experiences, intuitions, and haptic senses, which manifest in rich environmental and cultural contexts.[77] It is unclear that AI analytical models that focus on statistical information can adequately capture human vulnerability, suffering, fears, and hopes during one's illness journey.[78] Under datafication, our experiences are deemed more "objective" and worthy of consideration if they can be converted into numbers in predetermined categories that then produce predictive outputs via pseudo-diagnostic displays. In reality, the quantification of people's experiences in AI processes may impose additional systems of power and control on technology users by unilaterally redefining their self-identities.[79] Moreover, the ontological shift to treating our bodies as potential disease vessels that require continuous tracking, analyzing, and adjusting, even when we are otherwise feeling healthy, may pathologize the body and extend the very reach of medical power that DTC AI health monitoring claims to avoid.[80] While some variability of physiological indicators is normal and may resolve over time without medical intervention, the ongoing tracking and reporting of all data points by these technologies inadvertently renders health "a permanently imperilled biological state" that can only be maintained by continuous hypervigilance and constant adjustment, even when many DTC AI health applications have not been proven to have clinical value.[81]

In implying that authentic self-knowledge is achieved primarily through the lens of a tireless monitoring algorithm that is always ready to analyze, inform, and warn the user, despite the lack of strong efficacy data, DTC AI health platforms encourage hyperattention to or even obsession with one's personal variables,[82] ironically creating or exacerbating the paranoia and ceaseless anxiety that many people use self-monitoring to prevent in the first place. This may yield harmful downstream interventions based on false-positive judgments. One systematic review evaluating digital and online symptom checkers found that algorithm-based triage tended to be more risk averse than that of health professionals, most often referring users to visit their doctor, even though the diagnostic accuracy of these symptom checkers was generally low.[83] Patients who opt to share DTC app-generated information may also expect their health care providers to quickly review and respond to their inquiries, further disrupting clinical workflow and therapeutic relationships, especially if users and clinicians disagree about the clinical value of these algorithmic suggestions.[84]

The quantification of health also highlights another way in which DTC AI health monitoring may compromise users' self-governance. Many of these products convert users' data into simple graphics, presumably for ease of navigation and understanding. Nonetheless, this oversimplification in the name of democratizing health information may inadvertently undermine users' capacity to fully grasp their health situation. Moreover, most companies do not share information about the analytical methods used by their algorithms, such that users generally have no understanding of how these algorithms reach their findings or how accurate they are.[85] Even among younger and healthier population groups, who may have some familiarity with AI practices due to their high consumption of connected digital devices and services, many demonstrate limited medical, data, and statistical literacy. Instead of promoting users' understanding of how AI algorithms produce predictive outputs, nontransparent algorithmic practices and proprietary restrictions often prevent scrutiny of their processes. This can exploit and exacerbate users' lack of statistical literacy, reinforcing various fallacies that may influence their decisions. A scoping review of computerized algorithms that aim at helping users self-diagnose found that individuals who lack access to health care and/or have a stigmatizing condition are more likely to use these platforms, and that women and those with higher education are more likely to choose the correct diagnosis. These findings raise questions of whether expanded access to potentially inaccurate diagnoses for underserved populations may be counterproductive and exacerbate health inequity, or may affect therapeutic relationships if there is a disagreement between the physician and the DTC application output.[86]

Consider how DTC AI health technologies that aim at maximizing mass appeal often leave out pertinent information that is crucial for informed risk assessment and corresponding decision-making. For example, a good understanding of the true prevalence of a health outcome in the general population prior to data collection (i.e., knowing the base rate via prior distribution) is important as part of Bayesian reasoning for assessing a person's true likelihood of having that health outcome and determining the clinical value of tests or algorithmic outputs.[87] Incorporating both the prior distribution and the likelihood function using Bayes' theorem can update one's knowledge for more accurate inferences. Yet most users of DTC health products and algorithms are not domain experts and therefore lack this crucial knowledge—a gap that these products do little to remedy.[88] Even for DTC AI health platforms that are highly accurate—which is difficult to ascertain without robust clinical trials and transparent data availability—positive predictions are likely to be false positives for younger and healthier populations that are not predisposed to the conditions in question. Moreover, citing proprietary information privilege, developers generally do not disclose what model they are using to generate results (e.g., ML vs. other models),[89] the population composition of their training dataset, or how their algorithm utilizes various pieces of user-generated data in the predictive calculation, including the clinical relevance and relative weight of these heterogeneous types of data.[90] Users therefore do not have the tools to interpret DTC AI predictive outputs in the broader context, understand their true risks, and decide between accepting or rejecting algorithmic recommendations according to their health and other priorities.[91]

This is particularly concerning for wellness applications that do not have FDA approval but are nonetheless aggressively marketed as health-promoting technologies. Many DTC health algorithms frame themselves as tools for *detection* rather than *diagnosis* of health conditions, or as education rather than medical advice, to avoid regulatory scrutiny. For example, there is an expanding DTC market for computer algorithms that analyze photos of skin moles or rashes to detect changes over time that may suggest common skin cancers, even though various studies have raised questions regarding the reliability and validity of these algorithms for clinically relevant populations and the intended users of these platforms.[92] These products are mostly developed and driven by actors outside the traditional health care system (e.g., technology companies) whose interests and normative background assumptions may not coincide with the core premises of medical ethics or technology assessment.[93] While the Federal Trade Commission (FTC) has the authority to investigate complaints around deceptive advertising claims,[94] data security, or discriminatory algorithms,[95] it does not conduct proactive review for approval purposes, and even investigated companies are not obliged to provide proprietary information to defend their practices. As some commentators have noted, the regulatory framework of the FTC is poorly suited to address the fast-paced, ever-changing landscape of startups, many of which market devices that blur the line between medical and consumer products.[96]

DTC AI health technologies mostly appeal to low-risk individuals who are nonetheless sensitive to potential adverse health outcomes. Without education to enhance users' capacity to understand their true risks, these platforms may create or amplify the risk of false-positive judgments about users' health status. Similar concerns have been documented in DTC genetic and prenatal tests for rare conditions: False-positive results are rampant, yet companies advertise their findings as reliable and highly accurate, able to offer patients total confidence. These promotional messages strongly suggest to prospective parents that it would be in their rational self-interest to consent to these tests.[97] Though oversimplified outputs from wellness algorithms are not technically medical advice, the use of very precise statistical language in algorithmic predictions (e.g., "83.7 percent chance of disease"), even without proof of evidence, aims to imply scientific validity, which can lead people to overestimate the accuracy and actionability of these predictive outputs.[98] Moreover, there is no industry or regulatory threshold of sensitivity (the algorithm's ability to correctly identify positive cases) or specificity (the algorithm's ability to accurately identify negative cases) for a device to be approved or allowed on the market. As we have learned from criticisms of DTC genetic tests, where individuals send in cheek swabs to obtain genetic information regarding their risk of developing various conditions, these test results may not be clinically meaningful and can be misinterpreted.[99] However, due to the lack of an ongoing fiduciary relationship between DTC testing companies and the individuals undergoing DTC tests, the responsibility for interpreting possibly low-value results falls back on patients' physicians and genetic counselors, placing a potentially unwarranted and unfair burden on an already stretched medical system.[100] Similar concerns abound for AI health monitoring. Even FDA-approved DTC medical devices do not necessarily provide follow-up or counseling services, such that users still need guidance and further investigation from licensed practitioners if they have questions or concerns about their algorithmic findings. Thus, instead of increasing consumer knowledge when it is needed most and reducing the need for professional consultation, these technologies shift the cost and burden of educating users back to the beleaguered health system.[101] As users' faulty judgment may lead them to seek unnecessary tests and treatments, these DTC technologies may also result in overdiagnosis and overtreatment. Instead of enhancing user understanding and health outcomes, these devices may compromise users' well-being.[102]

3.2 Relational Self-Determination and the Proliferation of Pregnancy Platforms

In addition to potentially exacerbating health anxiety rather than promoting self-knowledge, DTC AI health technologies may shift power over health surveillance and data ownership from users to device companies, potentially compromising the former's self-determination in being able to control their data and information. While the presumably voluntary practice of participatory health monitoring allows people to contribute to data generation and gain access to health insights, the terms and measures for health monitoring are largely selected by the vendors, who own the data recorded on DTC health applications and can decide how to display, use, and share that data. Even as DTC AI health technologies engage in continuous data collection, analysis, and sharing, consumers generally have minimal knowledge of how their data is used for analytical and other commercial purposes.[103] Many apps require users to allow all data to be used by any undefined third parties to access any part of the services.[104] Indeed, parallels can once again be drawn to DTC genetic tests, whereby companies are building growing databases of customers' genetic and other personal details. While customers purchased these kits for their own purposes, companies mine the data for potential drug discovery and development, or for profit by selling datasets to other pharmaceutical companies.[105]

Despite collecting sensitive personal and health information, in the United States, device companies are not "covered entities" under Health Insurance Portability and Accountability Act (HIPAA) regulations, and are not bound by the same restrictions as other health care entities regarding data practices.[106] An analysis of health data protection in Apple and Google Play store policies also found that neither app store requires explicit consent for health data processing, with Google Play not even having rules on health apps and health data in general.[107] Another cross-sectional study looking at the privacy practices of more than 15,000 digital health apps found that these devices often collect other personal user information without adequate privacy disclosures, with 28 percent of the apps lacking any privacy policy information and more than 25 percent of user data transmissions violating the app's own stated policies.[108] The fact that digital technologies produce an unprecedented "net of surveillance" while also extending relatively unfettered medical power raises serious concerns regarding data security, privacy, and safety.[109] Moreover, these opaque commercial platforms are replacing medical professionals in determining which "risk factors" and "at-risk groups" are deemed eligible for indefinite targeting and warnings, ironically placing these technologies within a long history of medical surveillance and biopolitical governance.[110]

Echoing our discussions in the last chapter, the proliferation of DTC AI health technologies is also shifting responsibility for health management to laypeople in ways that reproduce rather than disrupt technological and medical power relations.[111] DTC AI health monitoring technologies do not simply generate, collect, analyze, and display information. Once such technological processes are implemented in the name of resisting or defying health deterioration through relentless projects of self-reflection, self-improvement, risk management, lifestyle maximization, and body optimization,[112] they can subtly manipulate users' behaviors in other ways, without the need to coerce compliance. Many devices impose discipline on users through constant reminders and alerts until the recommended behavioral change is achieved. These predictive and automated functions may alter the user's sense of identity to that of a (potentially) sick person in need of continuous tracking, warning, and nudging. While people may feel ambivalent about or overwhelmed by the endless obligation to comply with self-care routines, as prescribed by the algorithmic outputs,[113] their complex considerations are often glossed over in this growing socio-technological movement that promises control, self-improvement, and independence from institutional power.

Considering how DTC AI health monitoring may affect one's self-determination, a relational conception of autonomy looks beyond individual consent procedures to explore the external environment framing potential users' decisional motivations, including how the rules, conventions, and shared meanings of these health monitoring practices may affect people's opportunities to make and enact health maintenance choices based on their practical identities. This relational conception considers how the general character of one's socio-legal environment and culture may affect the range of available health monitoring options. Emerging AI technologies and the potentialities of their use can functionally change health monitoring practices by shifting individual and public expectations of what (and how) information can be collected, quantified, stored, utilized, and shared, and what types or levels of privacy and consent people are entitled to.

The manner in which these technological practices increasingly dominate in our social environment suggests a complex relational context that shapes people's freedom and opportunity to forgo or resist "voluntary" monitoring.[114] The proliferation of low-cost digital health monitoring tools, especially when aggressively marketed or deployed by health systems, insurance companies, or employers, has led not only to the opportunity to track and improve one's health, but also the expectation to do so, increasingly blurring the line between self-monitoring and being surveilled. As we saw in the last chapter, many health systems increasingly emphasize individual responsibility for self-management, such that those who are reluctant to be monitored, even out of concern for data privacy or accuracy, may be construed as being irresponsible. Moreover, in trying to reduce insurance costs and increase productivity, many employers have institutionalized health tracking by incentivizing employees to participate in corporate wellness programs,[115] offering bonuses or insurance discounts in exchange for the adoption of AI health apps that monitor and record employees' mood, exercise, smoking cessation activities, and other daily habits.[116] Employees gain access to tools that can help them engage in health promotion, while employers receive aggregated datasets of staff well-being across the organization to help predict sick leave, productivity, and general morale. The private insurance industry has also explored similar health tracking for mapping risks and setting premiums.[117] These practices, which have contributed to the growth of DTC AI wellness platforms, blur the distinction between individuals' private health data and corporate productivity and financial data,[118] commodifying people's information while camouflaging these activities as promoting users' self-knowledge and well-being.[119] They also reconfigure employer–employee relationships, and recast what would traditionally be considered private personal information that belongs to the employees as corporate wellness information that belongs to the company, which can then analyze the data for strategic planning without employee consent.

In other words, empowerment by DTC AI health monitoring increasingly takes the form of discipline and obligation, imposing expectations of how people should behave as part of individual responsibility and rational self-interest. This echoes Foucault's claim that biopower and biopolitics are not explicitly coercive; rather, they are even more effective at molding behavior by following the neoliberal modality of free choice and the promise of reward. People internalize the social norm by conforming to a predetermined and idealized standard of health and fitness that they are expected and incentivized to accept.[120]

The popularity of DTC AI pregnancy or prenatal platforms, which dominate the worldwide health-related DTC market, can help illustrate these issues and highlight how systemic and institutional patterns of structural privilege and oppression can constrain women's ability to exercise their agency in their pregnancy experience. In many parts of the world, women have been socialized to actively monitor, discipline, and modify their bodies in accordance with various social ideals, responding to and perpetuating objectifying norms that can have psychological and physical consequences,[121] from negative body image to anorexia nervosa.[122] As women manage their reproductive health and decisions, DTC AI pregnancy monitoring applications that continuously collect and analyze maternal-fetal information are often promoted as tools that give women a higher level of control over their pregnancy and fetal health. Engaging with pregnancy applications has become a routine and expected part of the maternity experience in the industrialized world.[123] For example, one pregnancy tracker, Velma, claims to be the first AI health app to reduce pregnancy risks and improve pregnancy health outcomes. In addition to using image recognition algorithms to automatically calculate the nutrition content of a meal from a photo, the app also tracks users' sleep quality, supplement intake, daily activities, weight, heart rate, fetal kick counts, and various symptoms to build a "unique health profile." It also claims to provide week-by-week guides curated by medical professionals and an intelligent chatbot to help women understand their "individual requirements for a healthy pregnancy lifestyle."[124]

However, for women who do not have high-risk pregnancies, the proliferation of AI DTC pregnancy monitoring, which quantifies women's embodied experience and encourages frequent data input, may needlessly intensify their health anxiety rather than promoting productive engagement.[125] This in turn can lead to overdiagnosis or overtreatment, harming and disempowering women in subtle but forceful ways.[126] These technologies continue to support a sex-gender system that configures women's wombs and other body parts as special biological and social problems requiring or legitimizing technological surveillance and interventions.[127] With the proliferation of DTC pregnancy platforms, women's fertility and intimate embodied experiences are increasingly medicalized and commercialized under the constant technological gaze. Such techno-medicalization perpetuates normative stereotypes and assumptions about women as sexual and reproductive subjects,[128] while also intersecting with the social and professional message that continuous monitoring of one's pregnancy is simply the rational and responsible thing for women to do.[129] Given the well-established power hierarchy in medicine and the presumption that DTC AI health monitoring is a desirable tool for self-management and early detection, there are questions of whether women truly have the freedom to decline technological options that they are expected or socially encouraged to accept.[130] Health-conscious prospective parents' understandings of parenthood, health, and identity are being redefined by the use of these technologies for "BabyVeillance."[131] Women who actively and intentionally reject self-surveillance or the medical gaze may be deemed irresponsible transgressors of the norms of motherhood,[132] which may ironically escalate intrusion by health care providers, pathologizing pregnancy and fortifying medical dominance.[133] Despite the pledge of promoting women's reproductive autonomy, DTC AI health monitoring may ultimately reinforce and reformulate oppressive gender roles, especially those around childbearing and motherhood, thereby compromising women's self-determination.

3.3 Self-Authorization and Agency

The intersecting relational analysis of self-governance and self-determination also sheds light on how DTC AI health monitoring affects people's self-authorization. A self-authorizing agent holds self-respect, self-trust, and self-esteem, and is socially recognized as autonomous by virtue of being accountable and answerable to others. Yet DTC AI health monitoring may ontologically shift people's practical identities in ways that ultimately undermine their self-authorization and epistemic credibility.

DTC AI health monitoring allows users greater access to their own information by interpellating them as rational and self-interested *consumers*. Instead of being vulnerable and passive *patients*, who may find themselves in a situation of involuntary or urgent need, with uncertain or limited knowledge, waiting for physicians to provide information and recommended care per their schedule, users as consumers are presumably well-informed and empowered to act voluntarily and decisively.[134] This image of a technologically enhanced consumer—one who freely, actively, and independently chooses DTC applications that allow them to manage and improve their physiological and mental well-being in ways they see fit—aligns with the liberal conception of a rational agent who acts strategically and is entirely responsible for their choices and consequences. Such access to one's own health information does not rely on traditional professional channels and may therefore boost users' self-confidence as well as equalize the therapeutic relationship if they decide to seek follow-up consultation with their physicians.

However, the ontological shift of turning patients into consumers may be self-serving for device manufacturers. By replacing the expectations of beneficence and non-maleficence, which are foundational to therapeutic relationships, with a rhetoric of consumer freedom and "buyer beware," device companies protect themselves from liability at the cost of users' self-determination and well-being. Clinicians are regulated and expected to only recommend interventions that have been scientifically proven to be effective, beneficial, or at least not harmful to patients; patients rely on these experts to watch out for their interests. They are also tasked with protecting patients' health-related information, which is presumed to be of exceptional sensitivity, as it can cause harm if misused.[135] The discourse around DTC AI health monitoring, however, puts the burden on users to inform themselves of the benefits and risks of these devices. As these platforms continuously collect health and other personal information, as well as link, transform, and reuse data in big data analyses, they normalize the collection and sharing of all data. Proponents justify these practices by claiming that self-authorizing consumers are "perfectly autonomous" and do not require paternalistic protections.[136] In theory, consumers' purchasing decisions will indirectly regulate the technologies coming onto the market, as device companies will develop and adjust their products according to consumer demands and preferences. Nonetheless, the lack of algorithmic transparency casts doubts on whether users can truly make informed decisions, and the absence of robust oversight of wellness algorithms may reinforce the informational and power asymmetry between device companies and general users while controlling users' perceptions of these products. Moreover, studies have found that many health apps lack validation of user input data, which can lead to incorrect output even if the algorithm performs as intended.[137] For example, a systematic assessment of smartphone apps for calculating insulin dose found that 91 percent lacked numeric input validation, and 59 percent allowed calculation even when one or more values were missing. Two-thirds of apps carried a risk of inappropriate output dose recommendations due to either violating basic clinical assumptions, not matching a stated formula, or failing to update dose recommendations in response to changing user inputs.[138] The lack of efficacy evidence for DTC AI health monitoring or protection against incorrect recommendations raises questions of whether these devices can provide meaningful information that will promote self-confidence.

There are also questions of whether DTC AI health platforms facilitate or hinder users' capacity to be answerable to others for their health behaviors. On the one hand, the ability of ordinary patients to bypass their clinicians in accessing information and health advice may help to equalize the power dynamic, as the expanded availability of health information may allow users to be more engaged, informed, and confident in explaining their reasons for seeking certain medical advice or treatment. Patients who can share their DTC AI health data with their health care team may also be epistemically advantaged and considered more trustworthy, as the use of these technologies may reduce confabulation, biases, illusions, false memories, and ignorance.[139]

On the other hand, given that many companies offer minimal evidence to support their claims of algorithmic authority,[140] the potential for misuse is concerning.[141] Paradoxically, patients may be increasingly expected to allow longitudinal surveillance and have data from these applications to support their claims; in other words, users' own testimony of their haptic sensations may be rendered less credible if their report or self-discovery cannot be supported by corresponding "objective" data. If the key to self-knowledge and epistemic authority requires the coupling of body and data, where biometrics from DTC AI health monitoring are presented as a source of instant truth,[142] then the authority of patients who want to rely on their own embodied experience without technologically mediated quantification might be questioned.[143] From a relational perspective, an overreliance on "objective" quantified data while dismissing the primacy of people's own experience may also exacerbate epistemic injustice, as it reinforces illegitimate social power and wrongs the user in their capacity as a knower.[144] The heavy promotion and expanding adoption of AI algorithmic predictions in the clinical setting and consumer market even when the information may not have clinical value may inflate the credibility of these technologies while further shifting epistemic power away from patients, whether they decide to use these platforms or resist them. Users themselves may not feel confident about their own embodied experience if it is not "validated" by machine judgment. Such concerns are heightened if clinicians prematurely dismiss or do not know how to address patient concerns that conflict with algorithmic outputs, or if patients feel disempowered to challenge their care provider and/or the AI predictive analytics.[145]

4. Conclusion

The potential benefits of DTC AI health monitoring are undeniably alluring. Emerging platforms promise to democratize health information, promote consumer autonomy, enhance preventive care, and provide more timely, accurate, convenient, comprehensive, and personalized health recommendations. They also claim to equalize power dynamics in therapeutic relationships and address unmet patient needs. At the same time, these technologies pose several risks that are underdiscussed in the current discourse. DTC AI health platforms are not subject to peer review or scientific testing of their validity, reliability, or safety, and there are no established best practices for evaluating their effects. Manufacturers' claims of proprietary information render algorithmic processes opaque and further impede efforts to evaluate health monitoring devices. Despite widespread industry enthusiasm, these platforms may ultimately disrupt care and therapeutic relationships, and shift power to technology companies. The expanding datafication of users' embodied experience may compromise their practical identity, create or exacerbate health anxiety, oversimplify health experiences, undermine users' epistemic authority and credibility, and pathologize or discipline users' bodies. At the broader professional and system levels, they may also lead to negative therapeutic relationships and overdiagnosis and overtreatment due to false positives, and exacerbate health inequity.

In addition to these risks, there are several other issues worth considering. First, much of the information collected, analyzed, and shared by DTC AI technologies is not actionable or clinically relevant, but may give the illusion of enhancing people's knowledge of their health status. Second, we have already seen that false positives can emerge due to faulty algorithms, but there is also the risk of intentional manipulation—after all, these products may not be deemed worthwhile by users if they fail to generate interactive messages and warnings.

Finally, in the case of AI wellness or even medical apps, data gathered or analyzed do not tell the whole story about one's health and need to be interpreted within the context of other variables. For example, an unusual ECG reading for an asymptomatic person with no other risk factors for heart disease (e.g., high blood pressure) can be clinically meaningless. However, in the absence of comprehensive patient and consumer education, healthy but anxious users who are alerted to potential issues by their DTC devices may flock to their physicians and seek additional testing based on ambiguous data. This can compromise therapeutic relationships, patient safety, and appropriate allocation of scarce medical resources, especially given the iatrogenic health risks from overdiagnosis and overtreatment. Due to the backlash against medical paternalism, clinicians may be reluctant to overtly dissuade their patients from using health-tracking devices. In the name of upholding patient autonomy and remaining hypervigilant about potential health concerns—no matter how statistically unlikely—physicians may feel pressured to practice "defensive medicine" and order further tests or low-value treatments that may carry other risks to avoid possible litigation. Transferring the costs of follow-up testing and care from for-profit device companies to health care systems that are already overstretched incurs wasteful spending and poses justice and equity considerations, despite these technologies' promise to democratize health care and reduce health disparities.

Notes

1. Stanford Medicine, *The Democratization of Health Care*, Stanford Medicine 2018 Health Trends Report, December 2018, https://med.stanford.edu/content/dam/sm/school/documents/Health-Trends-Report/Stanford-Medicine-Health-Trends-Report-2018.pdf.
2. Samantha McGrail, "88% of Providers Investing in Remote Patient Monitoring Tech," *mHealthIntelligence*, accessed February 9, 2022, https://mhealthintelligence.com/news/88-of-providers-investing-in-remote-patient-monitoring-tech.
3. "Managing Patient Care via Telehealth (OME)," Standards FAQs, The Joint Commission, last modified December 22, 2021, https://www.jointcommission.org/standards/standard-faqs/home-care/provision-of-care-treatment-and-services-pc/000002289/.
4. Simon P. Rowland et al., "What is the Clinical Value of mHealth for Patients?" *npj Digital Medicine* 3, no. 1 (January 2020): 4, https://doi.org/10.1038/s41746-019-0206-x.
5. IQVIA Institute, *Digital Health Trends, 2021*, July 21, 2021, https://www.iqvia.com/insights/the-iqvia-institute/reports/digital-health-trends-2021.
6. Eric J. Topol, "High-Performance Medicine: The Convergence of Human and Artificial Intelligence," *Nature Medicine* 25, no. 1 (January 2019): 44–56, https://doi.org/10.1038/s41591-018-0300-7.
7. However, many scholars have cautioned that habitual body monitoring may lead to body dissatisfaction. See Karen P. Grippo and Melanie S. Hill, "Self-Objectification, Habitual Body Monitoring, and Body Dissatisfaction in Older European American Women: Exploring Age and Feminism as Moderators," *Body Image* 5, no. 2 (June 2008): 173–82, https://doi.org/10.1016/j.bodyim.2007.11.003.
8. Arthur Willem Gerard Buijink, Benjamin Jelle Visser, and Louise Marshall, "Medical Apps for Smartphones: Lack of Evidence Undermines Quality and Safety," *Evidence-Based Medicine* 18, no. 3 (June 2013): 90–92, https://doi.org/10.1136/eb-2012-100885.
9. Boris Babic et al., "Direct-to-Consumer Medical Machine Learning and Artificial Intelligence Applications," *Nature Machine Intelligence* 3, no. 4 (April 2021): 283–87, https://doi.org/10.1038/s42256-021-00331-0.
10. Trishan Panch and Nikhil Bhojwani, "How AI Vendors Can Navigate the Health Care Industry," *Harvard Business Review*, May 17, 2021, https://hbr.org/2021/05/how-ai-vendors-can-navigate-the-health-care-industry.

11. Anita Ho, "Trusting Experts and Epistemic Humility in Disability," *IJFAB: International Journal of Feminist Approaches to Bioethics* 4, no. 2 (September 2011): 102–23, https://doi.org/10.3138/ijfab.4.2.102.
12. Ian Litchfield et al., "Test Result Communication in Primary Care: A Survey of Current Practice," *BMJ Quality & Safety* 24, no. 11 (November 2015): 691, https://doi.org/10.1136/bmjqs-2014-003712.
13. Lawrence P. Casalino et al., "Frequency of Failure to Inform Patients of Clinically Significant Outpatient Test Results," *Archives of Internal Medicine* 169, no. 12 (June 2009): 1123–29, https://doi.org/10.1001/archinternmed.2009.130.
14. J. Hickner et al., "Testing Process Errors and Their Harms and Consequences Reported from Family Medicine Practices: A Study of the American Academy of Family Physicians National Research Network," *Quality and Safety in Health Care* 17, no. 3 (June 2008): 194, https://doi.org/10.1136/qshc.2006.021915.
15. Annemarie Mol and John Law, "Embodied Action, Enacted Bodies: The Example of Hypoglycaemia," *Body & Society* 10, no. 2–3 (June 2004): 43–62, https://doi.org/10.1177/1357034X04042932.
16. "About Chronic Diseases," Centers for Disease Control and Prevention, last modified April 28, 2021, https://www.cdc.gov/chronicdisease/about/index.htm.
17. COVID-19 became one of the leading causes of death for parts of 2021, with particular burdens on people with pre-existing comorbidities. See https://www.healthsystemtracker.org/brief/covid-19-leading-cause-of-death-ranking/.
18. Sara Riggare and Maria Hägglund, "Precision Medicine in Parkinson's Disease—Exploring Patient-Initiated Self-Tracking," *Journal of Parkinson's Disease* 8, no. 3 (2018): 441–46, https://doi.org/10.3233/JPD-181314.
19. Btihaj Ajana, "Digital Health and the Biopolitics of the Quantified Self," *Digital Health* 3 (January 2017), https://doi.org/10.1177/2055207616689509.
20. Tamar Sharon, "Self-Tracking for Health and the Quantified Self: Re-Articulating Autonomy, Solidarity, and Authenticity in an Age of Personalized Healthcare," *Philosophy & Technology* 30, no. 1 (March 2017): 93–121, https://doi.org/10.1007/s13347-016-0215-5.
21. Ajana, "Digital Health."
22. Melanie Swan, "Health 2050: The Realization of Personalized Medicine through Crowdsourcing, the Quantified Self, and the Participatory Biocitizen," *Journal of Personalized Medicine* 2, no. 3 (September 2012): 93–118, https://doi.org/10.3390/jpm2030093.

23. I. Glenn Cohen et al., "Volume Introduction," in *The Future of Medical Device Regulation: Innovation and Protection*, ed. I. Glenn Cohen et al. (Cambridge: Cambridge University Press, 2022), 1–10, https://doi.org/10.1017/9781108975452.001.
24. Adam B. Cohen et al., "Direct-to-Consumer Digital Health," *The Lancet Digital Health* 2, no. 4 (April 2020): e163–65, https://doi.org/10.1016/S2589-7500(20)30057-1.
25. Sanket S. Dhruva et al., "Ensuring Patient Safety and Benefit in Use of Medical Devices Granted Expedited Approval," in *The Future of Medical Device Regulation: Innovation and Protection*, ed. I. Glenn Cohen et al. (Cambridge: Cambridge University Press, 2022), 217–28, https://doi:10.1017/9781108975452.017.
26. Aaron S. Kesselheim and Jerry Avorn, "New '21st Century Cures' Legislation: Speed and Ease vs Science," *Journal of the American Medical Association* 317, no. 6 (February 14, 2017): 581–82, https://doi: 10.1001/jama.2016.20640. PMID: 28056124.
27. In the European Union, the Council of the European Communities Directive 93/42/EEC concerning medical devices provides similar definitional guidance regarding medical devices. https://eur-lex.europa.eu/LexUriServ/LexUriServ.do?uri=CONSLEG:1993L0042:20071011:en:PDF.
28. Eric Wu et al., "How Medical AI Devices Are Evaluated: Limitations and Recommendations from an Analysis of FDA Approvals," *Nature Medicine* 27, no. 4 (April 2021): 582–84, https://doi.org/10.1038/s41591-021-01312-x.
29. "De Novo Classification Request," U.S. Food and Drug Administration, last modified January 3, 2022, https://www.fda.gov/medical-devices/premarket-submissions/de-novo-classification-request.
30. "Premarket Notification 510(k)," U.S. Food and Drug Administration, last modified March 13, 2020, https://www.fda.gov/medical-devices/premarket-submissions-selecting-and-preparing-correct-submission/premarket-notification-510k.
31. "Premarket Approval (PMA)," U.S. Food and Drug Administration, last modified May 16, 2019, https://www.fda.gov/medical-devices/premarket-submissions-selecting-and-preparing-correct-submission/premarket-approval-pma.
32. "FDA-Approved A.I.-Based Algorithms," *The Medical Futurist*, accessed January 6, 2022, https://medicalfuturist.com/fda-approved-ai-based-algorithms/.
33. Stan Benjamens, Pranavsingh Dhunnoo, and Bertalan Meskó, "The State of Artificial Intelligence-Based FDA-Approved Medical Devices and

Algorithms: An Online Database," *npj Digital Medicine* 3, no. 1 (September 2020): 118, https://doi.org/10.1038/s41746-020-00324-0.

34. "FDA Allows Marketing of First Direct-to-Consumer App for Contraceptive Use to Prevent Pregnancy," U.S. Food and Drug Administration, August 10, 2018, https://www.fda.gov/news-events/press-announcements/fda-allows-marketing-first-direct-consumer-app-contraceptive-use-prevent-pregnancy.
35. "FDA Allows Marketing," U.S. Food and Drug Administration.
36. Thea K. Kleinschmidt et al., "Advantages of Determining the Fertile Window with the Individualised Natural Cycles Algorithm over Calendar-Based Methods," *European Journal of Contraception & Reproductive Health Care* 24, no. 6 (November 2019): 457–63, https://doi.org/10.1080/13625187.2019.1682544.
37. E. Berglund Scherwitzl et al., "Perfect-Use and Typical-Use Pearl Index of a Contraceptive Mobile App," *Contraception* 96, no. 6 (December 2017): 420–25, https://doi.org/10.1016/j.contraception.2017.08.014.
38. Nicole Wetsman, "Birth Control Apps Show the Contradictions in FDA Device Oversight," *The Verge*, March 17, 2021, https://www.theverge.com/22335858/birth-control-app-clue-natural-cycles-fda; Natasha Lomas, "Clue Gets FDA Clearance to Launch a Digital Contraceptive," *TechCrunch*, March 1, 2021, https://techcrunch.com/2021/03/01/clue-gets-fda-clearance-to-launch-a-digital-contraceptive/.
39. Pippa Grenfell et al., "Fertility and Digital Technology: Narratives of Using Smartphone App 'Natural Cycles' While Trying to Conceive," *Sociology of Health & Illness* 43, no. 1 (January 2021): 116–32, https://doi.org/10.1111/1467-9566.13199.
40. "Tracking the States Where Abortion Is Now Banned," *New York Times*, last modified July 22, 2022, https://www.nytimes.com/interactive/2022/us/abortion-laws-roe-v-wade.html.
41. "Premarket Approval (PMA)," U.S. Food and Drug Administration.
42. Benjamens, Dhunnoo, and Meskó, "State of Artificial Intelligence."
43. Premarket Approval for Guardian Connect System, U.S. Food and Drug Administration, last modified January 3, 2022, https://www.accessdata.fda.gov/scripts/cdrh/cfdocs/cfpma/pma.cfm?id=P160007.
44. Nihaal Reddy, Neha Verma, and Kathleen Dungan, "Monitoring Technologies: Continuous Glucose Monitoring, Mobile Technology, Biomarkers of Glycemic Control," in *Endotext*, ed. Kenneth Feingold et al. (South Dartmouth, MA: MDText.com, 2000), https://www.ncbi.nlm.nih.gov/books/NBK279046/.

45. Heather Mack, "FDA Clears WellDoc's Non-RX Version of BlueStar, Its Mobile Diabetes Management Tool," *MobiHealthNews*, January 19, 2017, https://www.mobihealthnews.com/content/fda-clears-welldocs-non-rx-version-bluestar-its-mobile-diabetes-management-tool.
46. Babic et al., "Direct-to-Consumer Medical Machine Learning."
47. Marketing Authorization for Irregular Rhythm Notification Feature DEN180042, U.S. Food and Drug Administration, September 11, 2018, https://www.accessdata.fda.gov/cdrh_docs/pdf18/DEN180042.pdf.
48. Center for Devices and Radiological Health, "General Wellness: Policy for Low Risk Devices," U.S. Food and Drug Administration, FDA-2014-N-1039, September 26, 2019, https://www.fda.gov/regulatory-information/search-fda-guidance-documents/general-wellness-policy-low-risk-devices.
49. "Policy for Device Software Functions and Mobile Medical Applications: Guidance for Industry and Food and Drug Administration Staff," U.S. Food and Drug Administration, September 27, 2019, https://www.fda.gov/media/80958/download.
50. Buijink et al.,, "Medical Apps for Smartphones."
51. Niamh M. Hogan and Michael J. Kerin, "Smart Phone Apps: Smart Patients, Steer Clear," *Patient Education and Counseling* 89, no. 2 (November 2012): 360–61, https://doi.org/10.1016/j.pec.2012.07.016.
52. "Health2Sync App," accessed January 6, 2021, www.Health2sync.com/patients.
53. Natalie Stein, "Leading Chronic Disease Management and Prevention—An Interview with Lark VP of Growth, Cameron D. Jacox and Research2Guidance," Lark, July 6, 2019, https://www.lark.com/blog/leading-chronic-disease-management-and-prevention-an-interview-with-lark-vp-of-growth-cameron-jacox-and-research2guidanc/.
54. Hannah Chu-Han Huang and Dennis Ougrin, "Impact of the COVID-19 Pandemic on Child and Adolescent Mental Health Services," *BJPsych Open* 7, no. 5 (2021): e145, https://doi.org/10.1192/bjo.2021.976; Anna Maria Werling et al., "The Impact of the COVID-19 Pandemic on Mental Health Care of Children and Adolescents in Switzerland: Results of a Survey among Mental Health Care Professionals after One Year of COVID-19," *International Journal of Environmental Research and Public Health* 19, no. 6 (March 2022), https://doi.org/10.3390/ijerph19063252.
55. Maxime Taquet et al., "6-Month Neurological and Psychiatric Outcomes in 236 379 Survivors of COVID-19: A Retrospective Cohort Study Using Electronic Health Records," *Lancet Psychiatry* 8, no. 5 (May 2021): 416–27, https://doi.org/10.1016/S2215-0366(21)00084-5.

56. Anita Ho, "Can Public Health Investment and Oversight Save Digital Mental Health?," *AJOB Neuroscience* 13, no. 3 (July 2022): 201–3, https://doi.org/10.1080/21507740.2022.2082586; Joshua August Skorburg and Josephine Yam, "Is There an App for That?: Ethical Issues in the Digital Mental Health Response to COVID-19," *AJOB Neuroscience* 13, no. 3 (September 2022): 177–90, https://doi.org/10.1080/21507740.2021.1918284.
57. Scott Stonham, "AI, Wearable Tech and Mental Health Well-Being," *Well, That's Interesting Tech*, April 20, 2020, https://wellthatsinteresting.tech/ai-tech-mental-health-well-being/.
58. For more details, see https://wysa.io/.
59. Ajana, "Digital Health."
60. Ajana, "Digital Health."
61. Paul Krebs and Dustin T. Duncan, "Health App Use Among US Mobile Phone Owners: A National Survey," *JMIR mHealth and uHealth* 3, no. 4 (November 2015): e101, https://doi.org/10.2196/mhealth.4924.
62. Clarence Baxter et al., "Assessment of Mobile Health Apps Using Built-In Smartphone Sensors for Diagnosis and Treatment: Systematic Survey of Apps Listed in International Curated Health App Libraries," *JMIR mHealth and uHealth* 8, no. 2 (February 2020): e16741, https://doi.org/10.2196/16741.
63. According to the FDA, the AI technologies approved by the agency so far are generally called "locked" algorithms, which do not continually adapt or learn every time the algorithm is used. These locked algorithms are modified by the manufacturer at intervals, which includes "training" of the algorithm using new data, followed by manual verification and validation of the updated algorithm. See "Statement from FDA Commissioner Scott Gottlieb, M.D. on Steps toward a New, Tailored Review Framework for Artificial Intelligence-Based Medical Devices," U.S. Food and Drug Administration, April 2, 2019, https://www.fda.gov/news-events/press-announcements/statement-fda-commissioner-scott-gottlieb-md-steps-toward-new-tailored-review-framework-artificial.
64. Deborah Lupton, "Health Promotion in the Digital Era: A Critical Commentary," *Health Promotion International* 30, no. 1 (March 2015): 174–83, https://doi:10.1093/heapro/dau091. PMID: 25320120.
65. Deborah Lupton, "Quantified Sex: A Critical Analysis of Sexual and Reproductive Self-Tracking Using Apps," Culture, Health & Sexuality 17, no. 4 (April 2015): 440–53, https://doi.org/10.1080/13691058.2014.920528.

66. Peter Yobo, "How DTC Is Disrupting Health Care," Credera, May 1, 2020, https://www.credera.com/insights/how-dtc-is-disrupting-health-care.
67. Davey Winder, "How to Stop Your Smart Home Spying on You," *The Guardian*, March 8, 2020, https://www.theguardian.com/technology/2020/mar/08/how-to-stop-your-smart-home-spying-on-you-lightbulbs-doorbell-ring-google-assistant-alexa-privacy.
68. Deborah Lupton, "The Diverse Domains of Quantified Selves: Self-Tracking Modes and Dataveillance," *Economy and Society* 45, no. 1 (January 2016): 101–22, https://doi.org/10.1080/03085147.2016.1143726.
69. Deborah Lupton, "The Digitally Engaged Patient: Self-Monitoring and Self-Care in the Digital Health Era," *Social Theory & Health* 11, no. 3 (August 2013): 256–70, https://doi.org/10.1057/sth.2013.10.
70. Hannah van Kolfschooten, "The mHealth Power Paradox: Improving Data Protection in Health Apps through Self-Regulation in the European Union," in *The Future of Medical Device Regulation: Innovation and Protection*, ed. I. Glenn Cohen et al. (Cambridge: Cambridge University Press, 2022), 63–76, https://doi:10.1017/9781108975452.006.
71. Ajana, "Digital Health."
72. Helen Kennedy, Thomas Poell, and Jose van Dijck, "Data and Agency," *Big Data & Society* 2, no. 2 (December 2015), https://doi.org/10.1177/2053951715621569.
73. Eric Topol, *The Patient Will See You Now: The Future of Medicine Is in Your Hands* (New York: Basic Books, 2015).
74. Deborah Lupton, "Quantifying the Body: Monitoring and Measuring Health in the Age of mHealth Technologies," *Critical Public Health* 23, no. 4 (December 2013): 393–403, https://doi.org/10.1080/09581596.2013.794931; Sharon, "Self-Tracking for Health."
75. Sharon, "Self-Tracking for Health"; Lupton, "Quantifying the Body."
76. Yue You and Xinning Gui, "Self-Diagnosis through AI-Enabled Chatbot-Based Symptom Checkers: User Experiences and Design Considerations," *AMIA Annual Symposium Proceedings 2020* (January 2021): 1354–63, https://www.ncbi.nlm.nih.gov/pmc/articles/PMC8075525/.
77. Catherine D'Ignazio and Lauren F. Klein, *Data Feminism* (Cambridge, MA: MIT Press, 2020); Alison M. Darcy, Alan K. Louie, and Laura Weiss Roberts, "Machine Learning and the Profession of Medicine," *Journal of the American Medical Association* 315, no. 6 (February 2016): 551–52, https://doi.org/10.1001/jama.2015.18421; Antonio Maturo and Francesca Setiffi, "The Gamification of Risk: How Health Apps Foster Self-Confidence and Why This Is Not Enough," *Health, Risk & Society* 17, no. 7–8 (February 2016): 477–94, https://doi.org/10.1080/13698575.2015.1136599.

78. João V. Cordeiro, "Digital Technologies and Data Science as Health Enablers: An Outline of Appealing Promises and Compelling Ethical, Legal, and Social Challenges," *Frontiers in Medicine* 8 (July 2021): 647897, https://doi.org/10.3389/fmed.2021.647897.
79. Lupton, "Quantifying the Body."
80. Sharon, "Self-Tracking for Health."
81. Julian Sheather, "Selling Sickness to the Worried Well," BMJ Opinion, February 12, 2010, https://blogs.bmj.com/bmj/2010/02/12/julian-sheather-selling-sickness-to-the-worried-well/.
82. Shannon Vallor, *Technology and the Virtues: A Philosophical Guide to a Future Worth Wanting* (New York: Oxford University Press, 2016).
83. Duncan Chambers et al., "Digital and Online Symptom Checkers and Health Assessment/Triage Services for Urgent Health Problems: Systematic Review," *BMJ Open* 9, no. 8 (August 2019): e027743, https://doi.org/10.1136/bmjopen-2018-027743.
84. It is worth noting that just mentioning AI in product claims may improve a company's prospects, even when different methods can yield variable accuracy, such that companies indiscriminately advertise their algorithms as AI. See Ross J. Lordon et al., "How Patient-Generated Health Data and Patient-Reported Outcomes Affect Patient-Clinician Relationships: A Systematic Review," *Health Informatics Journal* 26, no. 4 (December 2020): 2689–706, https://doi.org/10.1177/1460458220928184.
85. Bertalan Meskó and Marton Görög, "A Short Guide for Medical Professionals in the Era of Artificial Intelligence," *npj Digital Medicine* 3, no. 1 (December 2020): 126, https://doi.org/10.1038/s41746-020-00333-z.
86. Stephanie Aboueid et al., "The Use of Artificially Intelligent Self-Diagnosing Digital Platforms by the General Public: Scoping Review," *JMIR Medical Informatics* 7, no. 2 (May 2019): e13445, https://doi.org/10.2196/13445.
87. Rens van de Schoot et al., "Bayesian Statistics and Modelling," *Nature Reviews Methods Primers* 1, no. 1 (January 2021): 1, https://doi.org/10.1038/s43586-020-00001-2.
88. Kimberly Lovett Rockwell, "Direct-to-Consumer Medical Testing in the Era of Value-Based Care," *Journal of the American Medical Association* 317, no. 24 (June 2017): 2485–86, https://doi.org/10.1001/jama.2017.5929.
89. Camille Nebeker, John Torous, and Rebecca J. Bartlett Ellis, "Building the Case for Actionable Ethics in Digital Health Research Supported by Artificial Intelligence," *BMC Medicine* 17, no. 1 (July 2019): 137, https://doi.org/10.1186/s12916-019-1377-7.

90. For example, the two aforementioned FDA-approved fertility tracking applications use very different methods to predict the user's fertility window, even though the second device was approved based on presumed substantial equivalency. See Dawn Moyer, "Your Fancy Proprietary AI Model Has No Value to Me," Medium, November 16, 2020, https://towardsdatascience.com/your-fancy-proprietary-ai-model-has-no-value-to-me-2a7d40dfd8ca.
91. Thomas Grote and Philipp Berens, "On the Ethics of Algorithmic Decision-Making in Healthcare," *Journal of Medical Ethics* 46, no. 3 (March 2020): 205, https://doi.org/10.1136/medethics-2019-105586.
92. Karoline Freeman et al., "Algorithm Based Smartphone Apps to Assess Risk of Skin Cancer in Adults: Systematic Review of Diagnostic Accuracy Studies," *BMJ* 368 (February 2020): m127, https://doi.org/10.1136/bmj.m127.
93. Bettina Schmietow and Georg Marckmann, "Mobile Health Ethics and the Expanding Role of Autonomy," *Medicine, Health Care, and Philosophy* 22, no. 4 (December 2019): 623–30, https://doi.org/10.1007/s11019-019-09900-y.
94. Bret S. Cohen et al., "FTC Authority to Regulate Artificial Intelligence," Reuters, July 8, 2021, https://www.reuters.com/legal/legalindustry/ftc-authority-regulate-artificial-intelligence-2021-07-08/.
95. Jennifer K. Wagner, "The Federal Trade Commission and Consumer Protections for Mobile Health Apps," *Journal of Law, Medicine & Ethics* 48, no. 1_suppl (March 2020): 103–14, https://doi.org/10.1177/1073110520917035.
96. Anna Wexler and Steven Joffe, "5 Ways to Address the Challenges of Direct-to-Consumer Health Products," STAT, April 2, 2019, https://www.statnews.com/2019/04/02/address-challenges-direct-to-consumer-health-products/.
97. Sarah Kliff and Aatish Bhatia, "When They Warn of Rare Disorders, These Prenatal Tests Are Usually Wrong," *New York Times*, January 1, 2022, https://www.nytimes.com/2022/01/01/upshot/pregnancy-birth-genetic-testing.html?action=click&module=Well&pgtype=Homepage&section=The%20Upshot.
98. Babic et al., "Direct-to-Consumer Medical Machine Learning."
99. Anita Ho and Oliver Quick, "Leaving Patients to Their Own Devices? Smart Technology, Safety and Therapeutic Relationships," *BMC Medical Ethics* 19 (2018), https://doi.org/10.1186/s12910-018-0255-8.
100. Alice K. Hawkins and Anita Ho, "Genetic Counseling and the Ethical Issues around Direct to Consumer Genetic Testing," *Journal of Genetic*

Counseling 21, no. 3 (June 2012): 367–73, https://doi.org/10.1007/s10897-012-9488-8.

101. Kristian Gottliebsen and Göran Petersson, "Limited Evidence of Benefits of Patient Operated Intelligent Primary Care Triage Tools: Findings of a Literature Review," *BMJ Health & Care Informatics* 27, no. 1 (May 2020): e100114, https://doi.org/10.1136/bmjhci-2019-100114.
102. Babic et al., "Direct-to-Consumer Medical Machine Learning"; Rockwell, "Direct-to-Consumer Medical Testing."
103. Marjolein Lanzing, "The Transparent Self," *Ethics and Information Technology* 18, no. 1 (March 2016): 9–16, https://doi.org/10.1007/s10676-016-9396-y.
104. van Kolfschooten, "mHealth Power Paradox."
105. Jessica Hamzelou, "DNA Firms Are Set to Profit from Your Data as Testing Demand Falls," *New Scientist*, February 7, 2020, https://www.newscientist.com/article/2232770-dna-firms-are-set-to-profit-from-your-data-as-testing-demand-falls/.
106. Thomas Germain, "Mental Health Apps Aren't All As Private As You May Think," *Consumer Reports*, March 2, 2021, https://www.consumerreports.org/health-privacy/mental-health-apps-and-user-privacy/.
107. van Kolfschooten, "mHealth Power Paradox."
108. Gioacchino Tangari et al., "Mobile Health and Privacy: Cross Sectional Study," *BMJ* 373 (June 2021): n1248, https://doi.org/10.1136/bmj.n1248.
109. Emma Rich and Andy Miah, "Mobile, Wearable and Ingestible Health Technologies: Towards a Critical Research Agenda," *Health Sociology Review* 26, no. 1 (January 2017): 84–97, https://doi.org/10.1080/14461242.2016.1211486; Chris Till, "Exercise as Labour: Quantified Self and the Transformation of Exercise into Labour," *Societies* 4, no. 3 (2014): 446–62 https://doi.org/10.3390/soc4030446.
110. Michel Foucault, *Discipline and Punish: The Birth of the Prison*, trans. Alan Sheridan (New York: Pantheon Books, 1977).
111. Lupton, "Digitally Engaged Patient."
112. Debbie Laliberte Rudman, "Shaping the Active, Autonomous and Responsible Modern Retiree: An Analysis of Discursive Technologies and Their Links with Neo-Liberal Political Rationality," *Ageing and Society* 26 (March 2006): 181–201, https://doi.org/10.1017/S0144686X05004253.
113. Lupton, "Digitally Engaged Patient."
114. Minna Ruckenstein and Natasha Dow Schüll, "The Datafication of Health," *Annual Review of Anthropology* 46, no. 1 (October 2017): 261–78, https://doi.org/10.1146/annurev-anthro-102116-041244.

115. Till, "Exercise as Labour."
116. Lanzing, "Transparent Self."
117. Ajana, "Digital Health."
118. David Nield, "Employee Wellness Programs Now One of Fitbit's Fastest Growing Areas," Digital Trends, April 19, 2014, https://www.digitaltrends.com/mobile/employee-wellness-programs-now-one-fitbits-fastest-growing-areas/#!bDRFJr.
119. Till, "Exercise as Labour."
120. Michel Foucault, "The Subject and Power," *Critical Inquiry* 8, no. 4 (1982): 777–95, http://www.jstor.org/stable/1343197.
121. Grippo and Hill, "Self-Objectification."
122. Mary Briody Mahowald, "To Be or Not Be a Woman: Anorexia Nervosa, Normative Gender Roles, and Feminism," *Journal of Medicine and Philosophy* 17, no. 2 (April 1992): 233–51, https://doi.org/10.1093/jmp/17.2.233.
123. Jo-Anne Patricia Hughson et al., "The Rise of Pregnancy Apps and the Implications for Culturally and Linguistically Diverse Women: Narrative Review," *JMIR mHealth and uHealth* 6, no. 11 (November 2018): e189, https://doi.org/10.2196/mhealth.9119.
124. "Velma: Pregnancy Tracker App," Apple App Store Preview, accessed February 9, 2022, https://apps.apple.com/us/app/velma-pregnancy-tracker-app/id1498760243.
125. Janice Hopkins Tanne, "Direct to Consumer Medical Tests Are Offered in United States," *BMJ* 333, no. 7557 (July 2006): 12, https://doi.org/10.1136/bmj.333.7557.12-a.
126. Matthieu Komorowski and Leo Anthony Celi, "Will Artificial Intelligence Contribute to Overuse in Healthcare?" *Critical Care Medicine* 45, no. 5 (May 2017): 912–13, https://doi.org/10.1097/CCM.0000000000002351.
127. Hilde Lindemann Nelson, "Feminist Bioethics: Where We've Been, Where We're Going," *Metaphilosophy* 31, no. 5 (October 2000): 492–508, https://doi.org/10.1111/1467-9973.00165.
128. Lupton, "Quantified Sex."
129. Anita Ho, "The Individualist Model of Autonomy and the Challenge of Disability," *Journal of Bioethical Inquiry* 5, no. 2 (June 2008): 193–207, https://doi.org/10.1007/s11673-007-9075-0.
130. Susan Sherwin, "A Relational Approach to Autonomy in Health Care," in *The Politics of Women's Health: Exploring Agency and Autonomy*, ed. Susan Sherwin (Philadelphia: Temple University Press, 1998), 19–47.

131. Veronica Barassi, "BabyVeillance? Expecting Parents, Online Surveillance and the Cultural Specificity of Pregnancy Apps," *Social Media + Society*, 3, no. 2 (2017), https://doi.org/10.1177/2056305117707188.
132. Laura R. Woliver, *The Political Geographies of Pregnancy* (Urbana: University of Illinois Press, 2002).
133. Bec Jenkinson, Sue Kruske, and Sue Kildea, "The Experiences of Women, Midwives and Obstetricians When Women Decline Recommended Maternity Care: A Feminist Thematic Analysis," *Midwifery* 52 (September 2017): 1–10, https://doi.org/10.1016/j.midw.2017.05.006.
134. Schmietow and Marckmann, "Mobile Health Ethics."
135. Schmietow and Marckmann, "Mobile Health Ethics."
136. Marc Lemire, "What Can Be Expected of Information and Communication Technologies in Terms of Patient Empowerment in Health?" *Journal of Health Organization and Management* 24, no. 2 (January 2010): 167–81, https://doi.org/10.1108/14777261011047336.
137. Saba Akbar, Coiera Enrico, and Farah Magrabi, "Safety Concerns with Consumer-Facing Mobile Health Applications and Their Consequences: A Scoping Review," *Journal of the American Medical Informatics Association* 27, no. 2 (February 2020): 330–40, https://doi.org/10.1093/jamia/ocz175.
138. Kit Huckvale et al., "Smartphone Apps for Calculating Insulin Dose: A Systematic Assessment," *BMC Medicine* 13, no. 1 (May 2015): 106, https://doi.org/10.1186/s12916-015-0314-7.
139. Lanzing, "Transparent Self."
140. Deborah Lupton and Annemarie Jutel, "'It's Like Having a Physician in Your Pocket!' A Critical Analysis of Self-Diagnosis Smartphone Apps," *Social Science & Medicine* 133 (May 2015): 128–35, https://doi.org/10.1016/j.socscimed.2015.04.004.
141. Annemarie Jutel and Deborah Lupton, "Digitizing Diagnosis: A Review of Mobile Applications in the Diagnostic Process," *Diagnosis* 2, no. 2 (June 2015): 89–96, https://doi.org/10.1515/dx-2014-0068.
142. Katja Franko Aas, "'The Body Does Not Lie': Identity, Risk and Trust in Technoculture," *Crime, Media, Culture* 2, no. 2 (August 2006): 143–58, https://doi.org/10.1177/1741659006065401.
143. Ajana, "Digital Health."
144. Miranda Fricker, *Epistemic Injustice: Power and the Ethics of Knowing* (Oxford: Oxford University Press, 2007).
145. Aboueid et al., "The Use of Artificially Intelligent Self-Diagnosing Digital Platforms."

4

A Digital Pill to Swallow

Artificial Intelligence Monitoring for Medication Adherence and Therapeutic Relationships

> Pharma cares about noncompliance, but why should patients care?
>
> —Vasudev Bailey, PhD, partner at Artis Ventures

In previous chapters, I explored how the expanding use of artificial intelligence (AI) health monitoring may affect users' relational autonomy and well-being even when they accept or initiate the utilization of these technologies. This chapter interrogates an emerging area for AI health monitoring, one in which users often explicitly resist continuous observation, thus rendering these technologies particularly fraught from the perspective of autonomy: medication dosage monitoring. In recent years, medication monitoring algorithms for tracking and predicting patients' medication intake patterns and physiological data have gained traction among clinicians and health systems as a means of promoting patient safety.[1] However, as these tools are generally recommended for patients whose self-reports of medication adherence are deemed incomplete, inaccurate, fabricated, ill-intentioned, or otherwise untrustworthy, medication monitoring algorithms may exacerbate paternalism and distrust, which can in turn compromise therapeutic relationships and reinforce an oppressive power hierarchy, thereby undermining patient autonomy.

The very concept of medication adherence has long been contested, and the last few decades have seen a shift from a clinician-centered framework to a patient-centered one.[2] In the 1970s and 1980s, *compliance*, which describes "the extent to which the patient's behavior (including medication-taking) coincides with medical or healthcare advice," was the common term.[3] But the paternalistic connotations of passive patients who blindly follow doctors' instructions prompted the World Health Organization (WHO) to call for a shift to the term *adherence*,[4] defined as the extent or degree to which the use of medication by the patient corresponds with the prescribed regimen recommended by the health care provider.[5] This newer term is generally considered more cognizant of patients' agency and the complex considerations behind their medication decisions.

In more recent years, further efforts have been made to change the term to *concordance* in order to denote treatment planning as a collaborative effort, whereby the patient's priorities and goals are incorporated into medication prescribing decisions.[6] Yet, despite evolving terminology, the growing phenomenon of using technologies to measure patients' medication intake and predict potential nonadherence appears to be going in the opposite direction, as it entails or even reinforces a power imbalance between doctors and patients.[7] As we will see throughout this chapter, AI medication monitoring generally measures patients' medication intake as compared to a prescribed or pre-identified threshold, rather than according to the patient's self-determined or collaboratively determined priorities around their quality of life or competing concerns. Moreover, the implementation of these technologies is mostly driven by clinicians' or health systems' perceived need to closely track certain patient populations' behavior, rather than by patients' own motivations and other contextual considerations. I will therefore use the term *adherence* in the general discussion here while also highlighting concerns around compliance expectations and potential steps towards patient-centered concordance.

Lack of adherence to a prescribed therapeutic regimen—whether by forgoing recommended pharmacotherapy altogether or by not taking the prescribed doses correctly or consistently—is a prevalent and complex individual and public health problem. In the context of chronic illnesses and mental health, medication adherence has become a major concern worldwide.[8] Medications are the primary clinical approach for treating many of these illnesses,[9] and a lack of adherence is often associated with suboptimal disease management, poor health outcomes, and heavy financial burdens on patients and health systems due to physician and emergency room visits and hospitalizations.[10] While the numbers and scales are widely variable, partly due to how adherence is defined and measured, some studies suggest that poor medication adherence contributes to 125,000 deaths and accounts for anywhere from $100 billion to $300 billion in health care costs in the United States each year.[11] In Canada, an estimated 5.4 percent of all hospitalizations are the result of medication nonadherence.[12]

To date, many strategies for measuring and facilitating better adherence have been labor intensive, complex, and ineffective, especially for patients with chronic comorbidities that require long-term or multiple medications. To promote more effective and efficient practices that can target patients with the highest likelihood of harm due to nonadherence to medication instructions, big data analytics and machine learning (ML) models that can develop medication adherence profiles have been increasingly incorporated into population health management to prevent major health complications and reduce preventable hospitalizations and health care costs.

While some of the AI home health and direct-to-consumer (DTC) monitoring technologies discussed in previous chapters may include medication tracking or reminders as ancillary functions, this chapter spotlights AI monitoring algorithms that have been specifically developed to identify and predict medication adherence at the individual patient level. Focusing on the examples of mental illness and opioid pain management outside of the acute or emergency care settings (i.e., outpatients), I explore how these emerging technologies, while promising to promote patient safety, patient autonomy, and personalized care, may in fact disempower patients in ways that compromise their relational autonomy. Section 1 defines key components of medication adherence and presents the scope of the complex and multidimensional concerns around suboptimal adherence from both individual and public health perspectives. Section 2 provides examples of how AI has been proposed or used to identify and predict medication adherence. It focuses on examples in mental health care and opioid for chronic non-malignant pain (CNMP) management to illustrate how AI medication adherence monitoring as a proposed practice is designed to address clinicians' distrust of patients and bypass patient testimonies. Section 3 explores how medication adherence monitoring expands medical authority and dismisses patients' subjective experiences and concerns in ways that violate their relational self-governance, self-determination, and self-authorization.

It is important to clarify that I am not arguing against the prescription or utilization of medications, and to acknowledge that AI medication adherence monitoring is not necessarily inherently harmful. I recognize the possibility that well-developed algorithms could radically improve treatment pathways for outpatients if they were trained or utilized to consider and incorporate patients' multifaceted contexts, and implemented to work collaboratively with patients to determine goal-concordant dosing. Nonetheless, most existing or emerging technologies as well as their (proposed) deployment focus almost exclusively on surveillance and discipline, judging adherence according to static or predetermined thresholds without careful consideration of patients' complex desires, motivations, and embodied experiences. As these tools by design prioritize pre-established dosage levels and physiological data over patients' self-reports, they may enact a form of epistemic injustice that perpetuates stigmatization and marginalization for certain patient populations and compromises their relational autonomy. Even if some patients may misreport their medication behavior or deviate from the prescribed dosage, implementation of AI medication monitoring without full understanding of the reasons behind these actions may reinforce bidirectional distrust rather than promote patient well-being or safety.

1. A Tough Bill/Pill to Swallow

Medication adherence generally refers to a patient's behavior as related to their prescribed regimen. It involves measuring the timing, dosage, and frequency of patients' medication intake.[13] The medication adherence threshold rate, above which the clinical outcome is satisfactory, is sometimes defined as using the medication as directed at least 75 to 80 percent of the time.[14] Nonetheless, this range itself is misleading, as the necessary degree of adherence to promote a desired level of health outcome differs greatly depending on the particular condition, the medications involved, and patient characteristics.[15] Some medications are prescribed to be taken intermittently to treat symptoms as needed, which can vary among patients or even for the same patient at different times. Examples include antihistamines for allergies and nonsteroidal anti-inflammatory drugs for reducing pain, fever, and inflammation. Other medications require consistent and relatively precise dosage for a designated period for health improvement. For example, with certain types of infections (e.g., gonorrhea, pneumonia), patients are advised to take the full course of prescribed antibiotics to prevent remaining illness-causing bacteria from multiplying and becoming resistant to the antibiotics in the future. In the case of antiretroviral therapy (ART) for HIV viral suppression, the necessary lifetime adherence threshold rate for patients to become and remain virologically suppressed is often cited as at least 90 percent or even 95 percent.[16] However, studies show that with newer, more effective ART medications, the threshold for viral suppression may be lower, at 75 percent or 78 percent, depending on regimen type.[17]

In other words, there is no single threshold that applies to all conditions or medications below which patients are categorically nonadherent, such that interpretation of adherence rates reported in medication behavior studies must be carried out with due care, as they may not be adjusted according to the particular drug class or condition. Even in studies utilizing the same methodology and investigating the same drug class, threshold variations abound. Moreover, a medication that is deemed clinically appropriate for a given condition may nonetheless be overall unsuitable for a particular patient due to their unique personal context and socio-structural factors (e.g., allergies, taking other medications, not having easy access to clean water). A review article exploring adherence to oral antipsychotics in schizophrenia patients found that definitions of an adherent patient varied from agreeing to take *any* medication to taking at least 90 percent of the medications as prescribed.[18] As we will see throughout this chapter, such variability raises questions about the epistemological and ethical consequences of using AI to identify and predict medication adherence based on a predefined threshold or pattern. Unlike decisions about a specific and time-limited procedural intervention, such as surgery, medication adherence can evolve over time, especially for patients with chronic and/or multiple conditions. Challenges or reluctance to adhere to the regimens may occur at various points in the patient's treatment pathway and for different reasons.[19]

Medication adherence is also a multistep process. *Initiation*, sometimes also called primary medication adherence, refers to the patient filling and picking up the prescription or an appropriate alternative within a defined number of days after the medication is first prescribed.[20] Evidence from a study looking at filled claims of e-prescriptions across various drug classes and chronic conditions indicated that a quarter of patients never fill a new prescription.[21] Some patients with cognitive impairment may forget, whereas others may have concerns about the medication but hesitate (or lack the opportunity) to discuss their reluctance with their physicians. A meta-analysis on primary medication nonadherence also revealed that the absence of social support played a key role in negatively affecting primary adherence among patients with chronic diseases.[22]

Implementation, which is closer to the aforementioned WHO definition of adherence, refers to the actual dose-taking as per professional recommendations and will be the focus of this chapter. A meta-analysis of 569 studies published in the second half of the twentieth century showed a nonadherence rate of approximately 25 percent.[23] Deviation from the prescribed regimen is particularly common among people with chronic illnesses and complex conditions that require multiple and long-term medications. Data from U.S. Medicare members with diabetes, hypertension, and/or high cholesterol revealed that 76 percent were nonadherent to one of the three medicines, while 32 percent were nonadherent to more than one target medication class.[24]

Persistence involves consistent adherence to the medication continuously over longer intervals. It includes measurement of secondary adherence (i.e., refills within an expected timeframe).[25] Even for patients who initially take their medications as prescribed, large studies across multiple chronic conditions and drug classes have shown that one in every two prescription doses is not taken as prescribed.[26] The extent to which patients who require prolonged adherence take their medication as instructed often decreases over time,[27] with approximately 40 percent of patients discontinuing medications within a year.[28] For patients with schizophrenia prescribed various antipsychotic pharmaceuticals, discontinuation rates jump from 42 percent in twelve months to 74 percent in eighteen months,[29] a phenomenon I will explore later in this chapter. It is worth noting that, in the United States, secondary adherence has become a major quality improvement target. For example, the Centers for Medicare and Medicaid Services considers secondary adherence-related measures as part of its star ratings program. Medicare Advantage and other prescription drug plans are required to publicly report their secondary adherence rates, and incentives such as quality bonus payments are tied in part to performance on medication adherence measures.[30]

Efforts to accurately capture patients' medication consumption to promote better adherence are not new. Traditionally, medication adherence data have come from direct measurement methods, such as observing the patient while taking the medication in the clinic, measuring the drug or its metabolite concentration in the patient's biological fluid (i.e., blood or urine), or evaluating the presence of a biological marker given with the drug.[31] Electronic medication event tracking systems, which record the date and time a pill bottle is opened, are increasingly used to remotely observe patients' behavior. The actual medication dosage is then indirectly inferred from the bottle opening. Other indirect measurement methods to determine patients' medication patterns include patient self-reporting, pill counting, and assessments of pharmacy refill rates or claims data.[32]

Though numerous measurement tools have been designed and validated for various conditions and circumstances, there is currently no gold standard for how to properly quantify medication adherence; all measurement methods have both benefits and drawbacks. Direct measures are generally more accurate, but they are labor intensive and intrusive. Indirect methods require fewer human resources but depend on potentially faulty inferences, assumptions, and recollections. For example, pill counts show dosage removal but can be complicated by medication from earlier time periods being added to current prescription bottles; this technique also does not confirm medication ingestion. Self-reporting, meanwhile, has merely a weak to moderate correlation with prescription refills and electronic measures.[33] Moreover, these methods can only address problems or intervene after dosages have been missed and/or when the patient presents to the pharmacy, clinic, or hospital, such that they are reactionary and have little preventive value.

For certain conditions or drug classes where health outcomes can differ significantly between high and low treatment adherence,[34] poor medication adherence can increase patients' risk of accelerated disease progression, irrevocable health complications, and mortality.[35] This is particularly the case for patients who may also lack access to non-pharmaceutical therapies and other social resources. At the population level, the prevalence of nonadherence can result in drug resistance, especially in the case of antibiotics for infectious diseases (e.g., pneumonia, tuberculosis, gonorrhea), which are increasingly difficult to treat as antibiotics become less effective.[36] For HIV, a high level of adherence is not only important for preventing drug resistance that can worsen existing patients' infection but is also important to avoid passing on a more virulent resistant virus to others and preventing expensive and consumed medications being wasted. For other noncommunicable diseases, such as cardiovascular disease and diabetes, poor outcomes and costly hospital admissions associated with medication nonadherence have been well documented.[37] As we will see shortly, similar concerns abound for patients with mental illnesses and CNMP.

Given these potentially catastrophic consequences, medication adherence may seem like the obvious, responsible individual choice, and the use of AI technologies to promote such adherence may be desirable from professional, institutional, and health system perspectives. However, many factors can affect patients' adherence to prescribed medications,[38] raising questions of whether or how medication adherence algorithms can address these complex issues. One systematic study identified eighty factors across five different categories that were associated with medication adherence in older adults, including patient factors, medication factors, physician factors, system factors, and other factors.[39] Other studies have reached similar conclusions regarding the number and complexity of factors contributing to poor medication adherence[40] while also revealing additional layers of external influences, such as the patient's support environment.[41]

Patient factors can include the person's understanding, desires, and motivations.[42] Some patients may lack the necessary cognitive ability or insight to understand the implications of their prescribed regimen due to their underlying conditions, or they may have temporary or ongoing impaired recall ability or forgetfulness. Patients with severe anxiety or psychosis with delusional beliefs may also be fearful or inherently distrustful of the medications. Others do not have cognitive impairments but may face barriers to adopting or maintaining the prescribed regimen, such as suboptimal health literacy, medication knowledge, behavioral skills, financial resources, or social and practical support.[43] One study showed that patients with minimal health literacy skills are ten to eighteen times less likely to adhere to or correctly identify their medication compared to patients with adequate health literacy skills. They may also be less likely to understand medication information, which can alter their motivational structure and deter adherence to prescribed medications.[44] Even patients who have the capacity to understand the benefits of their medications may decide to adjust or reject the prescribed regimen based on their priorities and concerns. Interestingly, one study comparing the degree of treatment adherence among physicians as patients versus non-physician patients suggests that physicians have only slightly better adherence rates for both low- and high-value care guidelines than non-physicians, indicating that medication intake is more complex than simply obtaining more (understandable) information.[45] It is also important to note that patients with certain cultural beliefs or who are more accepting of non-biomedical approaches to healing may also feel less inclined to adhere to pharmaceutical agents as prescribed.[46]

Medication factors that can affect adherence include complexity of dosing regimen, pill burden, side effects, and cost.[47] If a prescription requires a new dosing method that is perceived by the patient to be riskier or less convenient, such as a self-injectable, patients may also be reluctant to start on the medication. As we saw in previous chapters, for certain neurodegenerative conditions such as Parkinson's disease and Alzheimer's disease, even long-term pharmacotherapies may only provide some symptom relief rather than cure or reverse the condition, and medication adjustments are often required to minimize side effects. Medications for chronic but asymptomatic conditions, such as statins for high cholesterol, may also lead patients to question the necessity or benefits of prolonged utilization. Older adults who are prescribed multiple medications (i.e., polypharmacy) for various chronic and non-curable conditions may experience additional social or economic barriers that render these medications unaffordable to them. These patients may also worry that some of their prescribed medications will interact with each other (drug–drug interaction) or cause unexpected or additional side effects due to other conditions (drug–condition interaction). Some patients who are not actively rejecting medications may wish to conduct their own evaluation of the medicine's physical and psychological side effects before deciding whether they will accept or modify the prescribed dosage.[48]

Since physicians are generally responsible for prescribing and explaining the benefits and risks of medications at the point of care, physician factors can also influence patients' adherence patterns. While support from physicians for confidential and open discussions may facilitate adherence,[49] physician-related barriers include having inadequate time to guide patients through their pharmacotherapies or explore patients' priorities and concerns in determining the most appropriate treatment, ineffective communication regarding complex drug regimens and/or adverse effects, lack of compassionate communication (which can negatively impact patient self-motivation), and an unwillingness or failure to share decision-making with the patient and establish patient-centered care plans.[50] A qualitative study with older adults on multiple long-term medications found that some patients had negative experience with their physicians around medication decisions, citing unacceptable aspects of consultation style, including not listening to patients' legitimate concerns, which rendered patients feeling unable to discuss their worries.[51]

Because physicians prescribe within the operational and regulatory structure of a health system, broader external factors may also affect adherence. These include short consultation time, limited medical or drug insurance coverage, lack of continuity of care (e.g., provision of care by multiple clinicians outside of patient control), and inadequate follow-up consultation and/or health information technology to support patients through complex or unpleasant regimens. The increasing availability and use of virtual health care encounters, which saw a 6,000 percent increase between 2019 and 2020 in the United States in response to the COVID-19 pandemic,[52] may have promoted convenient access. Nonetheless, questions remain as to whether this format may limit physicians' ability to detect nuanced signs of medication challenges, which are more visible during in-person consultations. Moreover, for most pharmaceutical agents,[53] there are no formal consent requirements for prescribing medications as there are for performing medical procedures; filling and taking the medication is considered implied consent on the part of the patient. In other words, there is no designated process to ensure that patients are informed about and in agreement with the prescribed regimen.

2. The Surveillance Power of AI

As we can see, medication adherence is not simply an individual matter—it is a complex socio-systemic phenomenon and experience. In addition to the variable definitions of, thresholds for, and reasons for medication (non)adherence, there is also a lack of consensus on the best method and/or setting for corrective approaches—for example, whether the clinic, the pharmacy, or the patient's home is the best place for intervention implementation. As deviation from prescribed regimens and inaccurate self-reporting can happen at various points along the treatment pathway, it can be challenging for physicians to predict or address the complex range of factors contributing to patients' medication-related behavior during short consultations or clinic visits.[54] This is particularly concerning for conditions and medications where nonadherence may quickly lead to negative health outcomes, including certain drug classes for people with psychiatric illnesses. Various interventions have been developed to help measure and improve medication adherence, but they are often complex and involve multiple health care providers and components, rendering implementation challenging. A Cochrane review of 182 randomized controlled trials (RCTs) of interventions to improve adherence to prescribed medications found no apparent common intervention characteristics. Only five reviewed RCTs showed modest improvements in both adherence and clinical outcomes; none showed large improvements.[55]

With the expanding availability of large-scale and diverse data sources as well as computational power, many health systems and technology companies are hoping to harness the power of big data analytics and new monitoring technologies to help identify or forecast patients' medication adherence probabilities and inform proactive strategies accordingly. There is a growing interest among clinicians and health systems in using AI algorithms at the individual level to continuously track patient behavior and other collateral information to detect initiation, implementation, and persistence patterns throughout the patient's pharmacotherapy pathway. As the ongoing COVID-19 pandemic further reduces system capacity for direct observation of patients' medication intake as well as point-of-care consultation and education, remote and predictive strategies using big data analytics have been increasingly proposed as a replacement for or supplement to in-person monitoring and measurement. There is high hope among AI enthusiasts that these technologies can shed light on the complex interplay of factors contributing to nonadherence, enhance patient–provider communication, empower patients to engage in their progress, and increase adherence that can in turn improve patients' clinical outcomes and quality of life.[56]

Various AI models have been proposed or developed that combine historical and real-time data to identify and predict patients' initiation and persistence adherence—that is, whether the patient will fill, refill, and/or pick up their prescriptions.[57] AI predictive algorithms using administrative/claims data and the patient's demographic information can monitor and attempt to change patients' behavior even before they pick up their prescriptions, such as notifying them of the closest pharmacy locations, without their explicit consent or knowledge of algorithmic use. The information can be used by health care providers and clinics to send reminders to encourage initiation. AI medication monitoring technologies have also been used to automate the process of prescription refills for patients with hypertension and to determine whether a patient request is in protocol, out of protocol, a duplicate, erroneous, or other status.[58] There is optimism that such technology can help to promote patient safety at the point of prescribing and dispensing medications, as physicians and pharmacists may be able to use algorithmically derived information to alter the prescription or counsel patients accordingly.

Once a patient has picked up their prescription, other individual-level AI technologies can detect and predict implementation or dosage adherence. For example, smart pill bottles that issue message reminders have been developed to monitor and increase refill adherence in diabetic patients with suboptimal adherence.[59] There is high hope that if AI technologies are more accurate and efficient in identifying, predicting, and promoting clinically meaningful medication adherence, they can enhance health care providers' ability to assess a patient's treatment progress and adjust medications to optimize health outcomes.[60] These technologies may be particularly helpful for conditions that require a full course of treatment to be effective (e.g., hepatitis C, many bacterial infections) or demand diligent dosage adherence to prevent harmful effects (e.g., iatrogenic addiction, relapse).

More recently, dosage adherence algorithms that use data from remote real-time measurements of medication dosing, patients' primary diagnosis, demographics, and prior adherence indications have emerged as a potential tool to predict medication adherence, which in turn could facilitate proactive clinical interventions to optimize health outcomes.[61] However, given that these technologies are increasingly promoted as medication compliance monitoring tools, they are designed to impose further control over patients' medication use and raise an array of ethical questions regarding patient autonomy. These platforms target certain conditions or patients that have lower adherence but possibly higher clinical consequences for poor adherence, aiming to detect and predict identifiable intake behavior and patterns for individual patients. In particular, they have been proposed for patients whose ability or willingness to follow the prescribed regimen and accurately report their medication behavior is deemed questionable by their clinicians. Two broad examples include patients with certain psychiatric illnesses, such as schizophrenia, and patients on opioid medication for CNMP. These will be the main focus of my ethical analysis in the remainder of this chapter.

Schizophrenia is one of the most burdensome and severe psychiatric disorders, affecting up to 1 percent of the population worldwide.[62] This chronic and heterogeneous mental disorder distorts thinking, moods/feelings, intentions, actions, and movement. Many patients experience variable severity of psychosis, accompanied by delusions, hallucinations, and paranoia. Medication is often necessary to control debilitating symptoms,[63] yet suboptimal response to medications is ubiquitous in schizophrenia. Many psychiatrists believe that the most critical reason for suboptimal treatment outcome is nonadherence to these medications,[64] which has averaged 40 to 55 percent in the United States over the last half-century, despite extensive research efforts, adherence interventions, and new medications.[65] Intersecting factors such as poor insight, forgetfulness, cognitive impairments, substance use disorder, a negative attitude towards medication, concerns about side effects,[66] social isolation, stigma,[67] and a high intensity of delusional symptoms and suspiciousness are often associated with poor medication adherence.[68] Moreover, some patients with relatively stable symptoms may prefer to live with mild disease symptoms rather than face potentially ravaging side effects, such as metabolic disorders and neurological sequelae (e.g., extrapyramidal symptoms).[69] Paradoxically, distrust in the health system due to personal experiences and/or fear of involuntary hospitalization or compelled medication may lead some patients to shun their prescribed regimen, which in turn is a major predictor of relapse, disease progression, recurrence, hospitalization, and emergency department visits.[70] International studies have shown that patients who do not adhere to antipsychotic drug regimens or are only partially adherent are more likely to be hospitalized.[71] In one pharmacy record study looking at Medicaid beneficiaries in San Diego, California (a large and diverse county), rates of psychiatric hospitalization were lower for those who were adherent (14 percent) than for those who were nonadherent (35 percent), who were partially adherent (24 percent), or who had excess fills (25 percent).[72] Other studies have shown that 50 percent of patients with untreated or inadequately treated schizophrenia attempt suicide,[73] and biochemically verified incomplete adherence to antipsychotic pharmacotherapy was associated with markedly increased risks of completed suicide.[74]

Unfortunately, despite the potential health impacts of poor adherence, physicians often cannot correctly identify which patients are adherent or nonadherent with their prescribed antipsychotic medications:[75] Patient self-reports and clinician judgments both tend to overstate adherence.[76] In a recent psychiatry expert panel with fifty-eight experts on schizophrenia, bipolar disorder, and major depressive disorders, 37 percent of experts thought clinical assessment of adherence was not accurate at all, and 54 percent rated it as only somewhat accurate,[77] raising questions of whether the prescribed medications are not always effective in controlling behavioral symptoms. Such detection uncertainty prevents proactive reminders or interventions for targeted patients.[78] Given that patients with schizophrenia and other psychotic disorders often also experience cognitive impairment and unstable living environments, it is particularly challenging to acquire real-time, accurate adherence information from this patient population to identify and intervene when nonadherence begins. Physicians are thus often limited to providing reactionary responses after patients have already deviated from the prescribed regimen for an unknown period and deteriorated as a result. As the risk of hospitalization for some patients may increase within just a few days of not taking medication,[79] there is great interest among health care providers and health systems in using AI medication monitoring to alert health care providers to nonadherence so that they can be proactive in their intervention strategies for patients at high risk of relapse.

Dosage adherence algorithms have also been proposed to monitor opioid medication adherence for management of CNMP. An anticipated 5 to 8 million Americans with CNMP are currently utilizing opioids for pain relief.[80] Many long-term users were introduced to opioids through drugs prescribed to relieve acute pain from surgery, injury, or a chronic condition.[81] If the acute pain is inadequately treated, or if there is a diminished responsiveness to some therapies, the pain may transition to chronic pain, defined by the International Association for the Study of Pain (IASP) as prolonged and persistent pain lasting at least three to six months.[82]

While clinicians' adherence concerns for most chronic physical and mental conditions generally revolve around inadequate dosing, opioid medications for CNMP have the opposite problem due to their addictive properties and harmful effects when overused or diverted. Even though most studies have revealed that underuse of pain medication is much more common than overuse,[83] in the last two decades the conversation around long-term pain management has shifted from concerns about inadequate chronic pain control to worries about too much opioid pain medication, which may lead to unintended prolonged opioid use,[84] iatrogenic opioid use disorder, prescription opioid–related overdoses,[85] and other harms from side effects. In 2016, the US Centers for Disease Control and Prevention (CDC) published its first guidelines recommending avoiding opioid prescriptions when possible and keeping dosage below 90 morphine milligram equivalents (MME) per day.[86] The guidelines led to an accelerated decrease in both the total number of prescriptions and prescriptions per capita; they also contributed to lowered dosages for patients on stable, long-term, high-dose (≥90 MME) opioid therapy. Nonetheless, the decision spurred controversy, as overdose deaths have not decreased as a result of the CDC's recommendations or subsequent policies. Unfortunately, some patients with CNMP have become physically dependent on opioid medications, even if their pain is not well served by these prescriptions; when they lose access to medications they have become reliant on, they may experience amplified pain through a withdrawal-mediated mechanism that can lead to an immediate crisis situation.[87] A retrospective cohort study of 113,618 patients between 2008 and 2019 revealed that dose tapering, defined as "at least 15 percent relative reduction in mean daily dose during any of 6 overlapping 60-day windows within a 7-month follow-up period," increased the risks of overdose and mental health crisis by 28 percent and 74 percent, respectively.[88] Indeed, since 2015, the percentage of all U.S. deaths attributed to opioid overdoses has grown from 1.9 percent to 2.8 percent, further spiking after the start of the COVID-19 pandemic and reaching a record high of more than 93,000 overdose deaths in 2020, with over 60 percent of these cases involving synthetic opioids.[89]

Faced with this alarming scale of overdose deaths, as well as the difficulty of detecting whether a patient is taking opioid medications as prescribed or diverting medications until it is too late,[90] there has been a professional shift towards reflexively distrusting all patients requiring opioid pain medication and practicing "a rational approach"[91] of universal precautions in opioid prescribing.[92] The current policy environment is one in which opioid medications are tightly controlled and surveilled. Patients with acute pain and a (suspected) history of opioid use disorder as well as patients with chronic pain are increasingly required to sign opioid treatment agreements to receive their medication. These agreements generally outline drug surveillance and the consequences of breach, such as termination of the therapeutic relationship and loss of access to opioids. Nonetheless, the implementation of these contracts often relies on labor-intensive direct observation or drug testing, prompting efforts for developing automated and predictive solutions. Moreover, rigorous empirical evidence for the effectiveness of these agreements in improving adherence in CNMP therapy is lacking.[93] AI medication adherence monitoring at the individual patient level is thus increasingly proposed as part of pharmaco-vigilance, as a means of exercising extreme caution in prescribing opioid pain medications to prevent iatrogenic addiction and harm to unintended recipients of these medications.

In addition to ML algorithms that aim to predict patients' pain severity[94] and potential need for opioid use after surgeries,[95] or that forecast which patients may be at high risk for opioid use disorder,[96] emerging technologies for monitoring and predicting dosage adherence include Bluetooth pill boxes that can notify physicians each time the patient opens the pill box.[97] However, these methods do not provide direct evidence of medication ingestion; they assume that doses are taken, but the details of medication dosing events are incomplete and imprecise.[98] They also do not show if the patient may be taking additional doses from other sources. Going a step further to confirm that the monitored patients are indeed the ones who have taken the prescribed medication and at the right dosage, computer vision algorithms connected to smartphone cameras are increasingly touted as innovative tools to visually identify the patient, the drug, and the confirmed ingestion.[99] In addition, wearable wrist and neckband sensors that can recognize the motion of taking the drug out of its packaging and consuming or swallowing it are increasingly promoted as "noninvasive" tools for monitoring and improving individual-level adherence.[100] The hope is that, by continuously monitoring patients and recording every dose, these technologies can help decrease overconsumption, mitigate factors related to relapse, and detect potential overdose.[101]

A more radical technology, which has been proposed to optimize "objective" and precise detection of dose-taking and physiological responses to psychiatric and opioid medications, is the "smart" or digital pill. It involves ingestible sensors made from edible ingredients, which can be attached to any pill to detect and record medication intake and physiological information.[102] Once ingested, the stomach fluids act like a battery and break down the pill to activate the sensor, which sends the medicine ingestion date and time, as well as other physiological information, to a skin patch. The algorithmically analyzed data are then uploaded to a cloud server via Bluetooth and made accessible to the patient and physicians through a mobile application or internet portal.[103] Health care providers and health systems hope that digital pills can replace labor-intensive direct observation of medication intake to detect nonadherence in real time, predict future medication behavior,[104] and inform refill or other treatment decisions for patients with complex chronic conditions.[105]

The first-ever digital pill approved by the U.S. Food and Drug Administration (FDA; in 2017) was aripiprazole (Abilify Mycite), a well-established second-generation antipsychotic medication that is used in the treatment of schizophrenia and other psychotic conditions.[106] The eight-week usability study conducted by the company enrolled sixty-seven participants, forty-nine of whom completed the study. It focused on "mildly ill" patients,[107] with the digital pill broadly targeting the outpatient population whose medication habits are otherwise not directly or regularly monitored by medical professionals.[108] These patients generally are not in acute psychosis that may place themselves or others in imminent danger, but their symptoms may nonetheless deteriorate or relapse without consistent pharmacotherapies. The pill is accompanied by a skin patch that has a built-in activity tracker to monitor the person's physiological data (e.g., heart rate, blood pressure, blood glucose, respiratory rate), physical activities, and rests. The data can then be transmitted to a smartphone for storage and sharing with doctors, nurses, family members, or others upon the patient's consent. The smartphone application also allows patients to log their moods or reasons for not taking their medication, although no publicly available information indicates whether such data of patients' expressed motivations are incorporated into algorithmic analyses or ensuing prescribing decisions, or if those stated motivations change how the algorithm subsequently determines whether the patient's behavior constitutes adherence or nonadherence.[109] With messages that suggest empowerment and taking control of one's own health, the company promotes the system as an innovative and safe medication monitoring tool to help patients stay engaged in their treatment plan, alert clinicians when patients deviate from the plan, and guide clinicians in making the most appropriate medication decisions based on the patient's self-generated data.[110] The aforementioned expert panel in psychiatry noted that digital pills are most helpful for patients who have demonstrated recurrent adherence problems, are in transitional care situations (e.g., post-hospital discharge), show increasing symptoms, and/or have a history of substance use. However, the panel agreed that the utility of digital pills in promoting adherence may depend partly on the patient's cognitive and transitional barriers, as well as the presence (or absence) of daily routines that can facilitate accurate ingestion of medication.[111]

A similar digital pill system has been developed to measure opioid ingestion patterns in patients with acute fracture pain,[112] although this algorithm is still in the developmental research stage and is not yet on the market. The pill emits a radio signal to an electronic reader on a lanyard; the lanyard is not attached to the person's body and can be taken off by the user, which allows better privacy protection than the skin patch, with the tradeoff of not being able to collect certain physiological data that requires skin contact. The detection reader can then send ingestion information to a physician's smartphone application via Bluetooth. Developers hope that the reader will eventually be able to track medication intake for not only patients with acute pain but also patients with chronic pain who use opioids on a long-term basis and will be integrated into wearables, thereby melding with patients' everyday life.[113] If accurate, these tools may allow physicians to identify and predict adherence behaviors without having to rely on patients' own reports or other labor-intensive direct observations. They may also facilitate more efficient allocation of resources, helping physicians focus on patients who have been identified by the algorithm to be at a higher risk for nonadherence and allowing for more timely and targeted interventions to promote safe medication practices. Some practitioners in pain medicine comment that, once the technology is "perfected," "universal adoption by the physician community is predicted."[114]

3. Regulating Distrust Through AI Medication Monitoring

Certainly, promotion of beneficial medication adherence and corresponding patient safety is important from both clinical and public health perspectives. If AI medication dosing monitoring can provide accurate real-time and longitudinal data of patients' intake patterns, it may facilitate timely measurements and predictions to help patients take their medications appropriately or adjust their regimen as needed. It may be particularly helpful for patients who accept pharmacotherapies but somehow deviate from the prescribed dosage and have difficulty recalling or articulating their medication-related behaviors or intentions due to cognitive, linguistic, or other barriers.

However, for patients with psychiatric conditions and chronic pain, the rhetoric around using individual-level AI technologies to measure and predict adherence is increasingly grounded in distrust of patients' testimonies regarding their medication consumption, intentions, and/or self-care capabilities. If a patient is targeted for medication monitoring due to this distrust, possibly because they have already been regarded by another AI algorithm to be of high risk,[115] then any decision they make to adjust or forgo prescribed regimens is not considered an expression of autonomy based in potentially valid individual priorities or concerns. Rather, proposals to use these technologies indirectly label or categorize such decisions as a form of noncompliance that justifies further paternalistic interventions. These technologies discipline patients by means of continuous surveillance and govern the behavior and health of population groups that are judged to be possibly irresponsible, costly, or incapable of taking care of themselves.

Extending the relational autonomy analysis from previous chapters, I argue that AI medication monitoring may compromise patients' self-governance, self-determination, and self-authorization, exacerbating patients' vulnerability and ability to advocate for themselves. The increasing interest in these technologies among health care providers and health systems reinforces biotechnological powers and further stigmatizes patients who are disproportionately targeted for surveillance and labeling. Indeed, implementation of these technologies may suppress patients' ability to form and negotiate their illness identity along their treatment pathway, expand medical power and dominance in ways that compromise patients' freedom, and stifle patients' self-authorization to make medication decisions by adopting a default position of distrust and paternalism.

3.1 One Size Does Not Fit All

Recall that self-governance in a care planning context involves having the necessary skills and capacities to make decisions based on one's reflectively constituted practical identity. From a relational perspective, social and structural factors can hinder or promote the development of these capacities and skills. Here, I focus on how barriers to relational self-governance can be exacerbated by AI medication monitoring that exerts oppressive power and control over patients' overall goals and concerns. As these emerging technologies are increasingly proposed as surveillance tools, and because professionals and health systems are financially incentivized to implement them in patient care despite uncertain accuracy and effectiveness, they may compromise people's ability to form or negotiate their illness identity and associated medication considerations.

Admittedly, many patients recognize that their prescribed regimens are beneficial and want to adopt and adhere to them, but forgetfulness and poor insight may lead to passive and unintentional nonadherence. Some patients who suffer from severe chronic episodic mental illnesses when deviating from prescribed medications may even want to put in place contracts or other treatment plans while they are capable of making decisions in order to hold themselves to beneficial treatment regimens in the event of relapse and acute psychosis.[116] AI predictive reminders in these situations may promote patients' self-governance by enhancing their ability to uphold their priorities and follow through with their accepted tasks. However, for another group of patients, who may have multifaceted motivations for deviating from or actively rejecting the prescribed regimen at various points in their treatment pathway,[117] questions abound as to how AI dosage monitoring may restructure power and control over their identity, thereby affecting their relational self-governance. Some patients who are newly diagnosed, who understand the benefits and risks of various treatment options, and who trust their prescribers' judgment may want to immediately begin their prescribed regimen in an attempt to take control of their health. Others may not have accepted their condition and the accompanying medication regimen yet. For certain conditions that require long-term management, some patients may need time to actively weigh the different benefits and burdens of the recommended treatment according to their evolving illness identity to determine how or whether they can make life adjustments to integrate pharmacotherapy into their lives.[118] Some of these patients may also struggle with the potential chronicity of their condition and consider these medications an unwelcome confirmation of their illness that imposes an indefinite sick role on them.[119] Financial considerations may also play a role, as high drug prices and distrust of the pharmaceutical industry may heighten some patients' skepticism about long-term medication adherence.

A key problem with AI dosing adherence monitoring is that it takes patients' (indefinite) agreement, willingness, and readiness to take prescribed medications for granted and uses predetermined and static thresholds based on biomedical models of adherence, without considering patients' multifaceted clinical and contextual concerns. This can negatively impact a patient's relational self-governance, as such a practice imposes meanings or standards of how one must act, thereby restructuring people's relationships with medications. Some patients may feel that their lives are governed by the medication regimens they must follow, even if compliance (or lack thereof) may affect their quality of life.[120] Moreover, the concept of adherence presumes that medication regimen decisions are settled as soon as a patient indicates understanding and acceptance of a prescribed medication, such that patients who subsequently deviate from the regimen for any reason can be characterized as nonadherent. This presumption persists even when patients' perspectives, as well as their desire or ability to follow through on medication regimens, may have been left out of or only minimally incorporated into the original treatment plan. While burdens of prolonged medications for certain drug classes can be high, AI dosing adherence algorithms expound the predominant belief in Western biomedical frameworks that pharmacotherapies are unquestionably beneficial, and takes for granted that any prescribed dosage is optimal. According to this logic, AI surveillance to help increase adherence is conclusively justifiable, even when some patients may be more concerned about the burdens of prescribed medicines and how to reduce adverse impacts.[121]

It is also important to note that medication adherence is not an immutable characteristic of individual patients. In addition to the variability of required dosage adherence to achieve certain clinical outcomes among different conditions and drug classes, different patients may also have divergent notions of the desired or optimal outcome based on their broader context. For some patients, pharmacotherapy is an ongoing journey that involves weighing competing considerations, especially if they are prescribed multiple medications that require long-term consumption with severe adverse effects and uncertain efficacy. Medicines can lead to restrictions on social activities and personal life to the extent that, for some, life revolves exclusively around medicines.[122] Being prescribed medication for stigmatizing conditions such as mental illness and chronic pain can leave some patients feeling ambivalent and vulnerable. Many thus constantly weigh concerns of symptom control against the risk of disclosing their medical status to others through noticeable side effects.[123] For example, while a meta analysis of six placebo-controlled studies of antipsychotic treatment for active symptoms for schizophrenia showed that patients with high baseline symptom severity can derive the most clinical benefit from medications, patients with the mildest symptoms may see less improvement but experience the full adverse effects of antipsychotics.[124] It is thus understandable that patients sometimes intentionally miss an occasional dose, take a consistent but reduced dose, consume medication sporadically, test different dosing levels, discontinue their prescribed medications, and/or pursue alternative regimens in order to minimize unwanted consequences and control medication dependence.[125] They may want to create a medication practice that aligns with both their social and illness identities.[126] As choice, self-determination, and empowerment remain fundamental values for people with psychiatric conditions,[127] studies on antipsychotic utilization have shown that patients often purposefully adjust their medications to maximize the benefits and minimize adverse effects based on their subjective experiential knowledge and as a strategy to regain some autonomy in their illness and treatment pathways.[128] Medication adherence is thus a fluid product of the intersecting scientific, socio-relational, and professional networks within which patients function.[129] Meanwhile, the ongoing emphasis on pharmaceutical products and the assumption that improved adherence—rather than improved health outcomes or better quality of life—is the ideal target may distract from other non-pharmaceutical approaches to health care, including behavioral therapies, illness prevention, and public health interventions.[130]

In the case of schizophrenia, even though medications can help prevent relapse and hospitalization, they also bring persistent symptoms or suboptimal treatment response for many patients.[131] In addition, some antipsychotics can lead to involuntary limb movement, weight gain, sedation, sexual side effects,[132] cognitive impairment,[133] and emotional flattening.[134] These adverse effects may exacerbate stigma, familial disapproval or disappointment,[135] and social withdrawal, which in turn can negatively impact patients' self-identity and well-being. Psychiatric conditions and prescribed medications have particular sociocultural meanings, carry strong emotions, and are interwoven with people's individual and socio-relational narratives.[136] And as noted in the aforementioned study in San Diego County, 14 percent of patients who were adherent still required hospitalization, compared to 24 percent of patients who were partially adherent.[137] We can imagine that patients who suffer from mild to moderate symptoms but experience severe medication-induced side effects may reduce or skip their dosage, especially if the medications may not provide adequate clinical benefits and yet further compromise their quality of life. Nonetheless, proposals for AI dosage monitoring often neglect the cultural and symbolic meanings of medication taking and the social power of these technologies, narrowly focusing on whether patients have deviated from the prescribed regimens. To date, there has been little discussion of building learning algorithms that can adjust predictive outputs based on patients' multidimensional considerations and patterns, and to enhance effectiveness by providing parallel professional, institutional, and system support. If the algorithms are implemented with the simplistic assumption that all patients should unquestionably adhere to the same predefined threshold, regardless of their concerns, priorities, and context, this may hinder patients' ability to understand and re-create their self-identity in times of illness, increase negative social meanings of pharmacotherapies, deter discussions about other non-pharmaceutical strategies, and reinforce power over patients in ways that compromise their relational self-governance.

3.2 Coercive Disclosure and the Illusion of Choice

In addition to the concerns outlined above, as AI is increasingly touted as providing superior solutions for patient safety, there are also questions of whether patients who are targeted for medication monitoring truly can shape their own care plan or decline such surveillance as they navigate their illness journey in ways that align with their goals and priorities. I argue that AI medication monitoring as a professional or institutional practice intensifies medical power by imposing a duty of informational disclosure on patients while dismissing patients' own illness identities or concerns about pharmacotherapy. AI medication monitoring compromises people's freedom and opportunities to determine whether or how they would like their medication behavior to be monitored, how their medication decisions should be understood, and who can decide how medication adherence information will be incorporated into ongoing care management plans.

It is generally accepted in Western bioethics that patients who have decisional capacity have a right to relevant information regarding their health and treatment options. Given the informational power asymmetry between clinicians and patients in therapeutic relationships, the responsibility of disclosure about a patient's health status and treatment-related information generally falls on health care providers. Bioethical and regulatory discussions on this subject have mostly focused on ensuring that health care providers fulfill their duty of open communication, which can facilitate patients' ability to make voluntary and informed decisions. Patients, on the other hand, have a general right to privacy in their medical encounters and are not required or even expected to reveal intimate information that solely concerns the patient (as opposed to an at-risk third party).[138] In fact, regulations around confidentiality and de-identification in aggregate datasets are established to help patients who would otherwise be vulnerable to data misuse feel more comfortable sharing personal information with their care providers. Certainly, there are sound clinical reasons for self-interested patients to disclose their medication intentions and concerns: Disclosure can promote accurate assessment, patient-centered care plans, and appropriate follow-up care. Nonetheless, patients generally retain the practical authority to determine how much information they want to share and whether they will ultimately follow professionals' recommendations, including pharmacotherapies. Indeed, studies have found that lay patients do not always view pharmaceutical agents as something to be taken "as prescribed" but rather as one resource among many in their care management journey.[139] Except in emergency situations, where a person may be brought to a hospital by others without their knowledge or explicit consent, such as in cases of traumatic accidents or serious illnesses whereby a person loses consciousness or decisional capacity, patients are usually the ones who initiate care or explicitly accept follow-up care. Any information sharing or monitoring of patients' conditions and behaviors, including direct observation of medication adherence, is time bound and location specific (e.g., limited to the clinic or lab).

Certainly, patients who trust their care providers may be more willing to share information, and clinicians who take the time to explore their patients' concerns or engage in shared decision-making may be able to collaboratively determine goal-concordant treatment recommendations that align with both the physician's and patient's expectations, which in turn can result in higher levels of adherence. Nonetheless, some patients may want to be in charge of their own life and believe that being ill in itself should not require them to divulge all information, particularly if they judge that certain information is not crucial to their care goals. Others may worry that their physician will negatively judge them and therefore withhold potentially embarrassing information to preserve their doctor's respect.[140] This may be particularly true for patients in marginalized groups who have been underserved by the health care and/or social system, or have experienced implicit or explicit bias in health care encounters. Patients who are licensed/certified professionals (e.g., physicians, pilots), hold high executive positions, or face custody battles may also worry that their fitness for professional or parental duties may be questioned if they share their treatment-related behavior. In other words, self-determination in the context of disclosing one's medication adherence is a socio-relational experience rather than simply an individual phenomenon.

It is worth noting that even the most trusted clinicians generally have no authority or means to monitor their patients' medication behavior continuously and closely outside the formal clinical care environment, except through indirect and inferential methods such as subsequent consultation assessments, laboratory findings, or prescription databases. This means that patients maintain some default level of personal and informational privacy as well as "veto power" over clinician recommendations. They can deviate from the prescribed regimen and keep their medication information to themselves.[141] Such power to adjust one's medications for noninfectious conditions can be important for patients' self-determination, especially since even patients who are not ideologically opposed to the prescribed medications may nonetheless worry about side effects, cost, or social consequences of taking medications—concerns that may not be apparent when the regimen is first prescribed. While physicians often focus on decreasing disease-induced symptoms and avoiding adverse health outcomes by ensuring medication adherence, patients may have broader concerns about improving their overall well-being or quality of life.[142] Depending on whether there are opportunities to address these multifaceted concerns, patients' ability to adhere even to desired regimens may be limited.

AI medication adherence monitoring as an emerging socio-medical practice imposes a new expectation of information disclosure on patients. It allows medication dosage and other physiological information that was not previously available to the care team to be continuously collected, analyzed, and potentially used to impose further restrictions on patients. At the same time, these technologies may ironically silence patients, as information disclosure is done through automated biodata collection and algorithmic analysis, designed to replace self-reports that health care providers may deem unreliable or no longer necessary. In addition to breeding or perpetuating a culture of distrust, wherein physiological data are viewed as more credible and authoritative than patient testimony, health care providers may ignore information that patients feel is important and that they are willing to share (e.g., their embodied experience, illness identity, worries about medications). By replacing or reducing multilayered concerns to simple dosage measurements and predictions, these algorithms are not only intrusive but also neglect what matters most to those who are being monitored.

Such automated monitoring processes have an outsized impact on patients with stigmatized identities. People with psychiatric conditions, who are often presumed to be incapable, irrational, and noncredible by virtue of their diagnosis,[143] and whose adherence is often questioned by care providers, are sometimes advised or expected to accept some form of medication surveillance regardless of their desire or concerns. Given the longstanding stereotypical assumptions about people with mental illnesses, these patients' resistance to medication may be automatically inferred as evidence of poor insight or cognitive impairment and thus a further justification of paternalistic monitoring for the patient's own good—even though nonadherence is a universal phenomenon, not limited to psychiatric patients.[144] With a shift to ever more compulsion and control in Western psychiatry,[145] particularly around medication taking,[146] patients may feel powerless to refuse these technologies.

It is noteworthy that law and ethics presume that all adults have sufficient capacity to make decisions for their own medical treatments unless there is significant evidence to suggest otherwise. Even when a medical condition impairs a patient's decisional capacity, the patient may still be able to form and communicate their desires and participate in some aspects of decision-making.[147] In some states, such as California, patients with mental illness retain a high degree of legal authority regarding psychiatric medications. If these patients lack decisional capacity, surrogate decision-makers and health care providers can make decisions regarding *medical* treatments (e.g., cancer treatment, surgery) on behalf of patients based on their known wishes or best interests. However, they cannot administer involuntary psychiatric medications in non-emergency situations by appealing only to the patient's presumed best interest. Even when the patient has a serious mental illness that renders them gravely disabled and unable to discern the risks and benefits of psychiatric medications, if a patient adamantly refuses to take these medications, a court hearing is required to determine whether involuntary medication can be imposed. Certainly, one may argue that refraining from medicating patients with serious mental illnesses, especially in situations where no other support services are provided, poses harm rather than promoting autonomy. Nonetheless, for a patient population that also carries a disproportionate burden of unmet social needs (e.g., housing, outpatient medication support) and may have experienced various forms of personal and systemic trauma (e.g., abuse, structural racism), AI dosage adherence algorithms that identify medication patterns without addressing other social determinants of mental health may reify mistrust and discrimination. It may normalize suspicion of patients' intentions and reinforce social control and oppressive policies or practices over this population.

Similar concerns abound that AI opioid pain medication monitoring may compromise patients' relational self-determination, as such surveillance is increasingly proposed or required within a broader culture of pharmaco-vigilance that further exacerbates stigmatization and asymmetrical power relations in therapeutic relationships. In a biomedical culture that relies on objective indicators of disease processes, clinical assessment of inherently subjective chronic pain experiences and psychogenic suffering is difficult. In addition to substantial variability in people's needs for opioid pain medication, the pain-related pathology, even if known, does not always correspond to the severity or duration reported by the patient.[148] Moreover, while opioid therapy can be effective in treating acute pain and some types of persistent pain, there is weak evidence that long-term use provides clinically significant pain relief or improvement in quality of life or functioning for patients with CNMP.[149] The alarming rise of opioid-related deaths, concerns of medication diversion, and physicians' lack of time and skills to understand and treat these complex conditions highlight the challenges of providing optimal pain management. These multifaceted concerns have rendered pain an exceptional nexus of doubt and incredulity within the practice and politics of opioid prescription.[150]

Some research initiatives are already under way to integrate AI-based risk scores into patients' electronic health records (EHRs) to warn clinicians about high-risk patients and recommend risk mitigation strategies.[151] Even as AI medication tracking is mostly still an emerging technology, rather than an established one with high accuracy and validity, it is increasingly promoted through the language of freedom and choice. When patients with undermanaged pain agree to direct and continuous monitoring by algorithmic technologies, it allows them to prove adherence and thereby receive prescribed opioid medications. However, in practice, these technologies only grant patients conditional freedom based on algorithmic results.[152] Patients who are identified by the predictive algorithm as straying from predetermined requirements may be characterized as untrustworthy, potentially subjecting them to even more stringent surveillance or interventions,[153] even if their psychogenic pain or reasons for deviating may not be identified or well understood by the algorithm or care providers. While aforementioned concerns about morbidities associated with unintended prolonged opioid use and iatrogenic opioid use disorder are legitimate, algorithmic monitoring, which neglects how psychogenic suffering, trauma, and power imbalances can all contribute to patients' medication patterns, limits the freedom and opportunities necessary for self-determination. As these algorithms are mostly used to address worries about patients misreporting their dosage and reduce health care providers' potential liability,[154] rather than to fully understand patients' complex concerns to promote goal-concordant pain management,[155] it is unlikely that predictive dosing data will improve therapeutic interactions and opportunity conditions for self-determination. There are also signs that patients on opioid therapy to prevent withdrawal and reduce cravings—including patients who are fully aware of addiction risks and fully adherent—may strongly resist continuous and predictive monitoring. For example, according to publicly available records, a research trial using AI to monitor medication adherence in opioid agonist therapy, which received $1 million from the National Institute on Drug Abuse,[156] registered only nine participants, despite the original goal of recruiting fifty to one hundred participants.[157] Such low enrollment for a well-funded study raises questions of whether AI medication monitoring would be deemed acceptable to this patient population.

In previous chapters, we saw how AI health monitoring technologies can assume the form of Foucauldian disciplining acts, subtly but relentlessly compelling users to abide by various health goals as predetermined by professionals, health systems, and technology developers, regardless of people's own priorities and risk tolerance. Foucault's concept of the panopticon can shed further light on how AI medication adherence monitoring may compromise users' relational self-determination.[158] Informed by Jeremy Bentham's descriptions of prison architectural designs in eighteenth-century Britain, where a guard could watch every inmate from above without being seen by the detainees, Foucault illustrates how surveillance can impose disciplinary power,[159] especially when reinforced by social and cultural discourses, professional practices, and medical institutions. Such a concept can help to illustrate various concerns for our context here. AI medication dosage monitoring, which is often uncritically proclaimed to be more objective and accurate without conclusive evidence, increasingly serves as the new surveillance engine, or panopticon. It categorically reframes even deliberate decisions to deviate from prescribed regimens as evidence of nonadherence, rather than an exercise of self-determination, and decides how such problems will be managed from the clinician's, technologist's, and/or health system's perspectives.[160] These algorithmic panopticons aim to prevent patients from concealing their activities from doctors without trying to understand *why* patients may deviate from their prescribed regimens or feel the need to hide such information and concerns from their care providers in the first place.[161]

As we saw in the last chapter, even for DTC AI health monitoring products, where users initiate implementation and data sharing with health care providers, these technologies impose self-discipline on users by reinforcing the social message that constant self-tracking is simply the rational and responsible thing to do. Frequent alerts and updates fortify such message. Proposals to use medication monitoring algorithms on patients, which are often initiated by health care providers or health systems, compound medical power and reinforce oppression in ways that compromise self-determination, as consent to monitoring and self-disciplining may be expected or required for continuing access to freedom and services based on distrust. For example, a patient with chronic relapse may have to agree to continuous monitoring by technology or supervised treatment in the community, such as through compulsory community treatment orders, to stay out of involuntary admission to psychiatric hospitals. This is particularly problematic from a relational perspective, since medication adherence is not simply a matter of individual behavior but also a response to external and structural environments. Multilayer factors (e.g., medication, physician, and socio-systemic factors) influence patients' responses to the medications and their desire or ability to follow the prescribed regimen. Attending to these broader factors can reveal how deviation from the prescribed dosage of antipsychotics may have a serious impact on patients without other forms of support, but a potentially less severe or immediate impact on others with social and non-pharmaceutical support. Nonetheless, instead of addressing various social determinants of adherence that can lead to inequitable health resources and outcomes, medication surveillance systems mostly focus on analyzing and predicting the patient's dosage compliance. Moreover, these platforms are currently not designed as continuously learning systems that would iteratively adjust the predictive analysis according to the patient's physiological responses or other socio-structural barriers that may prevent them from being able to adhere to a desired regimen. These domineering and unidirectional surveillance technologies are implemented as "scientific" media of medical power, continuously enforcing the professional or "correct" pharmacotherapy pathway, as predefined by the technology.

In other words, the medicalization and institutionalization of these technologies blur the line between care, discipline, and surveillance, rendering it difficult to impossible for patients to refuse these technologies or even form their own self-conception regarding incessant monitoring,[162] even as they may feel an increasing loss of privacy, self-trust and trust by others, and autonomy by virtue of being under constant surveillance.[163] It is also worth cautioning that patients who self-discipline to stay within the bounds of the prescribed dosage but have unmet pain needs or adverse effects from their psychiatric medications may not receive follow-up evaluations to address these concerns because they have not been flagged by the algorithm, which focuses narrowly on quantitative adherence. In one study determining the prevalence of medication adherence with 281 patients with chronic pain, 32 percent and 14 percent showed underuse and overuse respectively.[164] If these algorithms are developed for the main purpose of preventing medication overuse, instead of creating opportunities for more personalized pharmacotherapy and care pathways to truly promote self-determination, they may lead to unintended abandonment of patients with under-controlled pain and further compromise patients' well-being.

3.3 Whose Authority Is It Anyway?

Overlapping with questions around people's ability to form their practical identity (self-governance) and exercise their freedom and opportunities (self-determination) are issues regarding whether or how AI medication monitoring may compromise self-authorization. Here, I explain how the implementation of AI medication monitoring technologies may perpetuate epistemic injustice by dismissing patients' experiential knowledge and undermining their confidence in their embodied experiences and self-trust in their practical identities. The enthusiasm towards AI medication monitoring sends the message that predetermined thresholds and algorithmic detections are more credible and relevant in a patient's pharmacotherapy journey than the patient's own self-report or narrative of their medication experience.

Despite promises that AI algorithms can offer more precise identification and prediction of patients' medication adherence, there is currently scant evidence that these technologies are accurate or acceptable to those who are targeted for monitoring. Marketing claims from technologists notwithstanding, existing AI medication adherence models and studies that allege favorable results often have small sample sizes and short trial durations,[165] raising questions about the reliability and validity of these studies. For example, even for the aforementioned FDA-approved digital aripiprazole, which costs about 85 times that of the generic aripiprazole,[166] there were no prospective, double-blind, randomized controlled trials to understand the acceptability or clinical impact of this digital pill compared to the original tablet or placebo.[167] While long-term use of aripiprazole may be necessary for some patients, the longest trial for this digital pill was only sixteen weeks.[168] It is also noteworthy that one of the trials conducted on healthy subjects showed a false-negative rate of more than 20 percent,[169] which could lead to patients overusing the medication and exacerbate physicians' distrust of patients based on algorithmic error. These are important clinical and ethical considerations that have been largely ignored in the current discourse. If intrusive strategies only promote a higher adherence rate but not necessarily better outcomes, they further compromise not only patients' autonomy but also their broader interests. It is perhaps telling that Proteus Digital Health, the company that created the sensor for Abilify Mycite, struggled to find a market for its product and filed for bankruptcy in June 2020.[170]

Similar concerns of low evidentiary standards apply to other dosage adherence algorithms. Many medication adherence predictive models use EHRs as training data, which have an inherent bias towards patients with high health care utilization—that is, patients who are sicker or who have insurance that allows such utilization.[171] Training data from psychiatric emergency facilities may also have disproportionately higher rates of Indigenous, Black,[172] and other underserved populations.[173] Algorithmic predictions may thus overestimate the health impact of adherence deviation for outpatient populations with lower health risks or overemphasize relapse in marginalized groups. Returning to the example of opioid medication adherence monitoring, a comprehensive review of clinical risk prediction models for opioid-related overdose in the United States showed that many models lack external validation and have high false-positive rates.[174] While ML algorithms appear to perform well in identifying low-risk subgroups with minimal probability of overdose following opioid prescriptions, positive predictive values for identifying high-risk patients are low,[175] as opioid-related overdose is rare in the general population compared to those who have been hospitalized.[176] None of the studies evaluated the risk prediction models or tools within active clinical practice; as such, there is little assurance that these non-validated models would have better accuracy or clinical value in the complex real-world context of opioid pain management. Two related feasibility studies of digital opioid pills that reported promising results had only sixteen participants for a one-week period and ten participants for twenty-one doses (also a one-week period) respectively.[177] This raises questions about the generalizability and transferability of these short-term studies to the real-world setting of long-term consumption. Even if larger studies could validate a model for low-risk patients, monitoring this patient population is unnecessary for clinical safety and may incur unwarranted privacy harm and further stigmatization. For high-risk patients, the higher error rates may reflect the complexity of opioid use disorders, which cannot be adequately captured by dosage patterns that exclude patients' testimonies of their multifaceted experiences and concerns.

The growing trend among health care providers and health systems to place more trust in emerging AI medication monitoring than in people's own self-reports, especially in the case of stigmatizing conditions, highlights a broader concern that patients' self-authorization may be further eroded by these technologies. The use of AI algorithms to override patients' embodied experiences and narratives about their concerns is a form of testimonial injustice that exacerbates marginalization and stigma, disempowers patients who may now hesitate to trust their symptoms or their implications, and violates their relational autonomy. Even though patients are the ones experiencing the effects of the medications and illnesses, tracking and evaluating their symptoms and providing their own care between sporadic consultations or formal treatments, their authority over their personal health information and decision-making can be revoked if they are deemed nonadherent by the algorithm, regardless of the reasons.[178]

AI adherence monitoring technologies may further deny patients' self-authorization by reinforcing dominant social and biomedical frameworks and prioritizing thresholds set by outside experts, such as clinicians, scientists, and technology developers, even when those thresholds fail to match patients' own experiences. This sends the message that patients' embodied experiences are irrelevant or inessential to understanding or forecasting medication consumption patterns. Despite the promise of personalized care plans grounded in real-time data and big data analytics, messages around medication adherence algorithms assume that quantitative physiological data and statistical modeling on their own provide more objective, reliable, and coherent models of the patient's world than the patient's own reports of their experiences and other concerns.[179] Even when patients may have complex reasons for deviating from the prescribed regimens, the algorithm may reduce or reframe these rich considerations as quantifiable individual problems of nonadherence. Echoing arguments from earlier chapters, such categorical and premature dismissal of patients' credibility and contribution to knowledge building in favor of "objective" algorithmic predictions, despite a lack of efficacy evidence, is a form of epistemic injustice that perpetuates oppressive disempowerment and compromises patients' self-authorization.

Intersecting with and exacerbating concerns about medical power and epistemic injustice is the use of AI medication adherence algorithms to regulate distrust of patients' motivations and self-reports. The aforementioned example of using AI medication monitoring for opioid pain medications is illustrative here. In most treatment contexts, concerns regarding trustworthiness focus on physicians' competence and goodwill towards their patients, demonstrated by their openness in disclosing and discussing relevant information with patients, as well as collaborating with them in determining appropriate care plans. Patients, who are self-interested in seeking the most beneficial care for themselves, are presumed to be truthful in their testimony without a heavy burden of proof to demonstrate trustworthiness;[180] patients' power and authority are generally accepted prima facie. Since pain is a subjective experience that is often refractory to objective assessment or may lack discernable causes, patients are the rightful "experts" and authorities on their own experiences and the effectiveness of various treatment courses in providing pain relief.[181] Nonetheless, in contemporary Western biomedical culture, which favors observation of physical phenomena, medical power is reinforced when clinicians' determination of the meaning, source, representation, and management of pain automatically takes precedence over the patient's perspective and becomes the model for algorithmic analysis (as in the case for AI expert systems).[182] This epistemic injustice is particularly problematic when we consider the limited physician education and training in both CNMP and addiction,[183] and how being distrusted by their clinicians regarding dosage adherence can cause patients further suffering.[184] With AI-based facial analytics systems now being developed to generate pain scores that purport to help clinicians make decisions about administering pain relief for nonverbal individuals (e.g., people with severe dementia),[185] we can imagine that these tools may be promoted in the near future for clinicians treating patients with CNMP, to validate or potentially override patients' claims of pain level in prescribing or dispensing opioid analgesics.

4. Conclusion

As we can see, medication adherence platforms are becoming yet another example of AI solutionism, where algorithms are touted as the superior technological solution to a complex social problem, despite a lack of efficacy evidence. Certainly, pharmacotherapies are helpful treatment modalities for many conditions when consumed appropriately, and when deliberate planning and shared decision-making with patients to facilitate adherence promote patient engagement and well-being. Attention to potential iatrogenic addiction and mental health relapse, which can be debilitating for many patients, is also important within the broader goal of promoting not only patient autonomy but also safety. If AI medication monitoring were to be used not as a means of surveillance but as a collaborative tool for determining goal-concordant dosing—that is, if algorithms could be taught to identify, understand, predict, and incorporate users' multifaceted concerns into their analysis and adjust to the patient's own routine, rather than simply predict adherence according to a predetermined (or labeled) outcome—then it could help to promote patient autonomy and safe treatment planning. For instance, if predictive models using ML could determine which intervention variables (e.g., dosing method, timing, drug content, cost) have the most impact on patients' acceptance of and adherence to a particular medication protocol, they could provide personalized support or recommend different dosing schedules or treatment modalities accordingly.

Some versions of this technology do exist. For example, a neural-network–based predictive model exploring the impact of patient demographics and social determinants of health on medication adherence for patients with chronic illnesses has been developed to predict which patients would benefit from additional outreach.[186] The algorithm is integrated with a conversational natural language processing (NLP) system to process patients' refill-related requests and provide text message reminders to AI-identified patients. This kind of tool, especially if combined with evidence-based interdisciplinary pain programs that utilize a biopsychosocial model,[187] offers a model for how AI medication monitoring could fulfill the optimistic promises of AI enthusiasts.

Unfortunately, even as doctors who intend to protect patient wellbeing face thorny cases that involve difficult medical tradeoffs, most existing medication monitoring algorithms remain firmly in the camp of discipline rather than collaborative care, oversimplifying and reducing complex causes of nonadherence to quantified measurements of individual behavioral problems. This risks turning AI medication monitoring into just another tool for reinforcing the traditional compliance model. In short, unexamined AI medication monitoring practices may compromise patients' relational autonomy and join other ill-fated efforts to promote patients' willingness and ability to follow appropriate pharmacotherapies.

Notes

1. Daniel L. Labovitz et al., "Using Artificial Intelligence to Reduce the Risk of Nonadherence in Patients on Anticoagulation Therapy," *Stroke* 48, no. 5 (May 2017): 1416–19, https://doi.org/10.1161/STROKEAHA.116.016281.
2. Elaine Lehane and Geraldine McCarthy, "Medication Non-Adherence—Exploring the Conceptual Mire," *International Journal of Nursing Practice* 15, no. 1 (February 2009): 25–31, https://doi.org/10.1111/j.1440-172X.2008.01722.x.
3. D. L. Sackett et al., "Patient Compliance with Antihypertensive Regimens," *Patient Counselling and Health Education* 1, no. 1 (January–March 1978): 18–21, https://doi.org/10.1016/s0738-3991(78)80033-0.
4. Eduardo Sabaté, ed., *Adherence to Long-Term Therapies: Evidence for Action* (Geneva: World Health Organization, 2003), https://apps.who.int/iris/bitstream/handle/10665/42682/9241545992.pdf?sequence=1&isAllowed=y.
5. Nawal Chanane et al., "Acceptance of Technology-Driven Interventions for Improving Medication Adherence," in *Future Network Systems*

and Security, ed. Robin Doss, Selwyn Piramuthu, and Wei Zhou (Cham: Springer International Publishing, 2017), 188–98.

6. Dawn I. Velligan et al., "Defining and Assessing Adherence to Oral Antipsychotics: A Review of the Literature," *Schizophrenia Bulletin* 32, no. 4 (October 2006): 724–42, https://doi.org/10.1093/schbul/sbj075.
7. Alejandra Hurtado-de-Mendoza, Mark L. Cabling, and Vanessa B. Sheppard, "Rethinking Agency and Medical Adherence Technology: Applying Actor Network Theory to the Case Study of Digital Pills," *Nursing Inquiry* 22, no. 4 (December 2015): 326–35, https://doi.org/10.1111/nin.12101.
8. Marilou Gagnon, Jean Daniel Jacob, and Adrian Guta, "Treatment Adherence Redefined: A Critical Analysis of Technotherapeutics," *Nursing Inquiry* 20, no. 1 (March 2013): 60–70, https://doi.org/10.1111/j.1440-1800.2012.00595.x.
9. Murtadha Aldeer, Mehdi Javanmard, and Richard P. Martin, "A Review of Medication Adherence Monitoring Technologies," *Applied System Innovation* 1, no. 2 (2018): 14, https://doi.org/10.3390/asi1020014.
10. Gagnon et al., "Treatment Adherence Redefined"; Sunanda Kane and Fadia Shaya, "Medication Non-Adherence Is Associated with Increased Medical Health Care Costs," *Digestive Diseases and Sciences* 53, no. 4 (April 2008): 1020–24, https://doi.org/10.1007/s10620-007-9968-0.
11. Aurel O. Iuga and Maura J. McGuire, "Adherence and Health Care Costs," *Risk Management and Healthcare Policy* 7 (February 2014): 35–44, https://doi.org/10.2147/RMHP.S19801; Jon J. Vlasnik, Sherry L. Aliotta, and Bonnie DeLor, "Medication Adherence: Factors Influencing Compliance with Prescribed Medication Plans," *Case Manager* 16, no. 2 (March 2005): 47–51, https://doi.org/10.1016/j.casemgr.2005.01.009.
12. Mark Lemstra et al., "Primary Nonadherence to Chronic Disease Medications: A Meta-Analysis," *Patient Preference and Adherence* 12 (2018): 721–31, https://doi.org/10.2147/PPA.S161151.
13. Aldeer et al., "Review of Medication Adherence Monitoring Technologies."
14. Azita Alipour, Stephen Gabrielson, and Puja B. Patel, "Ingestible Sensors and Medication Adherence: Focus on Use in Serious Mental Illness," *Pharmacy* 8, no. 2 (2020): 103, https://doi.org/10.3390/pharmacy8020103.
15. Pascal C. Baumgartner et al., "A Systematic Review of Medication Adherence Thresholds Dependent of Clinical Outcomes," *Frontiers in Pharmacology* 9 (2018): 1290, https://doi.org/10.3389/fphar.2018.01290.
16. David L. Paterson et al., "Adherence to Protease Inhibitor Therapy and Outcomes in Patients with HIV Infection," *Annals of Internal Medicine*

133, no. 1 (July 2000): 21–30, https://doi.org/10.7326/0003-4819-133-1-200007040-00004.

17. Kathy K. Byrd et al., "Antiretroviral Adherence Level Necessary for HIV Viral Suppression Using Real-World Data," *Journal of Acquired Immune Deficiency Syndromes* 82, no. 3 (November 2019): 245–51, https://doi.org/10.1097/QAI.0000000000002142.
18. Velligan et al., "Defining and Assessing Adherence."
19. Michael J. Stirratt et al., "Advancing the Science and Practice of Medication Adherence," *Journal of General Internal Medicine* 33, no. 2 (February 2018): 216–22, https://doi.org/10.1007/s11606-017-4198-4; Terrence F. Blaschke et al., "Adherence to Medications: Insights Arising from Studies on the Unreliable Link between Prescribed and Actual Drug Dosing Histories," *Annual Review of Pharmacology and Toxicology* 52 (2012): 275–301, https://doi.org/10.1146/annurev-pharmtox-011711-113247.
20. Wai Yin Lam and Paula Fresco, "Medication Adherence Measures: An Overview," *BioMed Research International* (2015): 217047, https://doi.org/10.1155/2015/217047.
21. Michael A. Fischer et al., "Primary Medication Non-Adherence: Analysis of 195,930 Electronic Prescriptions," *Journal of General Internal Medicine* 25, no. 4 (April 2010): 284–90, https://doi.org/10.1007/s11606-010-1253-9.
22. Lemstra, "Primary Nonadherence to Chronic Disease Medications."
23. M. Robin DiMatteo, "Variations in Patients' Adherence to Medical Recommendations: A Quantitative Review of 50 Years of Research," *Medical Care* 42, no. 3 (March 2004): 200–209, https://doi.org/10.1097/01.mlr.0000114908.90348.f9.
24. R. Scott Leslie et al., "Evaluation of an Integrated Adherence Program Aimed to Increase Medicare Part D Star Rating Measures," *Journal of Managed Care Pharmacy* 20, no. 12 (December 2014): 1193–203, https://doi.org/10.18553/jmcp.2014.20.12.1193.
25. Lam and Fresco, "Medication Adherence Measures."
26. Stirratt et al., "Advancing the Science."
27. Gagnon et al., "Treatment Adherence Redefined."
28. Sabaté, *Adherence to Long-Term Therapies.*
29. Rune A. Kroken et al., "Time to Discontinuation of Antipsychotic Drugs in a Schizophrenia Cohort: Influence of Current Treatment Strategies," *Therapeutic Advances in Psychopharmacology* 4, no. 6 (December 2014): 228–39, https://doi.org/10.1177/2045125314545614.
30. Alex J. Adams and Samuel F. Stolpe, "Defining and Measuring Primary Medication Nonadherence: Development of a Quality Measure," *Journal of*

Managed Care & Specialty Pharmacy 22, no. 5 (May 2016): 516–23, https://doi.org/10.18553/jmcp.2016.22.5.516.

31. Lam and Fresco, "Medication Adherence Measures."
32. Aldeer et al., "Review of Medication Adherence Monitoring Technologies."
33. Michael J. Stirratt et al., "Self-Report Measures of Medication Adherence Behavior: Recommendations on Optimal Use," *Translational Behavioral Medicine* 5, no. 4 (December 2015): 470–82, https://doi.org/10.1007/s13142-015-0315-2.
34. M. Robin DiMatteo et al., "Patient Adherence and Medical Treatment Outcomes: A Meta-Analysis," *Medical Care* 40, no. 9 (September 2002): 794–811, https://doi.org/10.1097/00005650-200209000-00009.
35. Aldeer et al., "Review of Medication Adherence Monitoring Technologies."
36. "Antibiotic Resistance," World Health Organization, July 31, 2020, https://www.who.int/news-room/fact-sheets/detail/antibiotic-resistance.
37. Aditi Babel et al., "Artificial Intelligence Solutions to Increase Medication Adherence in Patients with Non-Communicable Diseases," *Frontiers in Digital Health* 3 (2021): 69, https://doi.org/10.3389/fdgth.2021.669869.
38. Meera Viswanathan et al., "Interventions to Improve Adherence to Self-Administered Medications for Chronic Diseases in the United States: A Systematic Review," *Annals of Internal Medicine* 157, no. 11 (December 2012): 785–95, https://doi.org/10.7326/0003-4819-157-11-201212040-00538.
39. Angela Frances Yap, Thiru Thirumoorthy, and Yu Heng Kwan, "Systematic Review of the Barriers Affecting Medication Adherence in Older Adults," *Geriatrics & Gerontology International* 16, no. 10 (October 2016): 1093–101, https://doi.org/10.1111/ggi.12616.
40. Marie T. Brown and Jennifer K. Bussell, "Medication Adherence: WHO Cares?" *Mayo Clinic Proceedings* 86, no. 4 (April 2011): 304–14, https://doi.org/10.4065/mcp.2010.0575.
41. Vlasnik et al., "Medication Adherence."
42. Rena Brar Prayaga et al., "Impact of Social Determinants of Health and Demographics on Refill Requests by Medicare Patients Using a Conversational Artificial Intelligence Text Messaging Solution: Cross-Sectional Study," *JMIR mHealth and uHealth* 7, no. 11 (November 2019): e15771, https://doi.org/10.2196/15771.
43. Babel et al., "Artificial Intelligence Solutions"; Walid F. Gellad, Jerry L. Grenard, and Zachary A. Marcum, "A Systematic Review of Barriers to Medication Adherence in the Elderly: Looking Beyond Cost and Regimen Complexity," *American Journal of Geriatric Pharmacotherapy*

9, no. 1 (February 2011): 11–23, https://doi.org/10.1016/j.amjoph arm.2011.02.004.

44. Huda Wali and Kelly Grindrod, "Don't Assume the Patient Understands: Qualitative Analysis of the Challenges Low Health Literate Patients Face in the Pharmacy," *Research in Social & Administrative Pharmacy* 12, no. 6 (December 2016): 885–92, https://doi.org/10.1016/ j.sapharm.2015.12.003.
45. Michael Frakes, Jonathan Gruber, and Anupam Jena, "Is Great Information Good Enough? Evidence from Physicians as Patients," *Journal of Health Economics* 75 (January 2021): 102406, https://doi.org/10.1016/j.jheal eco.2020.102406.
46. Elizabeth L. McQuaid and Wendy Landier, "Cultural Issues in Medication Adherence: Disparities and Directions," *Journal of General Internal Medicine* 33, no. 2 (February 2018): 200–206, https://doi.org/10.1007/s11 606-017-4199-3.
47. Vlasnik et al., "Medication Adherence."
48. Nicky Britten, Ruth Riley, and Myfanwy Morgan, "Resisting Psychotropic Medicines: A Synthesis of Qualitative Studies of Medicine-Taking," *Advances in Psychiatric Treatment* 16, no. 3 (2010): 207–18, https://doi. org/10.1192/apt.bp.107.005165.
49. Kirsi Kvarnström et al., "Factors Contributing to Medication Adherence in Patients with a Chronic Condition: A Scoping Review of Qualitative Research," *Pharmaceutics* 13, no. 7 (July 2021), https://doi.org/10.3390/ pharmaceutics13071100.
50. Vlasnik et al., "Medication Adherence."
51. Janet Krska et al., "Issues Potentially Affecting Quality of Life Arising from Long-Term Medicines Use: A Qualitative Study," *International Journal of Clinical Pharmacy* 35, no. 6 (December 2013): 1161–69, https://doi.org/ 10.1007/s11096-013-9841-5.
52. "HHS Awards Nearly $55 Million to Increase Virtual Health Care Access and Quality Through Community Health Centers," U.S. Department of Health and Human Services, February 14, 2022, https://www.hhs.gov/ about/news/2022/02/14/hhs-awards-nearly-55-million-increase-virtual-health-care-access-quality-through-community-health-centers.html.
53. As we will see shortly, two notable exception are opioid medications and psychiatric medications, where some providers may require explicit patient consent to adhere to various instructions before prescribing or making other treatment decisions.
54. John F. Steiner et al., "Sociodemographic and Clinical Characteristics Are Not Clinically Useful Predictors of Refill Adherence in Patients with

Hypertension," *Circulation: Cardiovascular Quality and Outcomes* 2, no. 5 (September 2009): 451–57, https://doi.org/10.1161/CIRCOUTCOMES.108.841635.

55. Robby Nieuwlaat et al., "Interventions for Enhancing Medication Adherence," *Cochrane Database of Systematic Reviews*, no. 11 (November 2014): CD000011, https://doi.org/10.1002/14651858.CD000011.pub4.
56. Babel et al., "Artificial Intelligence Solutions."
57. "AllazoHealth Now Offers AI Optimized Therapy Initiation," AllazoHealth, February 1, 2021, https://blog.allazohealth.com/resources/ai-optimized-therapy-initiation.
58. Alexander Galozy and Slawomir Nowaczyk, "Prediction and Pattern Analysis of Medication Refill Adherence through Electronic Health Records and Dispensation Data," *Journal of Biomedical Informatics* 112S (2020): 100075, https://doi.org/10.1016/j.yjbinx.2020.100075.
59. Jacqueline G. Hugtenburg et al., "Definitions, Variants, and Causes of Nonadherence with Medication: A Challenge for Tailored Interventions," *Patient Preference and Adherence* 7 (July 2013): 675–82, https://doi.org/10.2147/PPA.S29549.
60. Vidya Koesmahargyo et al., "Accuracy of Machine Learning-Based Prediction of Medication Adherence in Clinical Research," *Psychiatry Research* 294 (December 2020): 113558, https://doi.org/10.1016/j.psychres.2020.113558.
61. Koesmahargyo et al., "Accuracy of Machine Learning-Based Prediction."
62. Olga Chivilgina, Bernice S. Elger, and Fabrice Jotterand, "Digital Technologies for Schizophrenia Management: A Descriptive Review," *Science and Engineering Ethics* 27, no. 2 (April 2021): 25, https://doi.org/10.1007/s11948-021-00302-z.
63. Velligan et al., "Defining and Assessing Adherence."
64. Ainslie Hatch et al., "Expert Consensus Survey on Medication Adherence in Psychiatric Patients and Use of a Digital Medicine System," *Journal of Clinical Psychiatry* 78, no. 7 (July 2017): e803–12, https://doi.org/10.4088/JCP.16m11252.
65. Martijn J. Kikkert and Jack Dekker, "Medication Adherence Decisions in Patients with Schizophrenia," *Primary Care Companion for CNS Disorders* 19, no. 6 (December 2017), https://doi.org/10.4088/PCC.17n02182.
66. Velligan et al., "Defining and Assessing Adherence."
67. Peter M. Haddad, Cecilia Brain, and Jan Scott, "Nonadherence with Antipsychotic Medication in Schizophrenia: Challenges and Management Strategies," *Patient Related Outcome Measures* 5 (2014): 43–62, https://doi.org/10.2147/PROM.S42735.

68. Saínza García et al., "Adherence to Antipsychotic Medication in Bipolar Disorder and Schizophrenic Patients: A Systematic Review," *Journal of Clinical Psychopharmacology* 36, no. 4 (August 2016): 355–71, https://doi.org/10.1097/JCP.0000000000000523.
69. Andrew Briggs et al., "Impact of Schizophrenia and Schizophrenia Treatment-Related Adverse Events on Quality of Life: Direct Utility Elicitation," *Health and Quality of Life Outcomes* 6, no. 1 (November 2008): 105, https://doi.org/10.1186/1477-7525-6-105.
70. Katherine Bogart et al., "Mobile Phone Text Message Reminders of Antipsychotic Medication: Is It Time and Who Should Receive Them? A Cross-Sectional Trust-Wide Survey of Psychiatric Inpatients," *BMC Psychiatry* 14 (January 2014): 15, https://doi.org/10.1186/1471-244X-14-15.
71. Martin Knapp et al., "Non-Adherence to Antipsychotic Medication Regimens: Associations with Resource Use and Costs," *British Journal of Psychiatry* 184 (June 2004): 509–16, https://doi.org/10.1192/bjp.184.6.509.
72. Todd P. Gilmer et al., "Adherence to Treatment with Antipsychotic Medication and Health Care Costs among Medicaid Beneficiaries with Schizophrenia," *American Journal of Psychiatry* 161, no. 4 (April 2004): 692–99, https://doi.org/10.1176/appi.ajp.161.4.692.
73. Cordellia E. Bright, "Measuring Medication Adherence in Patients With Schizophrenia: An Integrative Review," *Archives of Psychiatric Nursing* 31, no. 1 (February 2017): 99–110, https://doi.org/10.1016/j.apnu.2016.09.003; Haya Ascher-Svanum et al., "Medication Adherence and Long-Term Functional Outcomes in the Treatment of Schizophrenia in Usual Care," *Journal of Clinical Psychiatry* 67, no. 3 (March 2006): 453–60, https://doi.org/10.4088/jcp.v67n0317.
74. Jonas Forsman et al., "Adherence to Psychotropic Medication in Completed Suicide in Sweden 2006–2013: A Forensic-Toxicological Matched Case-Control Study," *European Journal of Clinical Pharmacology* 75, no. 10 (October 2019): 1421–30, https://doi.org/10.1007/s00228-019-02707-z.
75. Dawn I. Velligan et al., "Relationships among Subjective and Objective Measures of Adherence to Oral Antipsychotic Medications," *Psychiatric Services* 58, no. 9 (September 2007): 1187–92, https://doi.org/10.1176/ps.2007.58.9.1187.
76. Donald C. Goff, Michele Hill, and Oliver Freudenreich, "Strategies for Improving Treatment Adherence in Schizophrenia and Schizoaffective Disorder," *Journal of Clinical Psychiatry* 71, Suppl. 2 (2010): 20–26, https://doi.org/10.4088/JCP.9096su1cc.04.

77. Hatch et al., "Expert Consensus Survey on Medication Adherence." The authors stated that the panel members "were identified based on recent publication activity, funded research, previous participation in consensus surveys in psychiatry, and/or work on guidelines concerning psychiatric illnesses." No specific details were offered as to whether these "experts" were practicing clinicians.
78. Matthew J. Byerly et al., "Validity of Electronically Monitored Medication Adherence and Conventional Adherence Measures in Schizophrenia," *Psychiatric Services* 58, no. 6 (June 2007): 844–47, https://doi.org/10.1176/ps.2007.58.6.844.
79. Alipour et al., "Ingestible Sensors and Medication Adherence."
80. Kurt Kroenke et al., "Challenges with Implementing the Centers for Disease Control and Prevention Opioid Guideline: A Consensus Panel Report," *Pain Medicine* 20, no. 4 (April 2019): 724–35, https://doi.org/10.1093/pm/pny307.
81. Scott Clement and Lenny Bernstein, "One-Third of Long-Term Users Say They're Hooked on Prescription Opioids," *Washington Post*, December 9, 2016, https://www.washingtonpost.com/national/health-science/one-third-of-long-term-users-say-theyre-hooked-on-prescription-opioids/2016/12/09/e048d322-baed-11e6-91ee-1adddfe36cbe_story.html.
82. International Association for the Study of Pain, *Unrelieved Pain Is a Major Global Health-Care Problem* (Washington, DC: International Association for the Study of Pain, 2012).
83. L. Timmerman et al., "Prevalence and Determinants of Medication Non Adherence in Chronic Pain Patients: A Systematic Review," *Acta Anaesthesiologica Scandinavica* 60, no. 4 (April 2016): 416–31, https://doi.org/10.1111/aas.12697.
84. W. Michael Hooten et al., "A Conceptual Framework for Understanding Unintended Prolonged Opioid Use," *Mayo Clinic Proceedings* 92, no. 12 (December 2017): 1822–30, https://doi.org/10.1016/j.mayocp.2017.10.010.
85. Daniel Z. Buchman, Anita Ho, and Judy Illes, "You Present like a Drug Addict: Patient and Clinician Perspectives on Trust and Trustworthiness in Chronic Pain Management," *Pain Medicine* 17, no. 8 (August 2016): 1394–406, https://doi.org/10.1093/pm/pnv08;
86. Deborah Dowell, Tamara Haegerich, and Roger Chou, "No Shortcuts to Safer Opioid Prescribing," *New England Journal of Medicine* 380, no. 24 (June 2019): 2285–87, https://doi.org/10.1056/NEJMp1904190.

87. Douglas L. Gourlay and Howard A. Heit, "Universal Precautions Revisited: Managing the Inherited Pain Patient," *Pain Medicine* 10, Suppl. 2 (July 2009): S115–23, https://doi.org/10.1111/j.1526-4637.2009.00671.x.
88. Alicia Agnoli et al., "Association of Dose Tapering with Overdose or Mental Health Crisis among Patients Prescribed Long-Term Opioids," *Journal of the American Medical Association* 326, no. 5 (August 2021): 411–19, https://doi.org/10.1001/jama.2021.11013.
89. Jesse Baumgartner and David Radley, "The Drug Overdose Toll in 2020 and Near-Term Actions for Addressing It," The Commonwealth Fund, August 16, 2021, https://www.commonwealthfund.org/blog/2021/drug-overdose-toll-2020-and-near-term-actions-addressing-it.
90. Beth Jung and Marcus M. Reidenberg, "Physicians Being Deceived," *Pain Medicine* 8, no. 5 (August 2007): 433–37, https://doi.org/10.1111/j.1526-4637.2007.00315.x.
91. Douglas L. Gourlay, Howard A. Heit, and Abdulaziz Almahrezi, "Universal Precautions in Pain Medicine: A Rational Approach to the Treatment of Chronic Pain," *Pain Medicine* 6, no. 2 (April 2005): 107–12, https://doi.org/10.1111/j.1526-4637.2005.05031.x.
92. Scott M. Fishman, "Trust and Pharmaco-Vigilance in Pain Medicine," *Pain Medicine* 6, no. 5 (October 2005): 392, https://doi.org/10.1111/j.1526-4637.2005.00068.x.
93. Robert M. Arnold, Paul K. J. Han, and Deborah Seltzer, "Opioid Contracts in Chronic Nonmalignant Pain Management: Objectives and Uncertainties," *American Journal of Medicine* 119, no. 4 (April 2006): 292–96, https://doi.org/10.1016/j.amjmed.2005.09.019.
94. Emma Pierson et al., "An Algorithmic Approach to Reducing Unexplained Pain Disparities in Underserved Populations," *Nature Medicine* 27, no. 1 (January 2021): 136–40, https://doi.org/10.1038/s41591-020-01192-7.
95. "Artificial Intelligence Can Predict Patients at Highest Risk for Severe Pain Increased Opioid Use after Surgery," American Society of Anesthesiologists, October 4, 2020, https://www.asahq.org/about-asa/newsroom/news-releases/2020/10/artificial-intelligence-can-predict-patients-at-highest-risk-for-severe-pain-increased-opioid-use-after-surgery.
96. "New AI Tool," University of Florida College of Pharmacy.
97. Hugtenburg et al., "Definitions, Variants, and Causes."
98. Earle E. Bain et al., "Use of a Novel Artificial Intelligence Platform on Mobile Devices to Assess Dosing Compliance in a Phase 2 Clinical Trial in Subjects with Schizophrenia," *JMIR mHealth and uHealth* 5, no. 2 (February 2017): e18, https://doi.org/10.2196/mhealth.7030.

99. Babel et al., "Artificial Intelligence Solutions."
100. Haik Kalantarian et al., "A Wearable Sensor System for Medication Adherence Prediction," *Artificial Intelligence in Medicine* 69 (May 2016): 43–52, https://doi.org/10.1016/j.artmed.2016.03.004.
101. Charlotte Goldfine et al., "Wearable and Wireless MHealth Technologies for Substance Use Disorder," *Current Addiction Reports* 7, no. 3 (September 2020): 291–300, https://doi.org/10.1007/s40429-020-00318-8.
102. Andrea Martani et al., "Digital Pills: A Scoping Review of the Empirical Literature and Analysis of the Ethical Aspects," *BMC Medical Ethics* 21, no. 1 (January 2020): 3, https://doi.org/10.1186/s12910-019-0443-1.
103. Carl B. Roth et al., "Psychiatry in the Digital Age: A Blessing or a Curse?" *International Journal of Environmental Research and Public Health* 18, no. 16 (August 2021), https://doi.org/10.3390/ijerph18168302.
104. Bain et al., "Use of a Novel Artificial Intelligence Platform."
105. Jackson M. Steinkamp et al., "Technological Interventions for Medication Adherence in Adult Mental Health and Substance Use Disorders: A Systematic Review," *JMIR Mental Health* 6, no. 3 (March 2019): e12493–e12493, https://doi.org/10.2196/12493.
106. Lisa Rosenbaum, "Swallowing a Spy—The Potential Uses of Digital Adherence Monitoring," *New England Journal of Medicine* 378, no. 2 (January 2018): 101–3, https://doi.org/10.1056/NEJMp1716206. It is perhaps ironic that this surveillance technology was first approved for a drug used to treat paranoia.
107. Timothy Peters-Strickland et al., "Usability of a Novel Digital Medicine System in Adults with Schizophrenia Treated with Sensor-Embedded Tablets of Aripiprazole," *Neuropsychiatric Disease and Treatment* 12 (2016): 2587–94, https://doi.org/10.2147/NDT.S116029.
108. Jo Best, "Smart Pills and the Future of Medicine: Insights from Your Insides," ZDNet, February 23, 2021, https://www.zdnet.com/article/smart-pills-and-the-future-of-medicine-insights-from-your-insides/; Michael Chorost, "The Networked Pill," *MIT Technology Review*, March 20, 2008, https://www.technologyreview.com/2008/03/20/34958/the-networked-pill/.
109. Hurtado-de-Mendoza et al., "Rethinking Agency."
110. R. Scooter Plowman, Timothy Peters-Strickland, and George M. Savage, "Digital Medicines: Clinical Review on the Safety of Tablets with Sensors," *Expert Opinion on Drug Safety* 17, no. 9 (September 2018): 849–52, https://doi.org/10.1080/14740338.2018.1508447.
111. Hatch et al., "Expert Consensus Survey on Medication Adherence."

112. Peter R. Chai et al., "Digital Pills to Measure Opioid Ingestion Patterns in Emergency Department Patients With Acute Fracture Pain: A Pilot Study," *Journal of Medical Internet Research* 19, no. 1 (January 2017): e19, https://doi.org/10.2196/jmir.7050; Peter R. Chai et al., "Oxycodone Ingestion Patterns in Acute Fracture Pain with Digital Pills," *Anesthesia and Analgesia* 125, no. 6 (December 2017): 2105–12, https://doi.org/10.1213/ANE.0000000000002574.
113. Emily Mullin, "Digital Pills Track How Patients Use Opioids," *MIT Technology Review*, December 11, 2017, https://www.technologyreview.com/2017/12/11/147144/digital-pills-track-how-patients-use-opioids/.
114. Mark A. Young and Lauren DiMartino, "The Emergence of Trackable Pill Technology: Hype or Hope?" *Practical Pain Management* 18, no. 4 (April 2019), https://www.practicalpainmanagement.com/treatments/pharmacological/opioids/editorial-emergence-trackable-pill-technology-hype-hope.
115. Maia Szalavitz, "The Pain Was Unbearable. So Why Did Doctors Turn Her Away?" *Wired*, August 11, 2021, https://www.wired.com/story/opioid-drug-addiction-algorithm-chronic-pain/.
116. Harriet Standing and Rob Lawlor, "Ulysses Contracts in Psychiatric Care: Helping Patients to Protect Themselves from Spiralling," *Journal of Medical Ethics* 45, no. 11 (November 2019): 693–99, https://doi.org/10.1136/medethics-2019-105511.
117. J. F. Steiner and M. A. Earnest, "The Language of Medication-Taking," *Annals of Internal Medicine* 132, no. 11 (June 2000): 926–30, https://doi.org/10.7326/0003-4819-132-11-200006060-00026.
118. Britten et al., "Resisting Psychotropic Medicines"; Hugtenburg et al., "Definitions, Variants, and Causes."
119. Pandora Pound et al., "Resisting Medicines: A Synthesis of Qualitative Studies of Medicine Taking," *Social Science & Medicine* 61, no. 1 (July 2005): 133–55, https://doi.org/10.1016/j.socscimed.2004.11.063.
120. Krska et al., "Issues Potentially Affecting Quality of Life."
121. Krska et al., "Issues Potentially Affecting Quality of Life."
122. Krska et al., "Issues Potentially Affecting Quality of Life."
123. Lisa A. Hillman et al., "The Medication Experience: A Concept Analysis," *Pharmacy* 9, no. 1 (December 2020), https://doi.org/10.3390/pharmacy9010007.
124. Toshi A. Furukawa et al., "Initial Severity of Schizophrenia and Efficacy of Antipsychotics: Participant-Level Meta-Analysis of 6 Placebo-Controlled Studies," *JAMA Psychiatry* 72, no. 1 (January 2015): 14–21, https://doi.org/10.1001/jamapsychiatry.2014.2127.

125. J. A. Trostle, W. A. Hauser, and I. S. Susser, "The Logic of Noncompliance: Management of Epilepsy from the Patient's Point of View," *Culture, Medicine and Psychiatry* 7, no. 1 (March 1983): 35–56, https://doi.org/10.1007/BF00249998; Pound et al., "Resisting Medicines."
126. Peter Conrad, "The Meaning of Medications: Another Look at Compliance," *Social Science & Medicine* 20, no. 1 (January 1985): 29–37, https://doi.org/10.1016/0277-9536(85)90308-9.
127. Patricia E. Deegan and Robert E. Drake, "Shared Decision Making and Medication Management in the Recovery Process," *Psychiatric Services* 57, no. 11 (November 2006): 1636–39, https://doi.org/10.1176/ps.2006.57.11.1636.
128. Britten et al., "Resisting Psychotropic Medicines."
129. Karen Lutfey, "On Practices of 'Good Doctoring': Reconsidering the Relationship between Provider Roles and Patient Adherence," *Sociology of Health & Illness* 27, no. 4 (May 2005): 421–47, https://doi.org/10.1111/j.1467-9566.2005.00450.x.
130. Britten et al., "Resisting Psychotropic Medicines."
131. Kikkert and Dekker, "Medication Adherence Decisions."
132. Goff et al., "Strategies for Improving Treatment Adherence."
133. Anabel Martinez-Aran et al., "Treatment Nonadherence and Neurocognitive Impairment in Bipolar Disorder," *Journal of Clinical Psychiatry* 70, no. 7 (July 2009): 1017–23, https://doi.org/10.4088/JCP.08m04408.
134. J. Moncrieff, D. Cohen, and J. P. Mason, "The Subjective Experience of Taking Antipsychotic Medication: A Content Analysis of Internet Data," *Acta Psychiatrica Scandinavica* 120, no. 2 (August 2009): 102–11, https://doi.org/10.1111/j.1600-0447.2009.01356.x.
135. Kikkert and Dekker, "Medication Adherence Decisions."
136. Britten et al., "Resisting Psychotropic Medicines"; Chivilgina et al., "Digital Technologies for Schizophrenia Management."
137. Gilmer et al., "Adherence to Treatment with Antipsychotic Medication."
138. Tom Tomlinson, "Getting Off the Leash," *American Journal of Bioethics* 18, no. 9 (September 2018): 48–49, https://doi.org/10.1080/15265161.2018.1498938.
139. Pound et al., "Resisting Medicines."
140. Sally E. Thorne and Carole A. Robinson, "Reciprocal Trust in Health Care Relationships," *Journal of Advanced Nursing* 13, no. 6 (November 1988): 782–89, https://doi.org/10.1111/j.1365-2648.1988.tb00570.x.
141. Steiner and Earnest, "Language of Medication-Taking."
142. Britten et al., "Resisting Psychotropic Medicines."

143. Anna K. Swartz, "Smart Pills for Psychosis: The Tricky Ethical Challenges of Digital Medicine for Serious Mental Illness," *American Journal of Bioethics* 18, no. 9 (September 2018): 65–67, https://doi.org/10.1080/15265161.2018.1498948.
144. Britten et al., "Resisting Psychotropic Medicines."
145. Tom Burns, "Locked Doors or Therapeutic Relationships?," *Lancet Psychiatry* 3, no. 9 (September 2016): 795–96, https://doi.org/10.1016/S2215-0366(16)30185-7.
146. Pound et al., "Resisting Medicines."
147. Jonathan M. Marron et al., "Medical Decision-Making in Oncology for Patients Lacking Capacity," *American Society of Clinical Oncology Educational Book* 40 (May 2020): e186–96, https://doi.org/10.1200/EDBK_280279.
148. Anita Ho and Daniel Buchman, "Pain," in *Encyclopedia of Global Bioethics*, ed. Henk ten Have (New York: Springer, 2015), https://doi.org/10.1007/978-3-319-05544-2_322-1.
149. Meredith Noble et al., "Long-Term Opioid Management for Chronic Noncancer Pain," *Cochrane Database of Systematic Reviews* 1 (January 2010), https://doi.org/10.1002/14651858.CD006605.pub2.
150. Buchman et al., "You Present like a Drug Addict."; Lisa Victor and Steven H. Richeimer, "Trustworthiness as a Clinical Variable: The Problem of Trust in the Management of Chronic, Nonmalignant Pain," *Pain Medicine* 6, no. 5 (October 2005): 385–91, https://doi.org/10.1111/j.1526-4637.2005.00063.x.
151. "New AI Tool," University of Florida College of Pharmacy.
152. Adrian Guta, Jijian Voronka, and Marilou Gagnon, "Resisting the Digital Medicine Panopticon: Toward a Bioethics of the Oppressed," *American Journal of Bioethics* 18, no. 9 (September 2018): 62–64, https://doi.org/10.1080/15265161.2018.1498936.
153. Gagnon et al., "Treatment Adherence Redefined."
154. Hurtado-de-Mendoza et al., "Rethinking Agency."
155. Fishman, "Trust and Pharmaco-Vigilance in Pain Medicine."
156. Jonah Comstock, "AiCure Clinical Trial Seeks to Validate Smartphone Camera-Enabled Medication Adherence," MobiHealthNews, November 24, 2014, https://www.mobihealthnews.com/38512/aicure-clinical-trial-seeks-to-validate-medication-adherence.
157. "Using Artificial Intelligence to Monitor Medication Adherence in Opioid Replacement Therapy," ClinicalTrials.gov, NCT02243670, last modified September 12, 2017, https://clinicaltrials.gov/ct2/show/study/NCT02243670.

158. Black Hawk Hancock, "Michel Foucault and the Problematics of Power: Theorizing DTCA and Medicalized Subjectivity," *Journal of Medicine and Philosophy* 43, no. 4 (July 2018): 439–68, https://doi.org/10.1093/jmp/jhy010.
159. Michel Foucault, *Discipline and Punish: The Birth of the Prison*, trans. Alan Sheridan (New York: Pantheon Books, 1977).
160. Peter Conrad, "The Shifting Engines of Medicalization," *Journal of Health and Social Behavior* 46, no. 1 (March 2005): 3–14.
161. Hurtado-de-Mendoza et al., "Rethinking Agency"; Guta et al., "Resisting the Digital Medicine Panopticon."
162. Hurtado-de-Mendoza et al., "Rethinking Agency"; D. Holmes, "From Iron Gaze to Nursing Care: Mental Health Nursing in the Era of Panopticism," *Journal of Psychiatric and Mental Health Nursing* 8, no. 1 (February 2001): 7–15, https://doi.org/10.1046/j.1365-2850.2001.00345.x.
163. Britten et al., "Resisting Psychotropic Medicines."
164. Susan Broekmans et al., "Determinants of Medication Underuse and Medication Overuse in Patients with Chronic Non-Malignant Pain: A Multicenter Study," *International Journal of Nursing Studies* 47, no. 11 (November 2010): 1408–17, https://doi.org/10.1016/j.ijnurstu.2010.03.014.
165. Alipour et al., "Ingestible Sensors."
166. Alexander C. Egilman and Joseph S. Ross, "Digital Medicine Systems: An Evergreening Strategy or an Advance in Medication Management?" *BMJ Evidence-Based Medicine* 24, no. 6 (December 2019): 203, https://doi.org/10.1136/bmjebm-2019-111265.
167. Roth et al., "Psychiatry in the Digital Age."
168. Lisa Cosgrove et al., "Digital Aripiprazole or Digital Evergreening? A Systematic Review of the Evidence and Its Dissemination in the Scientific Literature and in the Media," *BMJ Evidence-Based Medicine* 24, no. 6 (December 2019): 231–38, https://doi.org/10.1136/bmjebm-2019-111204.
169. "Clinical Review: Aripiprazole + MIND1 System (Abilify Mycite)," Center for Drug Evaluation and Research, U.S. Food and Drug Administration, April 21, 2017, https://www.accessdata.fda.gov/drugsatfda_docs/nda/2017/207202Orig1s000MedR.pdf.
170. Heather Landi, "Proteus Digital Health Was Once Valued at $1.5B. It May Be Acquired in a $15M 'Stalking Horse' Bid," Fierce Healthcare, July 27, 2020, https://www.fiercehealthcare.com/tech/proteus-digital-health-could-exit-bankruptcy-15m-stalking-horse-from-otsuka.
171. Galozy and Nowaczyk, "Prediction and Pattern Analysis."

172. Lonnie R. Snowden, Ray Catalano, and Martha Shumway, "Disproportionate Use of Psychiatric Emergency Services by African Americans," *Psychiatric Services* 60, no. 12 (December 2009): 1664–71, https://doi.org/10.1176/ps.2009.60.12.1664.
173. "Differences in Crisis Services and Psychiatric Hospitalizations across Race and Ethnicity," Wisconsin Department of Health Services, last modified February 4, 2021, https://www.dhs.wisconsin.gov/library/p-02904.htm.
174. Iraklis Erik Tseregounis and Stephen G. Henry, "Assessing Opioid Overdose Risk: A Review of Clinical Prediction Models Utilizing Patient-Level Data," *Translational Research* 234 (August 2021): 74–87, https://doi.org/10.1016/j.trsl.2021.03.012.
175. Wei-Hsuan Lo-Ciganic et al., "Evaluation of Machine-Learning Algorithms for Predicting Opioid Overdose Risk among Medicare Beneficiaries with Opioid Prescriptions," *JAMA Network Open* 2, no. 3 (March 2019): e190968–e190968, https://doi.org/10.1001/jamanetworkopen.2019.0968.
176. Tseregounis and Henry, "Assessing Opioid Overdose Risk."
177. Chai et al., "Oxycodone Ingestion Patterns"; Chai et al., "Digital Pills."
178. Fishman, "Trust and Pharmaco-Vigilance in Pain Medicine."
179. Swartz, "Smart Pills for Psychosis."
180. B. A. Rich, "The Doctor as Double Agent," *Pain Medicine* 6, no. 5 (2005): 393–95.
181. Anita Ho, "Reconciling Patient Safety and Epistemic Humility: An Ethical Use of Opioid Treatment Plans," *Hastings Center Report* 47, no. 3 (May 2017): 34–35, https://doi.org/10.1002/hast.703.
182. Ho and Buchman, "Pain."
183. John D. Loeser and Michael E. Schatman, "Chronic Pain Management in Medical Education: A Disastrous Omission," *Postgraduate Medicine* 129, no. 3 (April 2017): 332–35, https://doi.org/10.1080/00325481.2017.1297668.
184. Buchman et al., "You Present like a Drug Addict."
185. Wendy A. Rogers, Heather Draper, and Stacy M. Carter, "Evaluation of Artificial Intelligence Clinical Applications: Detailed Case Analyses Show Value of Healthcare Ethics Approach in Identifying Patient Care Issues," *Bioethics* 35, no. 7 (September 2021): 623–33, https://doi.org/10.1111/bioe.12885.
186. Brar Prayaga et al., "Impact of Social Determinants of Health."
187. Loeser and Schatman, "Chronic Pain Management in Medical Education."

5

From One-Way Mirror to Two-Way Street

Realigning Goals and Practices of Artificial Intelligence Health Monitoring

The previous chapters have shown how decisions around artificial intelligence (AI) health monitoring are not simply individualized choices about particular technologies or health concerns. Rather, predictive computation intersects with sociocultural ideas about aging, independent living, care relationships, and treatment adherence. These norms have longstanding implications for how people are expected to behave or live, sometimes to the point where individuals—especially those who are part of historically oppressed groups or are subjected to oppressive social conditions—may struggle to conceive how their values and preferences could differ in other circumstances. As such, health monitoring processes and decisions reveal themselves as structural phenomena of power and domination that shape others' choices, whether intentionally or unintentionally. Put another way, they are products of the actions of many different parties occupying various social locations.[1] The evolving technological, professional, regulatory, and commercial practices around the use of AI are blurring the lines between health and wellness, and restructuring prospective patients' and consumers' motivations and expectations around how their bodies and daily activities are to be monitored, by themselves and others, in the name of maintaining and improving their health. Importantly, as health care becomes increasingly digitized, with an assortment of health, lifestyle, and personal data being collected, shared, and analyzed across platforms both inside and outside of formal care settings, health monitoring decisions now occur within broader socio-technological structures. AI applications have the potential to fundamentally alter these structures and change the contours of therapeutic and familial care relationships regardless of people's own comfort level with these technologies.[2] Moreover, as health systems increasingly collaborate with commercial entities to develop AI technologies both for clinical care and at-home patient monitoring, these technological processes are reframing health care providers' expectations of how far they can and should reach into prospective patients' everyday lives, how insistently they should recommend (or demand) that patients and their family members take on health monitoring and self-management responsibilities, and how they will incorporate predictive computing data into workflow planning and care plans.

While enthusiasts argue that AI-enhanced health monitoring allows for more user interaction and data involvement, which in turn facilitates tailored recommendations, data intensity does not necessarily translate into clinically meaningful or autonomous engagement or high-value care management. As we have seen in previous chapters, with nontransparent algorithmic processes and data sharing practices, even individuals who agree to use various AI health monitoring technologies often do not know how (much of) their data may be collected, stored, shared across platforms, or sold to third parties for related or unrelated commercial use, and whether the information (to be) collected is directly relevant for the particular purpose of that technology. Depending on how the technology is configured, implemented, and adopted, monitored users may not be able to opt out of various functions or conditions. For example, some direct-to-consumer (DTC) health applications that are embedded in smartphones may collect users' location information and contact list by default, even if such information is irrelevant to the algorithm's purpose and analysis, and users may not be fully aware of such data collection.[3] With the proliferation and normalization of these practices, users may internalize the expectations that they must accept comprehensive and automated monitoring as part of their new reality. If rapidly adopted on a large scale, new AI practices may render people's reflection on their own goals, priorities, and concerns regarding such monitoring pointless, especially if they are in marginalized groups and cannot act on their practical identity.

Granted, continuous use of digital monitoring, analysis, and automated interactions (e.g., alerts) outside of formal clinical care settings may reassure some users and/or their loved ones in certain narrow scenarios, such as for people who are at substantial risk of atrial fibrillation (assuming the algorithm is highly accurate in detecting associated symptoms). Nonetheless, most AI health monitoring algorithms are still in proof-of-concept stages. And despite the increasing ubiquity of commercial home health monitoring platforms and DTC devices, which are touted by developers as tools to promote preventive care and self-management, there remains a lack of efficacy evidence demonstrating that they can actually improve users' health outcomes and/or lower health care costs. In particular, many commercial algorithms are trained on a small number of participants who may not be representative of the broader user base, leading to biased output that may have different effects on different populations.

In the United States, even for AI algorithms and software that have been cleared by the U.S. Food and Drug Administration (FDA) as medical devices or recommended by clinicians, successful clinical applications or integration of AI health monitoring technologies into patients' care pathways remain limited due to the complexity of real-world conditions. For example, while smartphone sensors have been found to be feasible technologies for gathering real-time health and lifestyle data from users, large-scale implementations of digital monitoring strategies have revealed high dropout rates, with more than 90 percent of participants failing to complete a seven-day follow-up for a cardiovascular health study,[4] and 55 percent failing to complete follow-up data for a pregnancy monitoring program.[5] This raises questions of whether patients truly desire to be continuously tracked and recorded as part of their journey through health maintenance, and whether in the increasingly surveilled world, patients can still choose how they want to be observed.

Drawing on examples and ideas from previous chapters, this final chapter argues that the concept of relational autonomy can help to promote a systems approach or feedback loop to ensure that further development and utilization of predictive health monitoring will enhance rather than erode users' practical identities as they navigate their health maintenance and illness journeys. Given the increasing quantification of patients and consumers due to expanding AI and other digital health practices, this chapter proposes relational strategies to preserve therapeutic relationships and enhance patients' autonomous agency in this evolving digital age. Section 1 explains how the lens of relational autonomy can help strengthen therapeutic relationships and ensure that advancing health monitoring technologies will be used as collaborative tools to increase stakeholders' knowledge of patients' care priorities rather than surveillance mechanisms to regulate distrust or override patients' testimonies. Section 2 argues that multilevel dialogic engagement at the individual, technological, professional/institutional, and societal levels may help promote a responsible and responsive feedback loop to guide the development and implementation of AI health monitoring, holding technologists and decision-makers responsible for ensuring safe and valid technologies as well as providing transparent and accurate information. This in turn may improve the social determinants of health and digital literacy, thereby enhancing patients' capacity to understand their health situation and providing opportunities to make goal-concordant health monitoring decisions that can advance their autonomy.

1. AI Has a Relationship Problem

As we have seen, the concept of relational autonomy highlights how the broad acceptance of an expanding array of loosely regulated AI health monitoring technologies may reinforce power imbalances at the interpersonal/familial, professional/institutional, and system levels, which in turn can affect (prospective) users' self-governance, self-determination, and self-authorization. AI health monitoring is rapidly becoming part of the dominant biopolitical narrative of the democratization of health information, which reinforces personal responsibility for learning more about and taking care of one's health.[6] Yet the proliferation of these technologies and the increasing enthusiasm towards predictive health algorithms among technologists, medical professionals, health systems, and funders also send the paradoxical message that some patients cannot or should not be trusted to take control of their own health. Rhetoric around patient autonomy and paternalism notwithstanding, patients whose competence or credibility around their self-management responsibilities is deemed questionable by health care providers (or families) are increasingly proposed as appropriate subjects for monitoring and management by "objective" algorithms, even when many of these algorithms continue to have high error rates or low clinical value. As we saw in previous chapters, populations such as women of reproductive age, older or disabled adults, people with mental illnesses, or people with chronic non-malignant pain (CNMP) are sometimes required or expected to accept continuous monitoring and predictive analysis according to predefined professional or technological thresholds, both for their own rational interests and for health professionals' liability protection. At the same time, there are also questions of whether or how the increasing prominence of AI health monitoring algorithms and smart devices, particularly those promoted by commercial entities as tools to help laypersons bypass health care providers in receiving health information and wellness advice, may lower patients' reliance on and trust in their health care providers, especially if algorithmic and clinician recommendations diverge.

Using the framework of relational autonomy, I argue that refocusing on the therapeutic relationship and committing to epistemic justice can help us develop and implement AI health monitoring practices in ways that will promote monitored users' self-governance, self-determination, and self-authorization. Such an approach would allow health care providers to collaboratively determine with their patients the ideal health goals or targets that they are trying to reach, explore what types of data are most important in informing such goals, and determine whether or how data from digital monitoring may facilitate the formation and realization of goal-concordant care plans that align with patients' practical identities and broader contexts. In particular, an explicit acknowledgment of the epistemic limits of what algorithmic outputs from AI health monitoring can offer, as well as intentional invitations for patients to share the full scope of their experiences as part of multilevel dialogic engagement, may help to promote reciprocal trust, crystalize the ideal health target, and enhance users' relational autonomy.

As health care becomes increasingly digitized, with certain aspects of patient experiences progressively converted into quantified and computable data, there is widespread concern that AI health monitoring may further erode therapeutic relationships, isolate patients, and exacerbate the digital divide. AI enthusiasts pledge that predictive health monitoring technologies can assist physicians' clinical decision-making by triaging patients on their behalf, allowing them to focus on individuals with more complex and/or urgent needs, and practice the uniquely human aspects of medicine such as listening and empathizing.[7] This in turn can enhance therapeutic relationships and job satisfaction for health care providers. However, concerns abound that, despite promises of tailored or "personalized" care based on patient-generated data, an increasing reliance on AI health monitoring may actually further depersonalize the care experience.

Part of the issue is that even accurate predictive algorithms remain a form of artificial narrow intelligence (ANI) and are therefore limited in their purpose and scope. For example, a computer vision deep learning (DL) algorithm may be able to predict with high accuracy how much or how quickly a patient with Parkinson's disease will lose the ability to carry out specific activities of daily living. A medication management algorithm trained on prescription drug dispensing data and/or hospital utilization data from thousands of previously hospitalized patients with schizophrenia may also be more reliable than other techniques in predicting whether a patient with this condition will stop taking medication within the next month or need hospitalization. Nonetheless, narrow algorithmic outputs provide only part of the information needed to balance freedom and safety while pursuing *patients'* ideal targets; they may be inadequate in determining appropriate living arrangements and care management for the older adult with Parkinson's disease, or in optimizing quality of life for the person with schizophrenia. As AI health monitoring algorithms generally do not incorporate nuanced qualitative and sometimes pervasive contextual factors into their predictive analysis[8]—whether due to technological limitations or technologists' perceived irrelevance of these factors—there are often incomplete data to help understand patients' multifaceted goals and concerns. Even algorithms that are accurate for the targeted population in their narrowly designated tasks will not tell physicians what practical, social, economic, or emotional impact the knowledge of these health changes may have on the patient, or what care plan or living arrangement may best support the patient. While AI analytical tools may serve as "driver assistance," enhancing clinicians' ability to predict a monitored person's behavior and associated clinical outcomes based on narrow sets of physiological characteristics or behavioral circumstances,[9] they are not themselves communication tools or artificial general intelligence (AGI) that can address multifaceted concerns for patients facing complex situations.

In other words, algorithmic predictions do not automatically strengthen clinicians' empathetic engagement, promote their understanding of patients' motivations and barriers, or enrich their appreciation of patients' potential suffering so as to shape individualized care decisions, actions, and recommendations that can balance patients' various priorities and determine the most appropriate care plan.[10] Consider, for example, an AI algorithm mentioned in Chapter 1 that uses electronic health records (EHRs) and DL to calculate the probability that a flagged patient will die within a year.[11] Adoption of the algorithm may nudge a physician to start having serious illness conversations with the patient.[12] However, if the physician has not already been trained to have these conversations, the algorithmic output may not help the physician have compassionate conversations around the most intimate questions about the patient's hopes, expectations, worries, and goals, and what would bring them the most comfort as they weigh different care options. Worse yet, as end-of-life discussions are often emotionally challenging for physicians, these algorithms may prevent rather than promote discussions, if some physicians refrain from initiating these discussions until or unless prompted by the AI algorithm, even if there may be other signs that the patient can benefit from having these conversations before they are within the predetermined life-expectancy parameters set by the algorithm, such as if the patient starts talking about other family members' illness experiences or their own fears regarding their health decline. Unless clinicians recognize the epistemic limits of algorithmic analytics and intentionally seek out such contextual and deeply human information, an inflated confidence that ANI can provide overarching answers to care planning decisions may compromise clinicians' ability to explore patients' goals and provide tailored support that will promote patients' practical identity.

Given technological limitations, we need to be particularly careful in determining what types of automation and predictive analytics may enhance therapeutic relationships and patients' self-governance, and which ones may further threaten the humanistic aspects of care. Digital medicine is transforming how care is delivered and by whom, those individuals' professional relationships with each other (e.g., whether radiologists consult with colleagues regarding a patient's digital images, or whether nurses discuss anomalies regarding an electronic prescription), and their therapeutic relationships with patients.[13] In a study of 1,183 adult patients with chronic conditions in France regarding their perceptions of the potential benefits and risks of using biometric monitoring and AI interventions, only 50 percent of patients felt that these digital tools represented a helpful opportunity; 11 percent considered them a danger.[14] Even participants who were most ready to use AI technologies in their treatment plans and were hopeful that AI would enhance follow-up care thought that predictive tools should not replace human care for situations related to sensitive topics (e.g., cancer) or long-term interventions (e.g., chronic condition monitoring).

A refocus on maintaining strong therapeutic relationships will likely be necessary if AI health monitoring is to fulfill its potential of enhancing users' autonomy. The expanding market for health monitoring algorithms, especially DTC devices and applications, has created a paradox for therapeutic alliance. On the one hand, these products promise users more independence from, or more equal partnership with, health care providers through continuous and convenient data collection and self-monitoring.[15] Users can allegedly regain power and challenge medical dominance by behaving as self-responsible, knowledgeable, and self-sufficient actors; they can generate their own data and personalized outputs to monitor their own health and self-manage their symptoms confidently, thereby potentially avoiding unnecessary visits to a physician.[16] On the other hand, most AI health monitoring device makers do not provide further counseling or care management beyond AI-guided recommendations. Thus, instead of minimizing reliance on the health care system, as often suggested by

AI enthusiasts, these products may actually increase system burden. Some patients may have to consult their clinicians precisely *because of* predictive outputs, such as when the device offers ambiguous information or encourages asymptomatic users who otherwise were not concerned about their health to seek professional advice based on data that are ultimately not clinically meaningful.[17] If our current system is proliferating devices that neither improve patient outcomes nor reduce costs, it is problematic.[18]

Health systems and individual health care providers need to anticipate how these potentially opposing forces may restructure care relationships and patient expectations, especially bearing in mind that system inadequacy and patients' feelings of disempowerment may be driving their interest in using AI health monitoring in the first place. Health care providers who maintain or develop robust therapeutic relationships with their patients can promote autonomy and well-being by discussing with patients whether existing or desired algorithmic technologies can indeed enhance their care, helping patients interpret findings, or guiding them to access AI-recommended follow-up actions. At the same time, because commercial AI health monitoring algorithms are often touted as giving patients more control over their data and care, a strong therapeutic alliance is particularly important when patients bring forth AI-guided recommendations or request associated follow-up interventions that conflict with health care providers' own clinical judgment. Clinicians can help to promote patients' self-governance and self-determination by protecting them from misinformation, promoting health and digital literacy, clarifying the algorithmic findings and limitations,[19] and engaging in shared decision-making with their patients to collaboratively determine an appropriate care plan, rather than ordering low-value follow-up tests or interventions simply to avoid possible claims of paternalism or litigation.[20] Otherwise, these technological practices may further dehumanize the care delivery process, diminish the role of clinicians to technicians who mostly interpret and implement algorithmic outputs,[21] and lead patients to undergo unnecessary procedures that may incur other inconveniences or even iatrogenic harm.

It is worth noting that maintenance of strong therapeutic relationships in the evolving era of big data and algorithmic analytics is not simply an individual professional's endeavor or responsibility. A relational framework of autonomy highlights how health care providers' capacity to promote patients' self-governance at this technological juncture depends on the former's communication and digital training as well as other institutional and system workflow factors. Thus, promotion of autonomy-enhancing therapeutic relationships in the emerging AI era requires a systems approach. Given that endless data streams and alerts from heterogeneous devices may prompt monitored users to seek frequent follow-up contact with their care providers, physicians may have trouble keeping up with the rapidly expanding field. Without broader digital education, system support, financial incentives (e.g., fee codes for AI exploration), or health system reorganization, AI health monitoring algorithms may paradoxically reduce busy providers' inclination to fully engage with patients' perspectives,[22] disempowering both patients and clinicians. For example, a 2016 study found that medical digitization resulted in physicians spending two hours doing computer work for every in-person hour spent with a patient.[23] And in the growing environment for DTC genetic testing, genetic counselors have also been getting more requests in recent years from people who want help interpreting their own test results.[24] These trends signal how the increasing ubiquity of DTC AI health monitoring developed by lay technologists and entrepreneurs may impose a further burden on health care providers and the health system as a whole.

Even if a reorganized system, facilitated by more accurate and clinically valuable AI, could promote efficiency in the long run, in the context of profit- or cost-driven health systems that are trying to leverage AI health monitoring to reduce in-person consultations, it remains uncertain whether clinicians would be able to redistribute any potential time saved by AI processes to deeper exploration with the same patients, rather than appointments with additional patients.[25] It is also important to keep in mind that licensed clinicians remain the gatekeepers of prescriptions, laboratory tests, sick leave, and other resources.[26] If the growing adoption of AI health monitoring technologies—whether commercial devices or clinician-recommended platforms—is not paired with intentional systemic efforts to enhance collaborative therapeutic relationships and workflow efficiency, these technologies may further disempower patients and alienate their perspectives rather than enhance their autonomy.

It is not only patients' trust in health care providers and the health system that must be preserved; a commitment to enhancing therapeutic relationships and promoting autonomy in the evolving digital era also requires health care providers to direct their attention towards the grounds for trust in their patients.[27] In particular, this involves refraining from using AI technologies as surveillance mechanisms to regulate distrust, which may exacerbate an oppressive power hierarchy. Any AI monitoring algorithms adopted by health care providers should be validated, supported by evidence, and shown to be more reliable than other methods for achieving the explicitly stated target. Moreover, promotion of autonomy requires that recommendations, decisions, and implementation plans should meaningfully engage with users' perspectives and priorities. This commitment is especially important for patients who are flagged for continuous monitoring for their safety, such as older adults and people with psychiatric or pain conditions. Targeting certain populations or individuals for monitoring renders these people even more vulnerable to losing freedom and/or privacy within care relationships, which are already inherently asymmetrical. As norms about various patient groups and patient behaviors get encoded into these technologies, we need to be particularly vigilant about checking for biases in algorithms that may reinforce stigmas and other disadvantages.

As we have seen in the examples of home health and medication adherence monitoring, continuous observation of certain patients' activities is sometimes deemed justifiable or even necessary from health care providers' or family members' perspectives due to concerns about targeted users' credibility, either in terms of their intentions or competence (or both). However, when health care providers use AI technologies as tools for surveillance to manage concerns of distrust, they place undue confidence in the objectivity, accuracy, and broad applicability of these algorithms and in their own determination of the ideal care goal, which may prompt them to disregard or at least cast doubt on other significant information, including patients' own narratives and health targets.[28] This "prejudicial dysfunction in testimonial practice," as Miranda Fricker calls it,[29] is a form of epistemic injustice that can directly compromise distrusted and monitored users' self-governance, self-determination, and self-authorization, as health care providers who put undue faith in algorithmic outputs may not recognize the need to critically reflect on their potential prejudice. Health care providers who adopt a default position of distrust may presume that health monitoring algorithms are categorically more reliable and/or informative than patients' own reports, such that they may prematurely and unfairly dismiss any patient perspectives, concerns, or testimonies that conflict with algorithmic outputs. This in turn may compromise patients' care experience and ability to direct their own care plan according to their practical identities or to advocate for themselves. As we saw in the last chapter, using AI medication monitoring to regulate distrust may lead health care providers to adopt a myopic focus on actual dosing, categorize nonadherence as individual failure, and place moral blame on patients who are deemed untrustworthy and thus in need of surveillance. For example, in the context of managing CNMP, there is a worry that the focus on algorithmic outputs may replace rather than enhance conversations about the real dangers of over-valuing and under-delivering opioids for long-term pain relief, or detract from efforts to fully understand patients' broader goals and concerns to help determine more appropriate pain relief modalities accordingly.

It is worth emphasizing that putting faith in inaccurate algorithms instead of helping patients form optimal care plans based on their multifaceted concerns can further increase distrust towards the health care system among marginalized individuals, who are already wary of the therapeutic space and clinician recommendations.[30] Nonetheless, even if the algorithm's measurements and predictions are accurate, constantly being watched and analyzed may affect patients' own self-conception. Moreover, the framing of these technologies as primarily deception detectors may lead health care providers to miss other important factors influencing a patient's medication decisions, such as side effects, complicated treatment regimens, or poor social functioning.[31] Indeed, distrusting patients based on even accurate forecasts, rather than seeking to understand the contexts around patients' medication decisions and communication, may ironically sustain or even exacerbate treatment adherence problems instead of promoting clinically appropriate pharmacotherapy and goal-concordant treatment plans. In the context of distrust, patients may not have the opportunity or self-confidence to discuss their health beliefs or explore how to address their competing therapeutic considerations,[32] or they may be reluctant to divulge sensitive information because they do not believe that a physician who distrusts them would truly consider and advocate for their needs.[33] At the same time, clinicians may overlook significant contextual elements, such as high drug costs and lack of socio-familial support, that can affect medication behaviors. For example, AI medication dosage monitoring may aim to increase antipsychotic medication compliance. However, for some patients, medication compliance may incur such burdensome side effects that it outweighs any improvement in psychotic symptoms and fails to achieve patients' ideal target of optimizing well-being.[34] If the AI monitoring system's target is predetermined by technologists or health care providers without meaningful user input, it may not align with the patient's goals, such that recommendations may fail to enhance productive adherence or patient outcomes.

By contrast, a default stance of promoting reciprocal trust and acknowledging the limited role or utility of AI monitoring in determining appropriate care plans allows care providers to build rapport with patients and remain open to broader perspectives—ones that are not captured by algorithmic analysis but may be even more important in collaboratively determining and reaching the patient's care goal. For example, we have seen how medication decisions are dynamic behaviors, influenced by intersecting individual, medication, professional, and system considerations. When algorithmic outputs are used primarily as a point of embarkation to promote more conversations, with physicians inviting patients' own narratives to help interpret, evaluate, and situate AI algorithmic outputs, they can strengthen therapeutic relationships. They may optimize a bidirectional understanding of the nuanced but intertwining individual, socio-relational, and structural-environmental factors that may cause difficulties or distress, place burdens on patients, and affect their ability or desire to adhere to a standard pharmacotherapy regimen.[35] For example, using AI dosage measurements in a nonjudgmental, problem-solving manner to identify the patient's highest priorities and potential obstacles to adherence and well-being may facilitate goal-concordant and context-sensitive care that can optimize outcomes. Even in situations where there may be a lack of good reasons to trust the patient, the act of believing them, or at least expressing the possibility of such trust and allowing the recipient the opportunity to demonstrate that they can live up to expectations, may constructively influence the trusted person's behavior to be more collaborative.[36]

A default stance of reciprocal trust is essential for autonomy, as we cannot promote self-authorization or patient well-being if we do not acknowledge the patient as a moral agent, capable of understanding and making choices as well as being accountable for them.[37] It is worth noting that reciprocal trust may promote greater therapeutic success, insofar as patients who know that they are trusted, rather than doubted or disparaged based on predictive analysis, are likely to be more willing and confident to report their routines and express their concerns (e.g., regarding medications, pain, or addiction). Placing trust allows patients to see themselves as co-creators of knowledge around their practical identity and the various determinants of their health behavior, while also allowing health care providers to glean more insight into how to support patients in developing health managements skills or utilize available resources. The focus can then shift from locating problems of adherence in the individual, waiting to be detected and corrected by algorithms, to interrogating how intersecting and multidimensional factors may affect patients' ability to establish and follow goal-concordant care plans, including pharmacotherapies.

As AI technologists continue to refine existing algorithms and develop new ones, recognizing the importance of these broader factors may also help determine what other forms of data AI developers should collect and incorporate into algorithmic analysis to better understand the patient's context.[38] Instead of focusing only on dosage adherence or using algorithms merely to "catch" deception, if the ideal target is better health outcomes or quality of life as collaboratively defined by the health care provider and the patient, it may be more useful to develop AI algorithms that can identify risk factors and thereby help health care providers and health systems design multiprong strategies that truly support patients' care journeys. For example, studies have shown that for patients with mental illnesses, satisfaction level with the information given,[39] trust in the system providing health services,[40] lower socioeconomic status, minority ethnicity, and experience with barriers to care are all social and systemic determinants of their medication experience.[41] And in the area of pain management, patients who receive treatment from high-intensity opioid prescribers, or have inadequate education regarding iatrogenic addiction[42] and safe storage or proper disposal of unused medication,[43] are more likely to become long-term opioid users.[44] Population-level algorithms that incorporate these multifaceted sets of behavioral, clinical, and structural-level data may help to generate deeper and more comprehensive insights into professional and system gaps as well as patient experiences and concerns. They may inform professional education as well as responsive pharmacotherapeutic and other social support resources to optimize care delivery and holistic care.[45] As patients consider medication as one of the means to achieve the best possible outcome, rather than the ideal target in itself, incorporating correlations between different levels of adherence and health outcomes as well as quality of life may also help patients weigh the benefits and drawbacks of taking various doses of medication, and guide physicians to reframe the problem of nonadherence so as to respect patients' self-authorization and better support their priorities and needs.

2. Dialogic Engagement as a Feedback Loop for AI Health Monitoring

As we have seen, AI advances in health care are not morally neutral technological endeavors,[46] and the relevant autonomy considerations go beyond informed consent for specific technologies or health outcomes.[47] Patients who are required or expected to accept monitoring as part of care delivery and/or operational decisions may not truly have the option to refuse monitoring or data sharing. They also may not be able to access the health monitoring modality that is most aligned with their practical identity (e.g., subsidized in-person home health monitoring) if they reject AI health monitoring. As these expanding technological practices gradually restructure users' lives and care pathways, both at home and in formal care settings, they emerge as culturally and relationally complex phenomena, reflecting and potentially reinforcing various social and medical norms, including AI solutionism and the technological imperative, whereby AI health monitoring is presumed to be a superior practice. The implication is that rejecting these technologies signals suboptimal care,[48] irrationality, or even personal irresponsibility towards one's health. Certainly, with the expanding availability of high-quality and diverse datasets, as well as advancing computational techniques, AI health monitoring technologies will likely continue to improve. But from a relational autonomy perspective, it is important to ask whose voices and priorities will inform the investments, goals, methods, and implementation of AI health monitoring; how these algorithms and devices will be evaluated or governed to ensure secure data practices as well as safe utilization; and how concerns, uncertainties, and disagreements will be handled.

Given these intertwining considerations, if AI health monitoring hopes to enhance users' various dimensions of relational autonomy and promote high-value and equitable care, a multilevel dialogic engagement,[49] comprising the individual, technological, professional/institutional, and societal levels, will be necessary to hold a broad range of stakeholders answerable to critical perspectives on these health monitoring practices and to empower prospective users in their engagement and/or decision-making. These engagements can serve as a symbiotic bioethical-technical feedback loop to inform computer engineers, entrepreneurial developers, clinicians, and decision-makers on how these technologies should be conceptualized, developed, implemented, evaluated, and governed in order to optimize autonomy-enhancing care relationships, decision processes, and care pathways. In particular, inclusive and collaborative dialogic engagement tools, such as user surveys, patient advisory groups, professional curricula, independent reviews, data sharing registries, AI review boards, and audit systems, may enhance users' capacity and confidence in comprehending and exploring these technologies in the context of their practical identity. They can also help developers and decision-makers to truly understand, respect, and uphold users' priorities, allowing them to develop and implement user-centric technologies that promote people's self-governance, self-determination, and self-authorization along their health maintenance and care pathways.

From a relational perspective, multilevel dialogic engagement is especially important because heterogeneous stakeholders who occupy different social and epistemic locations in the evolving technological space potentially have divergent goals and concerns, which may in turn introduce or reinforce power asymmetry as well as health disparity. Moreover, commercial actors and technologists, though only loosely regulated, are increasingly driving the AI health agenda and exerting social authority in this realm by reframing how personal and health data are collected, utilized, analyzed, presented, and shared. For example, Amazon, the e-commerce giant, announced in July 2022 an almost $4 billion deal to purchase One Medical, a subscription-based and tech-focused primary care organization.[50] Amazon's AI platforms already track customers' purchasing activities, streaming preferences, home environment monitoring, and prescription patterns (through its purchase of online pharmacy PillPack). This latest acquisition raises further privacy and data governance questions of whether or how Amazon may access and use the medical records of One Medical's approximately 767,000 members to glean further insights about these patients as consumers.[51]

As AI health monitoring is increasingly ubiquitous and is gradually changing the entire self-management and health care delivery landscape, multilevel engagements and feedback loops can serve as critical components of the accountability structure to help promote prospective users' relational autonomy. By recognizing the importance of being socially prepared to answer users and relevant stakeholders who may have questions regarding these technological practices, and being open to revising their responses or strategies in light of this questioning, dialogic engagement can be both a collaborative and governance strategy. It can help to build stakeholders' understanding and appreciation of the issues at hand and hold them accountable to (prospective) users and clinicians, thereby promoting safe, effective, transparent, and empowering technological development and implementation.

2.1 User-First Approach Through Dialogic Engagement

At the individual user and family levels, we have seen throughout this book various ways in which big data and AI health development are gradually changing how individuals seek and receive ongoing health monitoring and who may be providing such observation. While predictive computation technologies offer exciting potential for more convenient, efficient, and accurate processes, at least for specific tasks in narrow contexts, their clinical value in promoting better health outcomes remains to be seen. In order to truly promote autonomy and facilitate stakeholders' meaningful participation, dialogic engagement is needed to elucidate how prospective users of diverse sociocultural and health backgrounds may perceive the utility, acceptability, and trustworthiness of AI health monitoring technologies for everyday care in light of their practical and illness identities.[52] For example, studies have shown that patients are reluctant to utilize even effective AI health algorithms when they perceive that their personal factors may not conform with standardized algorithmic outputs.[53] This is understandable, especially since each patient has a unique configuration of elements comprising their identity, illness experience, and physical, social, and environmental contexts.[54] Moreover, even "personalized" algorithmic outputs may have hidden biases, such as when diverse patients' input data are interpreted according to patterns taken from homogeneous training datasets,[55] as we saw in the examples of biased skin lesion and population health management algorithms.[56]

Dialogic engagement at the individual user level may also inform clinicians and technology developers of users' health and digital literacy levels, what types of personal and health data they would be willing to share for the purpose of algorithmic prediction and with whom (e.g., family, health care providers, device companies), their priorities and expectations of these technological practices, and how they may consider different privacy tradeoffs and algorithmic uncertainties. Engagement with the individuals and social groups who are the focus of such technologies is particularly important for establishing shared understandings of the physiological data, experiences, or phenomena subject to monitoring and intervention. For example, patient and community advisory groups as well as usability testing may help to shed light on the experiences and priorities of (prospective) users and those who may have to support the users being monitored (e.g., family caregivers). They may facilitate the development and refinement of user-centric algorithms and interfaces that truly support monitored individuals' goals,[57] and inform the advancement of technologies that can help family caregivers confidently and safely care for their loved ones.[58] It may also help health care providers and technologists to plan training or technological support that can promote users' capacity to learn to use the technology as they navigate changes in their health and illness identities. Otherwise, these technological practices may exacerbate the digital divide and leave users who are trying to prove their ability to manage their own health, such as older adults with early-stage dementia, feeling even more disempowered as they doubt their own capacity to operate, control, or interact with the system.[59]

Incorporating users' perspectives and experiences can improve not only the robustness of algorithmic models but also implementation plans. While users' willingness to adopt AI health monitoring is most likely based on utilitarian or instrumental considerations, the actual implementation of these technologies involves other normative, moral, and social meanings that prospective users may incorporate into their discernment, such as how being continuously monitored and analyzed by predictive technologies may affect their illness and relational identities as well as their ability to negotiate with others around their care priorities. For example, in a study assessing older adults' experience using a remote health monitoring system that collects biometric information and addresses health topics such as nutrition, diabetes, cardiac care, and medication compliance, the longer participants used the technology, the more they perceived that those important to them would want them to use it, regardless of their own wishes.[60] Knowledge of users' perspectives on and sensitivity to these power dynamics may help clinicians and health systems collaboratively determine how to navigate the impact of social influence on older adults' technology adoption and provide them more opportunities to control the timing and duration of monitoring, as well as when and how data may be shared with others. Given that being under the continuous gaze of technology may affect the social and normative meanings of independent living, as well as control over one's life and information, dialogic engagement can also help technologists and clinicians to appreciate how prospective users may weigh different considerations, such as the freedom to turn off tracking functions at various intervals, which may provide more privacy and control but forfeit certain levels of predictive accuracy due to interrupted data streams. Moreover, as health systems increasingly rely on patients' family members to facilitate remote home health monitoring, dialogic engagement at the user level may also help health care providers and health systems determine how to support family caregivers, who may have to navigate the moral meanings and practical implications of taking on additional care and financial responsibilities as a result of these evolving AI health monitoring practices.

Dialogic engagement at the user level can also help shift the focus from relying solely on individual consent for a particular technology to having a comprehensive understanding of individual *and* sociorelational determinants of behavior and choice that can help to support prospective users' self-conceptions and priorities.[61] This collaborative engagement may be particularly important in promoting accountability when users are expected or required to agree to being monitored, and/or when the technologies are targeting individuals whose capacity to (withdraw) consent to continuous observation and longitudinal data sharing may gradually decline, such as older adults with dementia.[62] Participatory and user-driven design processes may help to integrate the actual needs and resources of older users into the technology development and implementation plans. In short, dialogic engagement can minimize the potential for coercive paternalism by elucidating users' overall goals and concerns and clarifying whom prospective users believe should hold the power over usage, data sharing, and discontinuance in these situations. Such engagement with targeted users (or representative advisory groups) can also help to uncover divergent perspectives among stakeholders in different social locations and roles, so as to address how various strategies may empower or disempower monitored users. This may help stakeholders to collaboratively determine how to incorporate these respective priorities and concerns into technology and implementation designs to ensure autonomy-enhancing practices.

2.2 Technological Transparency as a Path to Relational Autonomy

Currently, the limited technological, evidential, and operational (i.e., business) transparency of various medical and wellness tracking algorithms prevents (prospective) users and independent parties from evaluating these algorithms, hampering their ability to build capacity and knowledge that are important for prospective users to explore how these technologies may fit with their health goals and priorities. Dialogic engagement at the technological level is necessary for enhancing users' technological literacy and holding developers and decision-makers accountable. From a relational perspective, in order to truly promote users' self-governance, it is also essential to minimize power asymmetry between technology companies and the users. Dialogic engagement at the technological level can help hold developers accountable for ensuring that their algorithm is accurately and equitably predicting its ideal target for the intended users,[63] and informing prospective users how their data may be protected, used, and/or shared.

As we work to ensure that the socio-technological processes behind AI development and implementation promote accountability and user autonomy, dialogic engagement involves computer engineers and technology implementers being transparent regarding the intentions, indications for use, goals of an AI application, data sources for development (e.g., what population groups), and evidence of safety and efficacy, so that potential users (including both individuals and health care organizations) are better enabled to exercise their evaluative and decisional autonomy.[64] In the arena of DTC AI health apps, app stores can play stronger roles in requiring and enforcing relevant standards.[65] While deep neural networks may limit the feasibility of algorithmic explainability, human beings have significant oversight over them and can remain "in the loop" throughout the designing and monitoring processes, such that dialogic engagement between technologists and decision-makers may help to determine appropriate standards on explainability.[66] Once the goal of the algorithm is known, dialogic engagement at the technological level places the burden on technology developers to explain what data are collected, why these data are necessary for analysis, whether the data will be shared with third parties for other purposes, and what technical solutions and oversight mechanisms they have for ensuring data safety and security.[67]

While AI technologists often claim that patient-generated data can help to democratize health data, users may need assurance that the promises of AI health monitoring technologies do not inadvertently lead to the collection and incorporation of irrelevant data in algorithmic analyses that may produce inaccurate results and further burden monitored users, family and professional caregivers, and health systems. With the expanding availability and use of digital "biomarkers," which are potential indicators of disease, professionals and policymakers need to establish clear guidance on how to prevent the phenomenon of "biomarkup," whereby technologists, health care providers, health systems, laboratory testing services, or even patients themselves advocate for more testing and intervention when the presence of these biomarkers (especially from sensitive detection platforms) may not indicate a health problem, or when there is no reliable evidence that further investigations would improve outcomes.[68] As we have learned from criticisms of DTC genetic tests, the information provided for many tested conditions is not clinically meaningful and can be misinterpreted, but simply suggesting the probability of a potential health problem can already shape users' perception of the technology's value, and further testing and procedures can yield financial benefits for technologists and service providers. As these technologies continue to be aggressively marketed to the masses, dialogic engagement at the technological level is necessary to help create space for users and health care providers to address how to interpret outputs in context to prevent intentional and nonintentional overtesting and overtreatment.

As part of the excitement about AI technologies, particularly DL algorithms, is their potential abilities to iteratively improve with new data and experiences, dialogic engagement at the technological level also requires clarification on whether a particular AI health monitoring system being marketed or recommended is "locked" versus "continuously learning." Locked systems involve algorithms whose function is fixed, providing the same result each time for the same input and requiring manual processes for updates and validation. By contrast, as we have already seen, "continuously learning" AI systems are autonomous systems whose behavior can adapt over time, which has the potential of optimizing device performance in real time without human intervention.[69] Currently, most FDA-cleared or -approved AI medical devices are locked prior to marketing; their functions do not change or improve based on new input data. Clarification on this feature is important, as clinician users and those who are monitored need to be aware of the implications. For example, if users are using a locked natural language processing (NLP) chatbot to track their mental health symptoms, they need to recognize that, if the system is producing ambiguous or incorrect answers, it will not iteratively provide better results based on further conversations of the same sort (e.g., same wording of various symptoms) until manual updates by the developer are provided.[70]

From a relational autonomy perspective, technological dialogic engagement provides a mechanism for developers to be answerable regarding the reliability and validity of the technology for intended populations, and the accuracy of promotional claims. Such engagement to promote answerability is necessary to minimize power asymmetry between technologists or entrepreneurial developers and users, since opacity regarding safety, effectiveness, and data practice can compromises users' motivational structure and ability to incorporate the health monitoring algorithm's benefits and risks into their own decision-making. Accountability at the technological level should go beyond providing company-sponsored study data, both to ensure critical evaluation and to equalize power relations. As technologists and entrepreneurial developers often control the data and the promotional messages that claim various connections to such data, answerability requires independent reviews to confirm validity and accuracy. The ongoing close connection between technical development, evaluation, and reporting—wherein studies are both conducted and reported by those who are commercially involved with the platforms—reveals a lack of safeguards against the effects of financial conflict and raises questions as to whether technologists are truly answerable to legitimate inquiries regarding their claims.[71] Dialogic engagement can help the public, decision-makers, and other stakeholders to determine if there should be information repositories or registries where the public can find out more about how the content of the platform is created, who performs this content creation, how often it is updated (e.g., for locked systems), the funders or sponsors of the developers, and how any personal data that are collected by these devices are used, stored, or shared. Such information can help prospective users determine whether these technological processes are aligned with their risk–benefit analysis.[72] For example, dialogic engagement may help to clarify whether pharmaceutical or device companies whose products are recommended are contributing to the content, allowing users to recognize that any claims of "objective" algorithmic analysis may be accompanied by other commercial interests.

Importantly, the need for technological dialogic engagement holds whether the health monitoring algorithm is considered a wellness or a medical device. This is because even platforms that do not fit the definition of a medical device for regulatory purposes are nonetheless making authoritative claims about their social and clinical value and their ability to promote people's autonomy, self-knowledge, and well-being. Moreover, DTC devices amass vast amounts of heterogeneous personal data from users, giving entrepreneurial developers further power over those who are continuously tracked. In the United States, while the Federal Trade Commission (FTC) investigates complaints about unsafe algorithms or deceptive marketing claims, such as whether companies are utilizing ambiguous or contradictory language to claim high value of their products while simultaneously insisting that their platforms are recreational rather than advisory, these reactive strategies may still fail to promote users' confidence or self-authorization. For example, users who suffer from any adverse effects may be confused about whether the company's marketing claims are actually violating FTC guidelines, or whether they themselves are at fault for believing the claims (albeit misleading ones) put forth by these companies. Dialogic engagement can help stakeholders clarify expectations regarding wellness devices that often make bold and misleading claims but currently do not require regulatory review.

2.3 It's Not Just the Tool but How You Use It: Professional/Institutional Decisions Around AI Implementation

At the professional/institutional level, health care providers, health systems, and funders (e.g., investors, health insurance companies, corporate wellness programs) play integral roles in determining the conceptualization, development, implementation, and incorporation of algorithmic analysis into health monitoring. Dialogic engagement at this level involves establishing mechanisms for stakeholders to collaboratively determine the criteria for AI health monitoring adoption, as well as processes for communicating these criteria and decisions to patients. Transparency about institutional decisions to adopt AI health monitoring and surrounding care delivery and data protection practices is particularly important from a relational perspective, given that these decisions may be operational, such that individual patients are often required to participate—nontransparent processes can reinforce the inherent power asymmetry in these situations. For example, as hospital discharge decisions are often made based on whether there is a safe discharge plan, a hospital's recommendation to send a patient home rather than to a long-term care facility may depend on a patient's willingness to be remotely and continuously monitored by AI-assisted devices. These recommendations can exert further control over patients or even their family members, as they can directly affect patients' ability to determine how they want to live and be monitored, even as they regain some level of health and functioning, and how the family may manage the patient's post-hospitalization care. Dialogic engagement at the institutional level requires organizations to be transparent about what outcomes the institutions want and expect to achieve with proposed technologies, how these desired outcomes align with patients' goals and interests, and how proposed algorithms are deemed superior to other monitoring modalities in achieving the desired outcomes. This may include explaining the types and levels of evidence supporting the validity and reliability of AI health monitoring technologies for the intended patients. In particular, institutions need to be transparent about whether the algorithms were trained on adequately representative data to allow for high confidence that the outputs will be accurate for intended populations, or whether there has been any trial period where the safety and efficacy of the algorithm was monitored in its implementation settings.[73] Summary statistics about the general characteristics of participants and their distribution can provide basic information for public scrutiny while still protecting privacy and companies' proprietary information.

It is worth noting that some of the risks and benefits of health monitoring technologies depend on the implementation plan, such as when and where in a patient's care pathway a medication monitoring algorithm may be proposed. For the increasing number of organizations that incentivize corporate wellness through continuing monitoring and behavioral nudging, they also need to be answerable to whether deployment of these technologies may compromise employees' privacy and reinforce power and domination, as companies may now gain access to employees' intimate information (e.g., pregnancy status, mental health concerns) that have generally been off limit to employers. Dialogic engagement may thus include disclosure of known/potential risks and burdens of the implementation of proposed technology and any institutional plans to mitigate such risks, such as mechanisms to minimize the chance that people will be identified via the plethora of data being collected. Given that deployment of AI health monitoring as an operational decision may already deny users some level of freedom to refuse participation, and that AI predictions are probabilistic rather than definitive, dialogic engagement to determine how users may dispute algorithmic outputs is also important to optimize users' self-determination and self-authorization.

AI requires intensive data for algorithmic training and testing, and responsible and responsive data collection and data sharing practices are necessary to ensure that patients of diverse backgrounds can benefit from scientific advances and a learning health care system.[74] Institutions and health systems thus need to develop community-informed governance mechanisms to balance data privacy and social good in AI monitoring research and development. In addition, health systems are increasingly collaborating with commercial partners to develop AI-assisted health monitoring technologies and are sharing de-identified EHR data with those partners. Cautions abound that companies and health care organizations that collect, combine, and share massive amounts of data in complex data flow do not always have clear and enforced policies of how they process and govern data,[75] leaving stakeholders in the dark while exerting additional power on them by using people's own data to influence or discipline their behavior. Dialogic engagement provides a valuable mechanism for determining how data sharing arrangements should be established, governed, and audited, including whether or how patients will have the opportunity to be informed of these agreements. As the Health Insurance Portability and Accountability Act (HIPAA) regulations in the United States protect identifiable data collected by covered entities, but not necessarily anonymized data for secondary usage, disclosure on how patient data will be stored and shared is important in promoting digital literacy and preserving patient autonomy. Health systems like the Mayo Clinic explain that these arrangements are part of a cycle of innovation, whereby privacy and progress are parallel goals in helping to develop more effective technologies.[76] Nonetheless, recent U.S. federal initiatives by the Department of Health and Human Services to increase patient access to EHR data via mobile apps have been met with fierce resistance from some health systems due to privacy concerns.[77]

Dialogic engagement may allow stakeholders to have a better understanding of research lifecycles in the context of big data, weigh divergent considerations, and determine well-balanced guidelines that protect patient data security without stalling innovations that may enhance health monitoring and care delivery. This may help institutions establish responsive governance bodies or data request review boards (e.g., similar to institutional review boards) to promote accountable institutional processes that balance data confidentiality/security and public benefits. These entities may help determine and communicate the criteria and procedures for evaluating requests for data sharing, how/if the post-sharing data use may be monitored, and what data security provisions are included in these endeavors. For example, health system decision-makers can clarify to concerned parties if the system is selling anonymized datasets to data brokers versus only sharing data with technology firms to co-develop technologies or train/test health monitoring algorithms that are intended for patients in the health system. These different arrangements may have divergent implications on who will retain control over the data, including whether commercial partners can still utilize the datasets for their own commercial purposes upon termination of these endeavors (e.g., partnerships between IBM Watson and various academic health centers discussed in the introductory chapter), and how patients may consider the social value of their data contribution and the legitimacy of these sharing practices. These dialogic mechanisms are particularly helpful when it is not feasible to seek individual consent, either because it may be unduly burdensome to seek consent or remove individual patients' data from massive datasets, or because doing so could result in unrepresentative datasets. When certain populations are more likely to opt out of having even their de-identified data shared for quality improvement purposes—whether due to historical distrust in the health system or other reasons—there may be consent bias in the dataset, as more trusting populations, who are often more privileged, are disproportionately represented. This representational imbalance may in turn lead to health data poverty and inequitable health benefits, whereby certain individuals, groups, or populations fail to benefit from an AI innovation due to a scarcity of representative data.[78] Dialogic engagement at this level may help health systems explain when bypassing individual consent may be necessary for accurate and equitable algorithmic development and what mechanisms are in place to ensure that these practices will not pose data risk or other harm to patients (e.g., through AI audit).

Because effective operationalization of AI health monitoring by health care organizations often requires upfront funding, significant training for relevant stakeholders (e.g., monitored users, informal caregivers, and clinicians), and behavioral change interventions throughout the organizational and system levels, dialogic engagement at the professional/institutional level can shed light on what professional and continuing education curricula and change management support will be necessary to prepare health care providers in the evolving technological era, and how various stakeholders perceive this investment and the accompanying (potentially disruptive) changes. Such meso-level engagement can also help institutions assess and communicate their broader priorities, weigh the workforce and workflow implications, and invest responsibly and responsively.

For example, the COVID-19 pandemic has accelerated the emergence of hospital-at-home programs, which allow hospitals to receive Medicare reimbursement for at-home care services for more than sixty conditions.[79] These programs harness remote monitoring in combination with AI analytics and human adjudication to allow patients to convalesce at home in a more intimate, familiar, and affordable environment. However, such technologies will undeniably influence institutional investment in technological and human resources, discharge planning, and labor relations in both the short term and beyond the pandemic.[80] They can have direct impact on whether patients truly have the opportunity to refuse these technologies and still uphold their health maintenance goals. Dialogic engagement with not only patients and families but also clinicians and other decision-makers will be important to critically explore their perspectives and concerns around these changes and adjust adoption, implementation, and evaluation plans accordingly. Such engagement can also provide the opportunity for meso-level stakeholders to collaboratively establish mechanisms or processes to decide whether or when predictive analytics may be used (or should be halted), how to measure the safety and efficacy of these technologies, and how to audit for quality assurance and improvement.

2.4 AI Should Not Be a Band-Aid: Using Dialogic Engagement to Address Structural Issues

At the fourth level, the societal level, intersecting technological, operational, and ethical questions abound. As relational autonomy attends to contextual and structural factors affecting people's ability to live and make health monitoring decisions according to their practical identities, it highlights how applying AI technologies to a disempowering system without attempting to correct the structure and/or its operation to explicitly enhance patients' capacity, freedom, and/or confidence to enact and attain their health management goals is unlikely to achieve significant transformation or promote patient autonomy.[81] In addition, given that there is already systemic inequality in health care, dialogic engagement at the societal level can shed light on whether or how increasing utilization of AI health monitoring technologies may exacerbate inequity, and help determine the best strategies to prevent such occurrence. The ongoing digital divide, where people with high digital literacy and access to technologies can benefit from AI innovations, but those who lack these opportunities are unable to utilize these services and may also lose traditional services that are gradually reduced, can further disenfranchise historically underserved populations. Moreover, since data from historical datasets are used to train AI systems, algorithms can magnify and exacerbate the aforementioned health data poverty and inequities by virtue of biased outputs, as we saw in the example of the population health management algorithm that assigned extra support to patients based on past health care utilization and spending data.[82] Centering promotion of relational autonomy, dialogic engagement at the societal level can shed light on how stakeholders can determine feasible strategies to hold decision-makers answerable and responsible for promoting accurate and equitable AI health monitoring practices.

Dialogic engagement at the societal level can also illuminate how system forces either help people to fulfill their health goals and priorities or hinder their efforts,[83] and how the broader utilization of AI health monitoring is positively and/or negatively affecting the general public's views about health, wellness, illness, and what it means to be a patient or family caregiver.[84] It can also help to determine whether existing governance and regulatory approaches are adequate in managing these evolving and disruptive socio-technological practices and holding relevant stakeholders accountable, or if new frameworks will be necessary to ensure that people truly have meaningful opportunities to explore, understand, access, and refuse various health monitoring options according to their practical identities. For example, in the United States, a AI Bill of Rights put forth by the White House in October 2022 encourages technology developers to take "proactive and continuous measures" to protect users based on five principles: ensure safe and effective systems; protect users from algorithmic discrimination; strengthen data privacy and user control over their data; notify and explain to users when AI systems are used and the potential impact; and allow users to opt out of AI systems and have human oversight over these systems.[85] Nonetheless, the bill is a nonbinding white paper, and there is currently no other legislation requiring entrepreneurial developers to provide privacy or data policy statements in their informational materials,[86] even though commercialization of data from medically related apps, platforms, and websites is an increasingly common and profitable practice.[87] When companies provide such information, the policies are often complex and verbose, and may confuse rather than promote understanding of implications. As big data analytics as well as the storage and trading of digital data raise further concerns about data security, dialogic engagement at the broader societal level may provide the opportunity for policymakers to involve diverse stakeholders across various social locations in determining how these technological practices should be governed to ensure trustworthiness. Such stakeholder engagement is important, since the burgeoning market for consumer devices that amass heterogeneous user data at least raises questions of whether consumers share the same levels of concerns as privacy experts regarding data sharing or data brokerage. Broader societal engagement through surveys, qualitative research, and townhall meetings can help to determine whether users are unaware of various implications of privacy and data security issues,[88] of if they are aware of these issues and have access to different health monitoring options, but truly accept the potential tradeoffs for perceived benefits of using these technologies.

Dialogic engagement may also help the public and decision-makers balance the proprietary rights of developers and the need to hold them accountable for the validity, safety, and/or clinical value of their algorithms for the intended users. In the United States, some efforts have already been put forth by the FDA to engage multilevel stakeholders in determining best practices for developing and governing AI health technologies that seek agency clearance or approval as medical devices,[89] including expectations of operational transparency and algorithmic explainability. However, further dialogic engagement can help to determine if entities similar to data safety and monitoring boards (DSMBs), which undertake periodic risk–benefit assessments throughout a clinical trial using gathered data during the study, may be helpful in monitoring the safety of new AI health monitoring devices. A societal-level dialogic engagement can also inform whether additional governance and/or regulations may be required for health monitoring algorithms that are not seeking FDA clearance. For this vastly expanding class of devices that claim to be merely wellness or recreational platforms, enthusiasts often tout these products as democratizing personal and health information and empowering people to take control over their health. Dialogic engagement can help to determine if these devices should at minimum be proactively answerable to regulatory bodies and consumer advocacy groups regarding the validity of their algorithms in performing the designated tasks, rather than only responding to formal complaints filed with regulatory agencies (e.g., FTC). Dialogic engagement may also help diverse stakeholders to determine whether there should be requirements of explicit disclaimers or prohibiting branding and other marketing tactics that may suggest clinical value or validity without corresponding evidence. As some have observed, many DTC wellness platforms bear names (e.g., "Virtual Doctor"), logos, and well-recognized symbols of the medical profession (e.g., stethoscope, white coat, red cross) that imply medical authority and credibility.[90] Dialogic engagement at the societal level may help to determine how to ensure that companies cannot avoid regulatory scrutiny by claiming not to be medical devices while also misleading consumers into believing that they hold a similar level of expertise or authority. Dialogic engagement at the societal level can also help to determine whether ethical, legal, and social issues (ELSI) analysis for all AI research and development should be required to support ethical AI development and implementation strategies. This would involve investing a small percentage of the research budget in ELSI research and has been the norm for government-funded genomic research over the past three decades.[91]

As AI health monitoring technologies are promoted partly on the premise of workforce constraint and changing demographics, dialogic engagement at the societal level also helps stakeholders to critically assess how enthusiasm and investment in AI health monitoring technologies may juxtapose with governments' commitment to health care workforce training and planning as well as support for familial or other informal caregivers. Recall from Chapter 2 that part of the argument for promoting AI health monitoring at the health system and societal level is predicated on the alleged dwindling workforce availability. It is, however, worth noting that the labor market is not static; low wages and poor working conditions that continue to oppress care providers—many of whom are immigrants or women of color—are partly responsible for the labor shortage for in-person health monitoring. If dialogic engagement at the societal level reveals a continuing desire for in-person health monitoring, such information may help policymakers to redistribute resources to enhance training and create a sustainable and meaningful work environment that will facilitate more labor availability for health monitoring. It may also help to inform how to support prospective family caregivers, whether via caregiver-centric AI or other critical resources to facilitate their important work.

Finally, societal-level dialogic engagement can help to determine what systemic or structural barriers may prevent certain population groups from accessing desired forms of health monitoring—AI-assisted or otherwise. Broader social dialogues on how to promote equitable access to appropriate health monitoring and follow-up care may help to ensure that automated and remote observation technologies do not intensify health inequities by exacerbating the digital divide or social isolation. Such accountability is particularly important in the evolving AI development landscape, as populations that perceive themselves as being unable to benefit from these technological processes and/or have been underserved by the system may be less willing to participate in data contribution, which may perpetuate data poverty, biased algorithms, and the cycle of unequal access to beneficial health monitoring.

3. Conclusion

As some have observed, despite great advances in AI technologies, there is not yet sound reason to believe that AI-powered health applications are, in and of themselves, exceptional,[92] even as hypes in promissory claims made by technologists and developers often suggest that AI is innovative and superior practice.[93] Some of the problems presented in this book can also be found in other non-AI health technologies. Nonetheless, as the vast amounts of data involved in this rapidly advancing field intersect with the opacity of some DL algorithms and business/operational practices, cautions abound that

AI health monitoring, if not developed, implemented, and regulated properly, may be ripe for "catastrophic failures" that can further disempower patients and lead to public backlash against AI development.[94]

At this critical socio-technological juncture, a relational feedback loop may help to iteratively inform technology development and broader policy dialogues regarding how AI health monitoring can be best implemented to enhance users' relational autonomy. Dialogic engagement acknowledges that monitored users, as moral agents who are most affected by the utilization/implementation of these technologies, may face various informational or decisional uncertainties as well as structural barriers that may compromise their ability to truly form and carry out their own practical identities as they consider various health monitoring options. Incorporating their perspectives into technology development and implementation can lead to more user-centered features and practices and, more importantly, enhance prospective users' ability to exercise their negotiating power to ensure these technologies and related practices will promote their autonomy and well-being.[95]

Despite the wide-ranging doubts and warnings about AI health monitoring outlined in this book, at least some of the potential benefits touted by AI enthusiasts are attainable—but only if future development and implementation are informed by dialogic engagement among stakeholders at all levels. Techno-utopianism and AI solutionism should be viewed with a healthy dose of skepticism, but the appropriate response to these emerging technologies is not necessarily wholesale banishment of AI from the realm of health care (nor would that be possible at this juncture). Instead, we must critically evaluate how power asymmetry and other systemic inadequacies may have prompted significant interests in these technologies in the first place, and how various development and implementation plans may exacerbate or correct these problems. Such awareness can help us to look for ways to develop and integrate AI health monitoring as part of our strategies to improve our health care structures and therapeutic relationships, treating these technologies as complementary to, rather than a replacement for, in-person care or structural corrections. Moreover, just as patients and clinicians must weigh the risks and benefits of various non-AI-related tools and interventions within the broader context of patients' complicated (and sometimes contradictory) priorities and identities, so too must we acknowledge that any AI health monitoring technology will entail both risks and rewards. The trick, then, is to promote users' self-governance and self-determination by ensuring that all relevant parties have access to pertinent resources to develop the skills and competence necessary to understand those risks and rewards, and meaningful freedom and opportunities to choose what to do with that information in managing their health accordingly. Such understanding and freedom will only emerge as a result of dialogic engagement that provides channels for ensuring that technologists, decision-makers, and entrepreneurial developers are answerable to those whose abilities to form and live according to their practical identities are most affected by these technologies and emerging practices. While a relational feedback loop may seem idealistic, bold technologies bearing a tremendous impact on individual and population health require equally audacious approaches to ensure accurate and equitable implementation. Moreover, setting up a feedback loop from the outset of development may help to ensure smooth pathways that can prevent downstream costs and problems.

Notes

1. Iris Marion Young, *Justice and the Politics of Difference* (Princeton, NJ: Princeton University Press, 1990).
2. Stephanie A. Kraft, "Respect and Trustworthiness in the Patient-Provider-Machine Relationship: Applying a Relational Lens to Machine Learning Healthcare Applications," *American Journal of Bioethics* 20, no. 11 (2020): 51–53, https://doi.org/10.1080/15265161.2020.1820108.
3. Soofia Tariq, "Nine out of 10 Health Apps Harvest User Data, Global Study Shows," *The Guardian*, June 17, 2021, https://www.theguardian.com/technology/2021/jun/17/nine-out-of-10-health-apps-harvest-user-data-global-study-shows.
4. Michael V. McConnell et al., "Feasibility of Obtaining Measures of Lifestyle from a Smartphone App: The MyHeart Counts Cardiovascular Health Study," *JAMA Cardiology* 2, no. 1 (January 2017): 67–76, https://doi.org/10.1001/jamacardio.2016.4395.

5. Jennifer M. Radin et al., "The Healthy Pregnancy Research Program: Transforming Pregnancy Research through a ResearchKit App," *npj Digital Medicine* 1 (2018): 45, https://doi.org/10.1038/s41746-018-0052-2.
6. Deborah Lupton, "Health Promotion in the Digital Era: A Critical Commentary," *Health Promotion International* 30, no. 1 (March 2015):174-83, https://doi:10.1093/heapro/dau091. PMID: 25320120.
7. Eric Topol, *The Patient Will See You Now: The Future of Medicine Is in Your Hands* (New York: Basic Books, 2015).
8. Kraft, "Respect and Trustworthiness."
9. Viet-Thi Tran et al., "Patients' Views of Wearable Devices and AI in Healthcare: Findings from the ComPaRe e-Cohort," *npj Digital Medicine* 2, no. 1 (June 2019): 53, https://doi.org/10.1038/s41746-019-0132-y.
10. Matthew Nagy and Bryan Sisk, "How Will Artificial Intelligence Affect Patient–Clinician Relationships?" *AMA Journal of Ethics* 22, no. 5 (May 2020): E395–E400, https://doi.org/10.1001/amajethics.2020.395.
11. Rebecca Robbins, "An Experiment in End-of-Life Care: Tapping AI's Cold Calculus to Nudge the Most Human of Conversations," STAT, July 1, 2020, https://www.statnews.com/2020/07/01/end-of-life-artificial-intelligence/.
12. Anand Avati et al., "Improving Palliative Care with Deep Learning," *BMC Medical Informatics and Decision Making* 18, no. 4 (December 2018): 122, https://doi.org/10.1186/s12911-018-0677-8.
13. Robert Wachter, *The Digital Doctor: Hope, Hype, and Harm at the Dawn of Medicine's Computer Age* (New York: McGraw Hill, 2017).
14. Tran et al., "Patients' Views of Wearable Devices."
15. Bettina Schmietow and Georg Marckmann, "Mobile Health Ethics and the Expanding Role of Autonomy," *Medicine, Health Care, and Philosophy* 22, no. 4 (December 2019): 623–30, https://doi.org/10.1007/s11019-019-09900-y.
16. Deborah Lupton and Annemarie Jutel, "'It's Like Having a Physician in Your Pocket!' A Critical Analysis of Self-Diagnosis Smartphone Apps," *Social Science & Medicine* 133 (May 2015): 128–35, https://doi.org/10.1016/j.socscimed.2015.04.004.
17. Lupton and Jutel, "It's Like Having a Physician in Your Pocket!"
18. Wendy Netter Epstein, "Disrupting the Market for Ineffective Medical Devices," in *The Future of Medical Device Regulation: Innovation and Protection*, ed. I. Glenn Cohen et al. (Cambridge: Cambridge University Press, 2022), 179–91, https://doi:10.1017/9781108975452.014.
19. Cautions abound, however, that physicians also may not have adequate understanding of self-learning, black box systems to explain various

algorithmic decisions. See Anthony P. Weiss and Barak D. Richman, "Professional Self-Regulation in Medicine: Will the Rise of Intelligent Tools Mean the End of Peer Review?" in *The Future of Medical Device Regulation: Innovation and Protection*, ed. I. Glenn Cohen et al. (Cambridge: Cambridge University Press, 2022), 244–55, https://doi:10.1017/9781108975452.019.

20. Anita Ho and Oliver Quick, "Leaving Patients to Their Own Devices? Smart Technology, Safety and Therapeutic Relationships," *BMC Medical Ethics* 19 (2018), https://doi.org/10.1186/s12910-018-0255-8.
21. Giovanni Rubeis, "The Disruptive Power of Artificial Intelligence. Ethical Aspects of Gerontechnology in Elderly Care," *Archives of Gerontology and Geriatrics* 91 (November 2020): 104186, https://doi.org/10.1016/j.archger.2020.104186.
22. Kraft, "Respect and Trustworthiness."
23. Atul Gawande, "Why Doctors Hate Their Computers," *New Yorker*, November 5, 2018, https://www.newyorker.com/magazine/2018/11/12/why-doctors-hate-their-computers.
24. Carina Storrs, "Patients Armed with Their Own Genetic Data Raise Tough Questions," *Health Affairs* 37, no. 5 (May 2018): 690–93. https://doi.org/10.1377/hlthaff.2018.0364.
25. Rubeis, "Disruptive Power of Artificial Intelligence."
26. Lupton and Jutel, "'It's Like Having a Physician in Your Pocket!'"
27. Wendy A. Rogers, "Is There a Moral Duty for Doctors to Trust Patients?" *Journal of Medical Ethics* 28, no. 2 (April 2002): 77–80, https://doi.org/10.1136/jme.28.2.77.
28. Thierry Pelaccia et al., "Do Emergency Physicians Trust Their Patients?" *Internal and Emergency Medicine* 11, no. 4 (June 2016): 603–8, https://doi.org/10.1007/s11739-016-1410-1.
29. Miranda Fricker, "Epistemic Injustice and a Role for Virtue in the Politics of Knowing," *Metaphilosophy* 34, no. 1/2 (2003): 154–73, https://www.jstor.org/stable/24439230.
30. Daniel Z. Buchman et al., "You Present Like a Drug Addict: Patient and Clinician Perspectives on Trust and Trustworthiness in Chronic Pain Management," *Pain Medicine* 17, no. 8 (August 2016): 1394–406, https://doi.org/10.1093/pm/pnv083.
31. Donald C. Goff et al., "Strategies for Improving Treatment Adherence in Schizophrenia and Schizoaffective Disorder," *Journal of Clinical Psychiatry* 71, Suppl. 2 (2010): 20–26, https://doi.org/10.4088/JCP.9096su1cc.04.

32. Jon J. Vlasnik et al., "Medication Adherence: Factors Influencing Compliance with Prescribed Medication Plans," *Case Manager* 16, no. 2 (March 2005): 47–51, https://doi.org/10.1016/j.casemgr.2005.01.009.
33. Buchman et al., "You Present Like a Drug Addict."
34. Goff et al., "Strategies for Improving Treatment Adherence."
35. Janet Krska et al., "Issues Potentially Affecting Quality of Life Arising from Long-Term Medicines Use: A Qualitative Study," *International Journal of Clinical Pharmacy* 35, no. 6 (December 2013): 1161–69, https://doi.org/10.1007/s11096-013-9841-5.
36. Rogers, "Is There a Moral Duty for Doctors to Trust Patients?"
37. Rogers, "Is There a Moral Duty for Doctors to Trust Patients?"
38. Marilou Gagnon et al., "Treatment Adherence Redefined: A Critical Analysis of Technotherapeutics," *Nursing Inquiry* 20, no. 1 (March 2013): 60–70, https://doi.org/10.1111/j.1440-1800.2012.00595.x.
39. Katherine Bogart et al., "Mobile Phone Text Message Reminders of Antipsychotic Medication: Is It Time and Who Should Receive Them? A Cross-Sectional Trust-Wide Survey of Psychiatric Inpatients," *BMC Psychiatry* 14 (January 2014): 15, https://doi.org/10.1186/1471-244X-14-15.
40. Dawn I. Velligan et al., "Relationships among Subjective and Objective Measures of Adherence to Oral Antipsychotic Medications," *Psychiatric Services* 58, no. 9 (September 2007): 1187–92, https://doi.org/10.1176/ps.2007.58.9.1187.
41. Saínza García et al., "Adherence to Antipsychotic Medication in Bipolar Disorder and Schizophrenic Patients: A Systematic Review," *Journal of Clinical Psychopharmacology* 36, no. 4 (August 2016): 355–71, https://doi.org/10.1097/JCP.0000000000000523.
42. Maureen V. Hill et al., "Wide Variation and Excessive Dosage of Opioid Prescriptions for Common General Surgical Procedures," *Annals of Surgery* 265, no. 4 (2016): 709–14, https://doi.org/10.1097/SLA.0000000000001993.
43. Alene Kennedy-Hendricks et al., "Medication Sharing, Storage, and Disposal Practices for Opioid Medications among U.S. Adults," *JAMA Internal Medicine* 176, no. 7 (2016): 1027–29, https://doi.org/10.1001/jamainternmed.2016.2543.
44. Michael L. Barnett et al., "Opioid-Prescribing Patterns of Emergency Physicians and Risk of Long-Term Use," *New England Journal of Medicine* 376 (2017): 663–73, https://doi.org/10.1056/NEJMsa1610524.

45. Marie T. Brown and Jennifer K. Bussell, "Medication Adherence: WHO Cares?" *Mayo Clinic Proceedings* 86, no. 4 (April 2011): 304–14, https://doi.org/10.4065/mcp.2010.0575.
46. Stacy M. Carter et al., "The Ethical, Legal and Social Implications of Using Artificial Intelligence Systems in Breast Cancer Care," *Breast* 49 (February 2020): 25–32, https://doi.org/10.1016/j.breast.2019.10.001.
47. Tamar Sharon, "Self-Tracking for Health and the Quantified Self: Re-Articulating Autonomy, Solidarity, and Authenticity in an Age of Personalized Healthcare," *Philosophy & Technology* 30, no. 1 (March 2017): 93–121, https://doi.org/10.1007/s13347-016-0215-5.
48. Wendy A. Rogers et al., "Evaluation of Artificial Intelligence Clinical Applications: Detailed Case Analyses Show Value of Healthcare Ethics Approach in Identifying Patient Care Issues," *Bioethics* 35, no. 7 (September 2021): 623–33, https://doi.org/10.1111/bioe.12885.
49. Andrea C. Westlund, "Rethinking Relational Autonomy," *Hypatia* 24, no. 4 (2009): 26–49, https://doi.org/10.1111/j.1527-2001.2009.01056.x.
50. Rachel Lerman and Hamza Shaban, "Amazon Will See You Now: Tech Giant Buys Health-Care Chain for $3.9 Billion," *Washington Post*, July 21, 2022, https://www.washingtonpost.com/business/2022/07/21/amazon-health-care/.
51. Associated Press, "Amazon Buys US Medical Provider as It Cements Move into Healthcare," *The Guardian*, July 21, 2022, https://www.theguardian.com/technology/2022/jul/21/amazon-buys-medical-provider-one-medical.
52. Lerman and Shaban, "Amazon Will See You Now"; Chaiwoo Lee and Joseph F. Coughlin, "Perspective: Older Adults' Adoption of Technology: An Integrated Approach to Identifying Determinants and Barriers," *Journal of Product Innovation Management* 32, no. 5 (September 2015): 747–59, https://doi.org/10.1111/jpim.12176.
53. Chiara Longoni et al., "Resistance to Medical Artificial Intelligence," *Journal of Consumer Research* 46, no. 4 (December 2019): 629–50, https://doi.org/10.1093/jcr/ucz013.
54. Carolyn Ells et al., "Relational Autonomy as an Essential Component of Patient-Centered Care," *International Journal of Feminist Approaches to Bioethics* 4, no. 2 (2011): 79–101, https://doi.org/10.2979/intjfemappbio.4.2.79.
55. Anita Ho, "Deep Ethical Learning: Taking the Interplay of Human and Artificial Intelligence Seriously," *Hastings Center Report* 49, no. 1 (2019): 38–41, https://doi.org/10.1002/hast.977.

56. Ziad Obermeyer et al., "Dissecting Racial Bias in an Algorithm Used to Manage the Health of Populations," *Science* 366, no. 6464 (October 2019): 447–53, https://doi.org/10.1126/science.aax2342.
57. Lianping Ti et al., "Towards Equitable AI Interventions for People Who Use Drugs: Key Areas That Require Ethical Investment," *Journal of Addiction Medicine* 15, no. 2 (April 2021): 96–98, https://doi.org/10.1097/ADM.0000000000000722.
58. Shannon Vallor, *Technology and the Virtues: A Philosophical Guide to a Future Worth Wanting* (New York: Oxford University Press, 2016).
59. Pireh Pirzada et al., "Ethics and Acceptance of Smart Homes for Older Adults," *Informatics for Health and Social Care* (July 2021): 1–28, https://doi.org/10.1080/17538157.2021.1923500.
60. Jarod T. Giger et al., "Remote Patient Monitoring Acceptance Trends among Older Adults Residing in a Frontier State," *Computers in Human Behavior* 44 (March 2015): 174–82, https://doi.org/10.1016/j.chb.2014.11.044.
61. Alistair Wardrope, "Relational Autonomy and the Ethics of Health Promotion," *Public Health Ethics* 8, no. 1 (April 2015): 50–62, https://doi.org/10.1093/phe/phu025.
62. Vimal Sriram et al., "Informal Carers' Experience of Assistive Technology Use in Dementia Care at Home: A Systematic Review," *BMC Geriatrics* 19, no. 1 (June 2019): 160, https://doi.org/10.1186/s12877-019-1169-0.
63. Emily Bembeneck et al., "To Stop Algorithmic Bias, We First Have to Define It," Brookings Institute, October 21, 2021, https://www.brookings.edu/research/to-stop-algorithmic-bias-we-first-have-to-define-it/.
64. Danton S. Char et al., "Identifying Ethical Considerations for Machine Learning Healthcare Applications," *American Journal of Bioethics* 20, no. 11 (November 2020): 7–17, https://doi.org/10.1080/15265161.2020.1819469.
65. Hannah van Kolfschooten, "The mHealth Power Paradox: Improving Data Protection in Health Apps through Self-Regulation in the European Union," in *The Future of Medical Device Regulation: Innovation and Protection*, ed. I. Glenn Cohen et al. (Cambridge: Cambridge University Press, 2022), 63–76, https://doi:10.1017/9781108975452.006
66. Barry Solaiman and Mark G. Bloom, "AI, Explainability, and Safeguarding Patient Safety in Europe: Toward a Science-Focused Regulatory Model," in *The Future of Medical Device Regulation: Innovation and Protection*, ed. I. Glenn Cohen et al. (Cambridge: Cambridge University Press, 2022), 91–102, https://doi:10.1017/9781108975452.008.
67. The European Union codified the right to personal data privacy in 2016 with the General Data Protection Regulation (GDPR), which became enforceable in 2018. The GDPR mandates that personal data must be

collected for specified, explicit, and legitimate purposes and not reused for other non-indicated purposes. There is currently no equivalent or unified federal data protection regulation in the United States, although various states have enacted their own regulations similar to that of the GDPR (e.g., California Consumer Privacy Act).

68. Kenneth D. Mandl and Arjun K. Manrai, "Potential Excessive Testing at Scale: Biomarkers, Genomics, and Machine Learning," *Journal of the American Medical Association* 321, no. 8 (February 2019): 739–40, https://doi.org/10.1001/jama.2019.0286.
69. U.S. Food and Drug Administration, "Artificial Intelligence/Machine Learning (AI/ML)-Based Software as a Medical Device (SaMD) Action Plan," January 2021, https://www.fda.gov/media/145022/download.
70. It is, however, important to recognize that, even though continuously learning algorithms that automatically update via inputs can presumably lead to more accurate predictions, if the system is deployed for very different populations than initially intended, they may lead to different output results than the originally tested algorithm. Since evaluating the safety, efficiency, and equity of these opaque and autonomous algorithms is more challenging, continuously learning systems also have their own drawbacks. See Char et al., "Identifying Ethical Considerations."
71. Rogers et al., "Evaluation of Artificial Intelligence Clinical Applications."
72. Lupton and Jutel, "'It's Like Having a Physician in Your Pocket!'"
73. Weiss and Richman, "Professional Self-Regulation in Medicine."
74. Bartha Maria Knoppers and Adrian Mark Thorogood, "Ethics and Big Data in Health," *Current Opinion in Systems Biology* 4 (August 2017): 53–57, https://doi.org/10.1016/j.coisb.2017.07.001.
75. Sophie Putka, "Meta, Hospitals Sued for Sharing Private Medical Info," Medpage Today, August 3, 2022, https://www.medpagetoday.com/special-reports/features/100050.
76. Candace Frates, "At Mayo Clinic, Sharing Patient Data with Companies Fuels AI Innovation—and Concerns about Consent," STAT, June 3, 2020, https://www.statnews.com/2020/06/03/mayo-clinic-patient-data-fuels-artificial-intelligence-consent-concerns/.
77. Deven McGraw and Kenneth D. Mandl, "Privacy Protections to Encourage Use of Health-Relevant Digital Data in a Learning Health System," *npj Digital Medicine* 4, no. 1 (January 2021): 2, https://doi.org/10.1038/s41746-020-00362-8.
78. Hussein Ibrahim et al., "Health Data Poverty: An Assailable Barrier to Equitable Digital Health Care," *Lancet Digital Health* 3, no. 4 (April 2021): e260–65, https://doi.org/10.1016/S2589-7500(20)30317-4.

79. "Acute Hospital Care at Home," Centers for Medicare and Medicaid Services, accessed January 31, 2022, https://qualitynet.cms.gov/acute-hospital-care-at-home.
80. Kat Jercich, "Nurse Unions Slam Kaiser's Advanced Care at Home Strategy," Healthcare IT News, November 8, 2021, https://www.healthcareitnews.com/news/nurse-unions-slam-kaisers-advanced-care-home-strategy.
81. Organization for Economic Cooperation and Development, "Trustworthy AI in Health: Background Paper for the G20 AI Dialogue, Digital Economy Task Force," April 2020, https://www.oecd.org/health/trustworthy-artificial-intelligence-in-health.pdf.
82. Ziad Obermeyer et al., "Dissecting Racial Bias in an Algorithm."
83. Sara Gerke et al., "The Need for a System View to Regulate Artificial Intelligence/Machine Learning-Based Software as Medical Device." *npj Digital Medicine* 3, no. 53 (April 2020). https://doi.org/10.1038/s41746-020-0262-2.
84. W. Ben Mortenson et al., "No Place Like Home? Surveillance and What Home Means in Old Age," *Canadian Journal on Aging* 35, no. 1 (March 2016): 103–14, https://doi.org/10.1017/S0714980815000549.
85. White House Office of Science and Technology Policy, "Blueprint for an AI Bill of Rights," October 2022, https://www.whitehouse.gov/ostp/ai-bill-of-rights/.
86. In comparison, in Europe, General Data Protection Regulation's (GDPR) provisions on personal data, consent, and purpose limitations impose some requirements for these technologies. See European Commission, "Regulation (EU) 2016/679 of the European Parliament and of the Council of 27 April 2016 on the Protection of Natural Persons with Regard to the Processing of Personal Data and on the Free Movement of Such Data, and Repealing Directive 95/46/EC (General Data Protection Regulation)," https://eur-lex.europa.eu/legal-content/EN/TXT/?uri=CELEX%3A02016R0679-20160504&qid=1532348683434. Moreover, the European Union has proposed an AI Act to regulate AI applications based on risk level, and a new bill, the AI Liability Directive, allows individuals and groups to sue for damages after being harmed by an AI system. See European Commission, "Laying Down Harmonised Rules on Artificial Intelligence (Artificial Intelligence Act) and Amending Certain union Legislative Act," https://eur-lex.europa.eu/legal-content/EN/TXT/?uri=CELEX%3A52021PC0206. Also see European Commission, "Proposal for a Directive of the European Parliament and of the Council on Adapting Non-Contractual Civil Liability Rules to Artificial Intelligence (AI Liability Directive),"

https://ec.europa.eu/info/sites/default/files/1_1_197605_prop_dir_ai_en.pdf

87. Lupton and Jutel, "'It's Like Having a Physician in Your Pocket!'"
88. Clara Berridge, "Breathing Room in Monitored Space: The Impact of Passive Monitoring Technology on Privacy in Independent Living," *Gerontologist* 56, no. 5 (October 2016): 807–16, https://doi.org/10.1093/geront/gnv034.
89. U.S. Food and Drug Administration, "Artificial Intelligence/Machine Learning (AI/ML)-Based Software as a Medical Device (SaMD) Action Plan."
90. Lupton and Jutel, "'It's Like Having a Physician in Your Pocket!'"
91. Tilman Hartwig et al., "Artificial Intelligence ELSI Score for Science and Technology: A Comparison between Japan and the US," *AI & Society* (January 2022), https://doi.org/10.1007/s00146-021-01323-9.
92. Char et al., "Identifying Ethical Considerations."
93. Rogers et al., "Evaluation of Artificial Intelligence Clinical Applications."
94. Char et al., "Identifying Ethical Considerations."
95. Wardrope, "Relational Autonomy and the Ethics of Health Promotion."

Epilogue

Since I first told my friend Jon about this book (see Preface), his mother Diane's dementia has progressed, and she recently moved to a memory care center. Intermittent COVID-19 restrictions at the facility have rendered it more challenging for visits, prompting Jon to seek low-barrier communication platforms that would allow him to have regular video calls with Diane. One device that allows family members to remotely connect with their older loved ones is a smart frame that does not require significant digital skills or training. The device is remotely managed by the family member, who can set up a list of authorized individuals who can make video calls to the older adult using a smartphone app. It has an auto-answer function, which allows the screen and the camera to come on automatically when an authorized person calls—the older adult does not need to navigate the screen or push any button to answer.[1] While the auto-answer function can be turned off, Jon left it on to ease communication. He determined that, due to Diane's progressive dementia, even if he were to tell her about the function, she would likely forget, and it would cause more confusion than promote her autonomy.

Staff members were initially worried about the device, not because they wondered whether Diane would want more control over whether to answer incoming video calls. Rather, some of the direct care staff members had low digital literacy and were uncomfortable with possibly having to help Diane operate the device. Some also expressed concerns that the device may capture their care activities while being in Diane's room. After further explanations, reassurances, and negotiation, the memory care center eventually approved of Jon's communication device within various parameters.

Interestingly, while the memory care facility was deciding on the device, a worry that Diane had previously expressed materialized. When she was in her assisted living apartment, she would sometimes forget having moved her own belongings. She suspected that the building manager or others might have entered her unit while she was out and rearranged her items—something that was never substantiated. But in her new memory care unit, which is not very well-lit, another resident with dementia, who may be confused about his surroundings, has indeed on occasions entered her room, leaving her startled and distressed. When Jon asked the staff about residents' bedroom security, they responded that residents' bedrooms are not locked for fire safety precautions and for preventing forgetful residents from locking themselves in or out of their room, even though the organization's decision around door locks might have been based on blanket assumptions around the diagnosis of dementia rather than each resident's assessed needs or functional abilities. The facility has 24-hour staffing, and caregivers would redirect wandering residents when they witness such behavior, but staff members are not always present when or where that occurs. Nonetheless, the facility did not seem overly concerned about Jon's inquiry, perhaps partly because staff members assumed that residents would weigh safety over privacy, or also because wandering behavior is not uncommon for people with dementia, even if the unwanted intrusion was upsetting to his mother.

There are currently no CCTV or computer vision technologies at the facility to provide continuous monitoring of residents' movement or behavior. However, as AI and other forms of passive monitoring gradually move into care facilities,[2] it is possible that some of these technologies will eventually be introduced at this and other memory care facilities, promoted as a safety- and autonomy-enhancing feature that allows residents more freedom to move around the facility.

Jon and I have wondered, if presented with the choice and assuming adequate cognitive capacity to understand the implications, whether Diane and other residents would accept continuous monitoring of hallways and room entrances to detect, predict, and/or prevent potential intrusion. How would residents prioritize the competing privacy and dignity concerns of being continuously monitored versus the unwanted interruption from another resident? Would passive computer vision monitoring that replaces human or CCTV monitoring provide a better sense of privacy for the residents, who could live like nobody was watching? Or would they feel even more isolated if staff members may check in on them less frequently if not alerted? And would algorithmic alerts further startle some residents with dementia? Intersecting with residents' potential concern, would staff members who are uncomfortable with video chat platforms welcome broader monitoring that likely requires higher digital literacy and exerts response expectations on the part of caregivers? And who owns the data, and how should such monitoring data be used for residents' ongoing care, and who should have access to such information that is collected in a quasi-communal setting?

As we have seen throughout this book, despite claims about AI solutionism, decisions around continuous AI health monitoring, particularly of individuals who are presumed to lack capacity to decide for themselves, are relationally complex, since even decisions motivated by paternalistic benevolence can reinforce power and domination on those being observed. It is unclear whether the management at the facility has considered staffing, architectural, environmental, or equipment adjustments to help alert and/or deter wandering behaviors, and if or how they solicit residents' concerns in their space planning or adjustment. But before entrepreneurial developers of CCTV cameras or other AI monitoring devices reach the management team with their promises of technological solutionism, perhaps they can first try brighter lightbulbs.

Notes

1. This device is not marketed as an AI-enabled device.
2. Clara Berridge, "Breathing Room in Monitored Space: The Impact of Passive Monitoring Technology on Privacy in Independent Living," *Gerontologist* 56, no. 5 (October 2016): 807–16, https://doi.org/10.1093/geront/gnv034.

Bibliography

AARP and National Alliance for Caregiving. *Caregiving in the U.S. 2020*. Washington, DC: AARP, 2020. https://www.aarp.org/content/dam/aarp/ppi/2020/05/full-report-caregiving-in-the-united-states.doi.10.26419-2Fppi.00103.001.pdf.

Aas, Katja Franko. "'The Body Does Not Lie': Identity, Risk and Trust in Technoculture." *Crime, Media, Culture* 2, no. 2 (August 2006): 143–58. https://doi.org/10.1177/1741659006065401.

Aboueid, Stephanie, Rebecca H. Liu, Binyam Negussie Desta, Ashok Chaurasia, and Shanil Ebrahim. "The Use of Artificially Intelligent Self-Diagnosing Digital Platforms by the General Public: Scoping Review." *JMIR Medical Informatics* 7, no. 2 (May 2019): e13445. https://doi.org/10.2196/13445.

Adams, Alex J., and Samuel F. Stolpe. "Defining and Measuring Primary Medication Nonadherence: Development of a Quality Measure." *Journal of Managed Care & Specialty Pharmacy* 22, no. 5 (May 2016): 516–23. https://doi.org/10.18553/jmcp.2016.22.5.516.

Adamson, Adewole S., and Avery Smith. "Machine Learning and Health Care Disparities in Dermatology." *JAMA Dermatology* 154, no. 11 (2018): 1247–48. https://doi.org/10.1001/jamadermatol.2018.2348.

Agnoli, Alicia, Guibo Xing, Daniel J. Tancredi, Elizabeth Magnan, Anthony Jerant, and Joshua J. Fenton. "Association of Dose Tapering with Overdose or Mental Health Crisis among Patients Prescribed Long-Term Opioids." *Journal of the American Medical Association* 326, no. 5 (August 2021): 411–19. https://doi.org/10.1001/jama.2021.11013.

Ahlin Marceta, Jesper. "A Non-Ideal Authenticity-Based Conceptualization of Personal Autonomy." *Medicine, Health Care and Philosophy* 22 (2019): 387–95. https://doi.org/10.1007/s11019-018-9879-1.

Ajana, Btihaj. "Digital Health and the Biopolitics of the Quantified Self." *Digital Health* 3 (January 2017). https://doi.org/10.1177/2055207616689509.

Akbar, Saba, Coiera Enrico, and Farah Magrabi. "Safety Concerns with Consumer-Facing Mobile Health Applications and Their Consequences: A Scoping Review." *Journal of the American Medical Informatics Association* 27, no. 2 (February 2020): 330–40. https://doi.org/10.1093/jamia/ocz175.

Alashwal, Hany, Mohamed El Halaby, Jacob J. Crouse, Areeg Abdalla, and Ahmed A. Moustafa. "The Application of Unsupervised Clustering Methods to Alzheimer's Disease." *Frontiers in Computational Neuroscience* 13 (2019). https://doi.org/10.3389/fncom.2019.00031.

Aldeer, Murtadha, Mehdi Javanmard, and Richard P. Martin. "A Review of Medication Adherence Monitoring Technologies." *Applied System Innovation* 1, no. 2 (2018): 14. https://doi.org/10.3390/asi1020014.

Alipour, Azita, Stephen Gabrielson, and Puja B. Patel. "Ingestible Sensors and Medication Adherence: Focus on Use in Serious Mental Illness." *Pharmacy* 8, no. 2 (2020): 103. https://doi.org/10.3390/pharmacy8020103.

Aljbawi, Wafaa, Sami O. Simmons, and Visara Urovi. "Developing a Multi-Variate Prediction Model for the Detection of COVID-19 from Crowd-Sourced Respiratory Voice Data." arXiv (preprint). September 8, 2022. https://arxiv.org/abs/2209.03727.

AllazoHealth. "AllazoHealth Now Offers AI Optimized Therapy Initiation." February 1, 2021. https://blog.allazohealth.com/resources/ai-optimized-therapy-initiation.

Al-Shaqi, Riyad, Monjur Mourshed, and Yacine Rezgui. "Progress in Ambient Assisted Systems for Independent Living by the Elderly." *SpringerPlus* 5 (2016): 624. https://doi.org/10.1186/s40064-016-2272-8.

Alzheimer's Association. "2021 Alzheimer's Disease Facts and Figures." *Alzheimer's and Dementia* 17, no. 3 (March 2021): 327–406. https://doi.org/10.1002/alz.12328.

American Society of Anesthesiologists. "Artificial Intelligence Can Predict Patients at Highest Risk for Severe Pain Increased Opioid Use after Surgery." October 4, 2020. https://www.asahq.org/about-asa/newsroom/news-releases/2020/10/artificial-intelligence-can-predict-patients-at-highest-risk-for-severe-pain-increased-opioid-use-after-surgery.

Anderson, Jeffrey P., Jignesh R. Parikh, Daniel K. Shenfeld, Vladimir Ivanov, Casey Marks, Bruce W. Church, Jason M. Laramie, et al. "Reverse Engineering and Evaluation of Prediction Models for Progression to Type 2 Diabetes: An Application of Machine Learning Using Electronic Health Records." *Journal of Diabetes Science and Technology* 10, no. 1 (2015): 6–18. https://doi.org/10.1177/1932296815620200.

Anderson, Joel, and Axel Honneth. "Autonomy, Vulnerability, Recognition, and Justice." In *Autonomy and the Challenges to Liberalism: New Essays*, edited by John Christman and Joel Anderson, 127–49. Cambridge: Cambridge University Press, 2005.

Anyoha, Rockwell. "The History of Artificial Intelligence." Science in the News. Harvard University. August 28, 2017. https://sitn.hms.harvard.edu/flash/2017/history-artificial-intelligence/.

Arias, Elizabeth, and Jiaquan Xu. "United States Life Tables, 2017." *National Vital Statistics Reports* 68, no. 7 (2019): 1–66.

Arnold, Robert M., Paul K. J. Han, and Deborah Seltzer. "Opioid Contracts in Chronic Nonmalignant Pain Management: Objectives and Uncertainties." *American Journal of Medicine* 119, no. 4 (April 2006): 292–96. https://doi.org/10.1016/j.amjmed.2005.09.019.

Aronson, Jay E. "Expert Systems." In *Encyclopedia of Information Systems*, edited by Hossein Bidgoli, 277–89. Cambridge, MA: Academic Press, 2003. https://doi.org/10.1016/B0-12-227240-4/00067-8.

Ascher-Svanum, Haya, Douglas E. Faries, Baojin Zhu, Frank R. Ernst, Marvin S. Swartz, and Jeff W. Swanson. "Medication Adherence and Long-Term Functional Outcomes in the Treatment of Schizophrenia in Usual Care." *Journal of Clinical Psychiatry* 67, no. 3 (March 2006): 453–60. https://doi.org/10.4088/jcp.v67n0317.

Asghar, Ikram, Shuang Cang, and Hongnian Yu. "A Systematic Mapping Study on Assistive Technologies for People with Dementia." *9th International Conference on Software, Knowledge, Information Management and Applications (SKIMA)* (2015): 1–8. https://doi.org/10.1109/SKIMA.2015.7399989.

Associated Press. "Amazon Buys US Medical Provider as It Cements Move into Healthcare." *The Guardian*. July 21, 2022. https://www.theguardian.com/technology/2022/jul/21/amazon-buys-medical-provider-one-medical.

Auriemma, Catherine L., Scott D. Halpern, Jeremy M. Asch, Matthew Van Der Tuyn, and David A. Asch. "Completion of Advance Directives and Documented Care Preferences During the Coronavirus Disease 2019 (COVID-19) Pandemic." *JAMA Network Open* 3, no. 7 (2020): e2015762. https://doi.org/10.1001/jamanetworkopen.2020.15762.

Avati, Anand, Kenneth Jung, Stephanie Harman, Lance Downing, Andrew Ng, and Nigam H. Shah. "Improving Palliative Care with Deep Learning." *BMC Medical Informatics and Decision Making* 18, no. 4 (December 2018): 122. https://doi.org/10.1186/s12911-018-0677-8.

Babel, Aditi, Richi Taneja, Franco Mondello Malvestiti, Alessandro Monaco, and Shaantanu Donde. "Artificial Intelligence Solutions to Increase Medication Adherence in Patients with Non-Communicable Diseases." *Frontiers in Digital Health* 3 (2021): 69. https://doi.org/10.3389/fdgth.2021.669869.

Babic, Boris, Sara Gerke, Theodoros Evgeniou, and I. Glenn Cohen. "Direct-to-Consumer Medical Machine Learning and Artificial Intelligence Applications." *Nature Machine Intelligence* 3, no. 4 (April 2021): 283–87. https://doi.org/10.1038/s42256-021-00331-0.

Bain, Earle E., Laura Shafner, David P. Walling, Ahmed A. Othman, Christy Chuang-Stein, John Hinkle, and Adam Hanina. "Use of a Novel Artificial Intelligence Platform on Mobile Devices to Assess Dosing Compliance in a Phase 2 Clinical Trial in Subjects with Schizophrenia." *JMIR mHealth and uHealth* 5, no. 2 (February 2017): e18. https://doi.org/10.2196/mhealth.7030.

Barassi, Veronica. "BabyVeillance? Expecting Parents, Online Surveillance and the Cultural Specificity of Pregnancy Apps." *Social Media + Society* 3, no. 2 (2017). https://doi.org/10.1177/2056305117707188

Barnett, Michael L., Andrew R. Olenski, and Anupam B. Jena. "Opioid-Prescribing Patterns of Emergency Physicians and Risk of Long-Term Use." *New England Journal of Medicine* 376 (2017): 663–73. https://doi.org/10.1056/NEJMsa1610524.

Baumgartner, Jesse, and David Radley. "The Drug Overdose Toll in 2020 and Near-Term Actions for Addressing It." Commonwealth Fund. August 16, 2021. https://www.commonwealthfund.org/blog/2021/drug-overdose-toll-2020-and-near-term-actions-addressing-it.

Baumgartner, Pascal C., R. Brian Haynes, Kurt E. Hersberger, and Isabelle Arnet. "A Systematic Review of Medication Adherence Thresholds Dependent of Clinical Outcomes." *Frontiers in Pharmacology* 9 (2018): 1290. https://doi.org/10.3389/fphar.2018.01290.

Baxter, Clarence, Julie-Anne Carroll, Brendan Keogh, and Corneel Vandelanotte. "Assessment of Mobile Health Apps Using Built-In Smartphone Sensors for Diagnosis and Treatment: Systematic Survey of Apps Listed in International Curated Health App Libraries." *JMIR mHealth and uHealth* 8, no. 2 (February 2020): e16741. https://doi.org/10.2196/16741.

Beauchamp, Tom, and James Childress. *Principles of Biomedical Ethics*. 7th ed. New York: Oxford University Press, 2012.

Bembeneck, Emily, Rebecca Nissan, and Ziad Obermeyer. "To Stop Algorithmic Bias, We First Have to Define It." Brookings Institute. October 21, 2021. https://www.brookings.edu/research/to-stop-algorithmic-bias-we-first-have-to-define-it/.

Benjamens, Stan, Pranavsingh Dhunnoo, and Bertalan Meskó. "The State of Artificial Intelligence-Based FDA-Approved Medical Devices and Algorithms: An Online Database." *npj Digital Medicine* 3, no. 1 (September 2020): 118. https://doi.org/10.1038/s41746-020-00324-0.

Berridge, Clara. "Breathing Room in Monitored Space: The Impact of Passive Monitoring Technology on Privacy in Independent Living." *Gerontologist* 56, no. 5 (October 2016): 807–16. https://doi.org/10.1093/geront/gnv034.

Berridge, Clara, and Terrie Fox Wetle. "Why Older Adults and Their Children Disagree about In-Home Surveillance Technology, Sensors, and Tracking." *Gerontologist* 60, no. 5 (July 2020): 926–34. https://doi.org/10.1093/geront/gnz068.

Berruti, Federico, Pieter Nel, and Rob Whiteman. "An Executive Primer on Artificial General Intelligence." McKinsey. April 29, 2020. https://www.mckinsey.com/business-functions/operations/our-insights/an-executive-primer-on-artificial-general-intelligence.

Best, Jo. "Smart Pills and the Future of Medicine: Insights from Your Insides." ZDNet. February 23, 2021. https://www.zdnet.com/article/smart-pills-and-the-future-of-medicine-insights-from-your-insides/.

Birchley, Giles, Richard Huxtable, Madeleine Murtagh, Ruud ter Meulen, Peter Flach, and Rachael Gooberman-Hill. "Smart Homes, Private Homes? An

Empirical Study of Technology Researchers' Perceptions of Ethical Issues in Developing Smart-Home Health Technologies." *BMC Medical Ethics* 18, no. 1 (April 2017): 23. https://doi.org/10.1186/s12910-017-0183-z.

Bisen, Vikram Singh. "What Is Human in the Loop Machine Learning: Why and How Used in AI?" Medium. May 20, 2020. https://medium.com/vsinghbisen/what-is-human-in-the-loop-machine-learning-why-how-used-in-ai-60c7b44eb2c0.

Blaschke, Terrence F., Lars Osterberg, Bernard Vrijens, and John Urquhart. "Adherence to Medications: Insights Arising from Studies on the Unreliable Link between Prescribed and Actual Drug Dosing Histories." *Annual Review of Pharmacology and Toxicology* 52 (2012): 275–301. https://doi.org/10.1146/annurev-pharmtox-011711-113247.

Bleicher, Ariel. "Demystifying the Black Box That Is AI." *Scientific American*. August 9, 2017. https://www.scientificamerican.com/article/demystifying-the-black-box-that-is-ai/.

Bogart, Katherine, Sook Kuan Wong, Christine Lewis, Anthony Akenzua, Daniel Hayes, Athanasios Prountzos, Chike Ify Okocha, and Eugenia Kravariti. "Mobile Phone Text Message Reminders of Antipsychotic Medication: Is It Time and Who Should Receive Them? A Cross-Sectional Trust-Wide Survey of Psychiatric Inpatients." *BMC Psychiatry* 14 (January 2014): 15. https://doi.org/10.1186/1471-244X-14-15.

Bose, Eliezer, and Kavita Radhakrishnan. "Using Unsupervised Machine Learning to Identify Subgroups among Home Health Patients with Heart Failure Using Telehealth." *Computers, Informatics, Nursing* 36, no. 5 (2018): 242–48. https://doi.org/10.1097/CIN.0000000000000423.

Briggs, Andrew, Diane Wild, Michael Lees, Matthew Reaney, Serdar Dursun, David Parry, and Jayanti Mukherjee. "Impact of Schizophrenia and Schizophrenia Treatment-Related Adverse Events on Quality of Life: Direct Utility Elicitation." *Health and Quality of Life Outcomes* 6, no. 1 (November 2008): 105. https://doi.org/10.1186/1477-7525-6-105.

Bright, Cordellia E. "Measuring Medication Adherence in Patients with Schizophrenia: An Integrative Review." *Archives of Psychiatric Nursing* 31, no. 1 (February 2017): 99–110. https://doi.org/10.1016/j.apnu.2016.09.003.

Britten, Nicky, Ruth Riley, and Myfanwy Morgan. "Resisting Psychotropic Medicines: A Synthesis of Qualitative Studies of Medicine-Taking." *Advances in Psychiatric Treatment* 16, no. 3 (2010): 207–18. https://doi.org/10.1192/apt.bp.107.005165.

Brodwin, Erin, and Nicholas St. Fleur. "FDA Issues Alert on 'Limitations' of Pulse Oximeters, without Explicit Mention of Racial Bias." STAT. February 19, 2021. https://www.statnews.com/2021/02/19/fda-issues-alert-on-limitations-of-pulse-oximeters-without-explicit-mention-of-racial-bi/.

Broekmans, Susan, Fabienne Dobbels, Koen Milisen, Bart Morlion, and Steven Vanderschueren. "Determinants of Medication Underuse and Medication Overuse in Patients with Chronic Non-Malignant Pain: A Multicenter

Study." *International Journal of Nursing Studies* 47, no. 11 (November 2010): 1408–17. https://doi.org/10.1016/j.ijnurstu.2010.03.014.

Brown, Marie T., and Jennifer K. Bussell. "Medication Adherence: WHO Cares?" *Mayo Clinic Proceedings* 86, no. 4 (April 2011): 304–14. https://doi.org/10.4065/mcp.2010.0575.

Buchman, Daniel Z., Anita Ho, and Judy Illes. "You Present Like a Drug Addict: Patient and Clinician Perspectives on Trust and Trustworthiness in Chronic Pain Management." *Pain Medicine* 17, no. 8 (2016): 1394–406. https://doi.org/10.1093/pm/pnv083.

Buijink, Arthur Willem Gerard, Benjamin Jelle Visser, and Louise Marshall. "Medical Apps for Smartphones: Lack of Evidence Undermines Quality and Safety." *Evidence-Based Medicine* 18, no. 3 (June 2013): 90–92. https://doi.org/10.1136/eb-2012-100885.

Burns, Tom. "Locked Doors or Therapeutic Relationships?" *Lancet Psychiatry* 3, no. 9 (September 2016): 795–96. https://doi.org/10.1016/S2215-0366(16)30185-7.

Byerly, Matthew J., Ann Thompson, Thomas Carmody, Rhiannon Bugno, Thomas Erwin, Michael Kashner, and A. John Rush. "Validity of Electronically Monitored Medication Adherence and Conventional Adherence Measures in Schizophrenia." *Psychiatric Services* 58, no. 6 (June 2007): 844–47. https://doi.org/10.1176/ps.2007.58.6.844.

Byrd, Kathy K., John G. Hou, Ron Hazen, Heather Kirkham, Sumihiro Suzuki, Patrick G. Clay, Tim Bush, et al. "Antiretroviral Adherence Level Necessary for HIV Viral Suppression Using Real-World Data." *Journal of Acquired Immune Deficiency Syndromes* 82, no. 3 (November 2019): 245–51. https://doi.org/10.1097/QAI.0000000000002142.

Cain, Carol H., Estee Neuwirth, Jim Bellows, Christi Zuber, and Jennifer Green. "Patient Experiences of Transitioning from Hospital to Home: An Ethnographic Quality Improvement Project." *Journal of Hospital Medicine* 7, no. 5 (June 2012): 382–87. https://doi.org/10.1002/jhm.1918.

Calasanti, Toni, and Neal King. "Successful Aging, Ageism, and the Maintenance of Age and Gender Relations." In *Successful Aging as a Contemporary Obsession: Global Perspectives*, edited by Sarah Lamb, 27–40. New Brunswick, NJ: Rutgers University Press, 2017.

California Future Health Workforce Commission. "Meeting the Demand for Health: Final Report of the Future Health Workforce Commission." February 2019. https://futurehealthworkforce.org/wp-content/uploads/2019/03/MeetingDemandForHealthFinalReportCFHWC.pdf.

Carin, Lawrence. "On Artificial Intelligence and Deep Learning within Medical Education." *Academic Medicine* 95, no. 11S (2020): S10–S11. https://doi.org/10.1097/ACM.0000000000003630.

Carter, Stacy M., V. A. Entwistle, and M. Little. "Relational Conceptions of Paternalism: A Way to Rebut Nanny-State Accusations and Evaluate Public

Health Interventions." *Public Health* 129, no. 8 (August 2015): 1021–29. https://doi.org/10.1016/j.puhe.2015.03.007.

Carter, Stacy M., Wendy Rogers, Khin Than Win, Helen Frazer, Bernadette Richards, and Nehmat Houssami. "The Ethical, Legal and Social Implications of Using Artificial Intelligence Systems in Breast Cancer Care." *Breast* 49 (2020): 25–32. https://doi.org/10.1016/j.breast.2019.10.001.

Casalino, Lawrence P., Daniel Dunham, Marshall H. Chin, Rebecca Bielang, Emily O. Kistner, Theodore G. Karrison, Michael K. Ong, et al. "Frequency of Failure to Inform Patients of Clinically Significant Outpatient Test Results." *Archives of Internal Medicine* 169, no. 12 (June 2009): 1123–29. https://doi.org/10.1001/archinternmed.2009.130.

Castaneda, Ruben. "Creative Ways Hospitals Reach Diverse Populations." *US News & World Report*. January 23, 2017. https://health.usnews.com/wellness/slideshows/creative-ways-hospitals-reach-diverse-populations.

Center for Devices and Radiological Health. "General Wellness: Policy for Low Risk Devices." U.S. Food and Drug Administration. FDA-2014-N-1039. September 26, 2019. https://www.fda.gov/regulatory-information/search-fda-guidance-documents/general-wellness-policy-low-risk-devices.

Centers for Medicare and Medicaid Services. "Acute Hospital Care at Home." Accessed January 31, 2022. https://qualitynet.cms.gov/acute-hospital-care-at-home.

Centers for Medicare and Medicaid Services. "Chronic Conditions Charts: 2018." Last modified December 1, 2021. https://www.cms.gov/Research-Statistics-Data-and-Systems/Statistics-Trends-and-Reports/Chronic-Conditions/Chartbook_Charts.html.

Chai, Peter R., Stephanie Carreiro, Brendan J. Innes, Brittany Chapman, Kristin L. Schreiber, Robert R. Edwards, Adam W. Carrico, and Edward W. Boyer. "Oxycodone Ingestion Patterns in Acute Fracture Pain with Digital Pills." *Anesthesia and Analgesia* 125, no. 6 (December 2017): 2105–12. https://doi.org/10.1213/ANE.0000000000002574.

Chai, Peter R., Stephanie Carreiro, Brendan J. Innes, Rochelle K. Rosen, Conall O'Cleirigh, Kenneth H. Mayer, and Edward W. Boyer. "Digital Pills to Measure Opioid Ingestion Patterns in Emergency Department Patients with Acute Fracture Pain: A Pilot Study." *Journal of Medical Internet Research* 19, no. 1 (January 2017): e19. https://doi.org/10.2196/jmir.7050.

Chambers, Duncan, Anna J. Cantrell, Maxine Johnson, Louise Preston, Susan K. Baxter, Andrew Booth, and Janette Turner. "Digital and Online Symptom Checkers and Health Assessment/Triage Services for Urgent Health Problems: Systematic Review." *BMJ Open* 9, no. 8 (August 2019): e027743. https://doi.org/10.1136/bmjopen-2018-027743.

Chanane, Nawal, Farhaan Mirza, M. Asif Naeem, and Asfahaan Mirza. "Acceptance of Technology-Driven Interventions for Improving Medication Adherence." In *Future Network Systems and Security*, edited by Robin Doss,

Selwyn Piramuthu, and Wei Zhou, 188–98. Cham: Springer International Publishing, 2017.

Char, Danton S., Michael D. Abràmoff, and Chris Feudtner. "Identifying Ethical Considerations for Machine Learning Healthcare Applications." *American Journal of Bioethics* 20, no. 11 (November 2020): 7–17. https://doi.org/10.1080/15265161.2020.1819469.

Char, Danton S., Nigam H. Shah, and David Magnus. "Implementing Machine Learning in Health Care—Addressing Ethical Challenges." *New England Journal of Medicine* 378, no. 11 (March 2018): 981–83. https://doi.org/10.1056/NEJMp1714229.

Chivilgina, Olga, Bernice S. Elger, and Fabrice Jotterand. "Digital Technologies for Schizophrenia Management: A Descriptive Review." *Science and Engineering Ethics* 27, no. 2 (April 2021): 25. https://doi.org/10.1007/s11948-021-00302-z.

Chorost, Michael. "The Networked Pill." MIT Technology Review. March 20, 2008. https://www.technologyreview.com/2008/03/20/34958/the-networked-pill/.

Christensen, Kaare, Gabriele Doblhammer, Roland Rau, and James W. Vaupel. "Ageing Populations: The Challenges Ahead." *Lancet* 374, no. 9696 (October 2009): 1196–208. https://doi.org/10.1016/S0140-6736(09)61460-4.

Clarke, Janice L., Scott Bourn, Alexis Skoufalos, Eric H. Beck, and Daniel J. Castillo. "An Innovative Approach to Health Care Delivery for Patients with Chronic Conditions." *Population Health Management* 20, no. 1 (2017): 23–30. https://www.doi.org/10.1089/pop.2016.0076.

Clement, Scott, and Lenny Bernstein. "One-Third of Long-Term Users Say They're Hooked on Prescription Opioids." *Washington Post*. December 9, 2016. https://www.washingtonpost.com/national/health-science/one-third-of-long-term-users-say-theyre-hooked-on-prescription-opioids/2016/12/09/e048d322-baed-11e6-91ee-1adddfe36cbe_story.html.

ClinicalTrials.gov. "Using Artificial Intelligence to Monitor Medication Adherence in Opioid Replacement Therapy." Last modified September 12, 2017. https://clinicaltrials.gov/ct2/show/study/NCT02243670.

Cohen, Adam B., Simon C. Mathews, E. Ray Dorsey, David W. Bates, and Kyan Safavi. "Direct-to-Consumer Digital Health." *Lancet Digital Health* 2, no. 4 (April 2020): e163–65. https://doi.org/10.1016/S2589-7500(20)30057-1.

Cohen, Bret S., James Denvil, Filippo A. Raso, and Stevie Degroff. "FTC Authority to Regulate Artificial Intelligence." Reuters. July 8, 2021. https://www.reuters.com/legal/legalindustry/ftc-authority-regulate-artificial-intelligence-2021-07-08/.

Cohen, I. Glenn. "Informed Consent and Medical Artificial Intelligence: What to Tell the Patient?" *Georgetown Law Journal* 108 (2020): 1425–69. https://doi.org/10.2139/ssrn.3529576.

Cohen, I. Glenn, Timo Minssen, W. Nicholson Price II, Christopher Robertson, and Carmel Shachar. "Volume Introduction." In *The Future of*

Medical Device Regulation: Innovation and Protection, edited by I. Glenn Cohen, Timo Minssen, W. Nicholson Price II, Christopher Robertson, and Carmel Shachar, 1–10. Cambridge: Cambridge University Press, 2022. https://doi.org/10.1017/9781108975452.001.

Comstock, Jonah. "AiCure Clinical Trial Seeks to Validate Smartphone Camera-Enabled Medication Adherence." MobiHealthNews. November 24, 2014. https://www.mobihealthnews.com/38512/aicure-clinical-trial-seeks-to-validate-medication-adherence.

Conrad, Peter. "The Meaning of Medications: Another Look at Compliance." *Social Science & Medicine* 20, no. 1 (January 1985): 29–37. https://doi.org/10.1016/0277-9536(85)90308-9.

Conrad, Peter. "The Shifting Engines of Medicalization." *Journal of Health and Social Behavior* 46, no. 1 (March 2005): 3–14. https://doi.org/10.1177%2F002214650504600102.

Corbyn, Zoë. "The Future of Elder Care Is Here—and It's Artificial Intelligence." *The Guardian*. June 3, 2021. https://www.theguardian.com/us-news/2021/jun/03/elder-care-artificial-intelligence-software.

Cordeiro, João V. "Digital Technologies and Data Science as Health Enablers: An Outline of Appealing Promises and Compelling Ethical, Legal, and Social Challenges." *Frontiers in Medicine* 8 (July 2021): 647897. https://doi.org/10.3389/fmed.2021.647897.

Cosgrove, Lisa, Ioana Alina Cristea, Allen F. Shaughnessy, Barbara Mintzes, and Florian Naudet. "Digital Aripiprazole or Digital Evergreening? A Systematic Review of the Evidence and Its Dissemination in the Scientific Literature and in the Media." *BMJ Evidence-Based Medicine* 24, no. 6 (December 2019): 231–38. https://doi.org/10.1136/bmjebm-2019-111204.

Coughlin, Steven S., Jessica L. Stewart, Lufei Young, Vahé Heboyan, and Gianluca De Leo. "Health Literacy and Patient Web Portals." *International Journal of Medical Informatics* 113 (2018): 43–48. https://doi.org/10.1016/j.ijmedinf.2018.02.009.

Coughlin, Steven S., Marlo Vernon, Christos Hatzigeorgiou, and Varghese George. "Health Literacy, Social Determinants of Health, and Disease Prevention and Control." *Journal of Environment and Health Sciences* 6, no. 1 (2020). https://www.ncbi.nlm.nih.gov/pmc/articles/PMC7889072/.

Dahlke, Deborah Vollmer, and Marcia G. Ory. "Emerging Opportunities and Challenges in Optimal Aging with Virtual Personal Assistants." *Public Policy & Aging Report* 27, no. 2 (May 2017): 68–73. https://doi.org/10.1093/ppar/prx004.

Darcy, Alison M., Alan K. Louie, and Laura Weiss Roberts. "Machine Learning and the Profession of Medicine." *Journal of the American Medical Association* 315, no. 6 (2016): 551–52. https://doi.org/10.1001/jama.2015.18421.

Deegan, Patricia E., and Robert E. Drake. "Shared Decision Making and Medication Management in the Recovery Process." *Psychiatric*

Services 57, no. 11 (November 2006): 1636–39. https://doi.org/10.1176/ps.2006.57.11.1636.

Delahoz, Yueng Santiago, and Miguel Angel Labrador. "Survey on Fall Detection and Fall Prevention Using Wearable and External Sensors." *Sensors* 14, no. 10 (October 2014): 19806–42. https://doi.org/10.3390/s141019806.

Depp, Colin A., and Dilip V. Jeste. "Definitions and Predictors of Successful Aging: A Comprehensive Review of Larger Quantitative Studies." *American Journal of Geriatric Psychiatry* 14, no. 1 (January 2006): 6–20. https://doi.org/10.1097/01.JGP.0000192501.03069.bc.

Dhruva, Sanket S., Jonathan J. Darrow, Aaron S. Kesselheim, and Rita F. Redberg. "Ensuring Patient Safety and Benefit in Use of Medical Devices Granted Expedited Approval. In *The Future of Medical Device Regulation: Innovation and Protection*, edited by I. Glenn Cohen, Timo Minssen, W. Nicholson Price II, Christopher Robertson, and Carmel Shachar (Cambridge: Cambridge University Press, 2022), 217–28. https://doi:10.1017/9781108975452.017

D'Ignazio, Catherine, and Lauren F. Klein. *Data Feminism*. Cambridge, MA: MIT Press, 2020.

DiMatteo, M. Robin. "Variations in Patients' Adherence to Medical Recommendations: A Quantitative Review of 50 Years of Research." *Medical Care* 42, no. 3 (March 2004): 200–209. https://doi.org/10.1097/01.mlr.0000114908.90348.f9.

DiMatteo, M. Robin, Patrick J. Giordani, Heidi S. Lepper, and Thomas W. Croghan. "Patient Adherence and Medical Treatment Outcomes: A Meta-Analysis." *Medical Care* 40, no. 9 (September 2002): 794–811. https://doi.org/10.1097/00005650-200209000-00009.

Doekhie, Kirti D., Mathilde M. H. Strating, Martina Buljac-Samardzic, and Jaap Paauwe. "Trust in Older Persons: A Quantitative Analysis of Alignment in Triads of Older Persons, Informal Carers and Home Care Nurses." *Health & Social Care in the Community* 27, no. 6 (November 2019): 1490–506. https://doi.org/10.1111/hsc.12820.

Donlan, Andrew. "Kaiser Permanente, Mayo Clinic, Johns Hopkins and Others Form 'Advanced Care at Home Coalition.'" Home Health Care News. October 14, 2021. https://homehealthcarenews.com/2021/10/kaiser-permanente-mayo-clinic-johns-hopkins-and-others-form-advanced-care-at-home-coalition/.

Dorsey, E. Ray, Floris P. Vlaanderen, Lucien Jlpg Engelen, Karl Kieburtz, William Zhu, Kevin M. Biglan, Marjan J. Faber, and Bastiaan R. Bloem. "Moving Parkinson Care to the Home." *Movement Disorders* 31, no. 9 (2016): 1258–62. https://doi.org/10.1002/mds.26744.

Dowell, Deborah, Tamara Haegerich, and Roger Chou. "No Shortcuts to Safer Opioid Prescribing." *New England Journal of Medicine* 380, no. 24 (June 2019): 2285–87. https://doi.org/10.1056/NEJMp1904190.

Durán, Juan Manuel, and Karin Rolanda Jongsma. "Who is Afraid of Black Box Algorithms? On the Epistemological and Ethical Basis of Trust in Medical AI." *Journal of Medical Ethics* 47, no. 5 (2021): 329–35. https://doi.org/10.1136/medethics-2020-106820.

Eckert, J. Kevin, Leslie A. Morgan, and Namratha Swamy. "Preferences for Receipt of Care among Community-Dwelling Adults." *Journal of Aging & Social Policy* 16, no. 2 (2004): 49–65. https://www.doi.org/10.1300/J031v16n02_04.

Egilman, Alexander C., and Joseph S. Ross. "Digital Medicine Systems: An Evergreening Strategy or an Advance in Medication Management?" *BMJ Evidence-Based Medicine* 24, no. 6 (December 2019): 203. https://doi.org/10.1136/bmjebm-2019-111265.

Ells, Carolyn, Matthew R. Hunt, and Jane Chambers-Evans. "Relational Autonomy as an Essential Component of Patient-Centered Care." *International Journal of Feminist Approaches to Bioethics* 4, no. 2 (2011): 79–101. https://doi.org/10.2979/intjfemappbio.4.2.79.

Entwistle, Vikki A., Rebecca C. H. Brown, Heather M. Morgan, and Zoë C. Skea. "Involving Patients in Their Care." *Current Breast Cancer Reports* 6, no. 3 (September 2014): 211–18. https://doi.org/10.1007/s12609-014-0151-2.

Epstein, Wendy E. "Disrupting the Market for Ineffective Medical Devices." In *The Future of Medical Device Regulation: Innovation and Protection*, edited by I. Glenn Cohen, Timo Minssen, W. Nicholson Price II, Christopher Robertson, and Carmel Shachar (Cambridge: Cambridge University Press, 2022), 179–91. https://doi:10.1017/9781108975452.014.

Esteva, Andre, Brett Kuprel, Roberto A. Novoa, Justin Ko, Susan M. Swetter, Helen M. Blau, and Sebastian Thrun. "Dermatologist-Level Classification of Skin Cancer with Deep Neural Networks." *Nature* 542 (2017): 115–18. https://doi.org/10.1038/nature21056.

European Commission. "Council Directive 93/42/EEC Concerning Medical Devices." Last amended 2007. https://eur-lex.europa.eu/LexUriServ/LexUriServ.do?uri=CONSLEG:1993L0042:20071011:en:PDF.

European Commission. "Laying Down Harmonised Rules on Artificial Intelligence (Artificial Intelligence Act) and Amending Certain Union Legislative Act." https://eur-lex.europa.eu/legal-content/EN/TXT/?uri=CELEX%3A52021PC0206.

European Commission. "Proposal for a Directive of the European Parliament and of the Council on Adapting Non-Contractual Civil Liability Rules to Artificial Intelligence (AI Liability Directive)." https://ec.europa.eu/info/sites/default/files/1_1_197605_prop_dir_ai_en.pdf.

European Commission. "Regulation (EU) 2016/679 of the European Parliament and of the Council on the Protection of Natural Persons with Regard to the Processing of Personal Data and on the Free Movement of Such Data, and Repealing Directive 95/46/EC (General Data Protection

Regulation).” 2016. https://eur-lex.europa.eu/legal-content/EN/TXT/?uri=CELEX%3A02016R0679-20160504&qid=1532348683434.

Faden, Ruth R., Nancy E. Kass, Steven N. Goodman, Peter Pronovost, Sean Tunis, and Tom L. Beauchamp. “An Ethics Framework for a Learning Health Care System: A Departure from Traditional Research Ethics and Clinical Ethics.” *Hastings Center Report* 43, no. 1 (2013): S16–S27. https://doi.org/10.1002/hast.134.

Fausset, Cara Bailey, Andrew J. Kelly, Wendy A. Rogers, and Arthur D. Fisk. “Challenges to Aging in Place: Understanding Home Maintenance Difficulties.” *Journal of Housing for the Elderly* 25, no. 2 (2011): 125–41. https://www.doi.org/10.1080/02763893.2011.571105.

Fineman, Martha. *The Autonomy Myth: A Theory of Dependency*. New York: New Press, 2004.

Fischer, Michael A., Margaret R. Stedman, Joyce Lii, Christine Vogeli, William H. Shrank, M. Alan Brookhart, and Joel S. Weissman. “Primary Medication Non-Adherence: Analysis of 195,930 Electronic Prescriptions.” *Journal of General Internal Medicine* 25, no. 4 (April 2010): 284–90. https://doi.org/10.1007/s11606-010-1253-9.

Fisher, Celia B., and Deborah M. Layman. “Genomics, Big Data, and Broad Consent: A New Ethics Frontier for Prevention Science.” *Prevention Science* 19, no. 7 (October 2018): 871–79. https://doi.org/10.1007/s11121-018-0944-z.

Fishman, Scott M. “Trust and Pharmaco-Vigilance in Pain Medicine.” *Pain Medicine* 6, no. 5 (October 2005): 392. https://doi.org/10.1111/j.1526-4637.2005.00068.x.

Fogel, Alexander L., and Joseph C. Kvedar. “Artificial Intelligence Powers Digital Medicine.” *npj Digital Medicine* 1 (2018). https://doi.org/10.1038/s41746-017-0012-2.

Fontana, Luigi, Brian K. Kennedy, Valter D. Longo, Douglas Seals, and Simon Melov. “Medical Research: Treat Ageing.” *Nature* 511 (2014): 405–7. https://doi.org/10.1038/511405a.

Forsman, Jonas, Heidi Taipale, Thomas Masterman, Jari Tiihonen, and Antti Tanskanen. “Adherence to Psychotropic Medication in Completed Suicide in Sweden 2006-2013: A Forensic-Toxicological Matched Case-Control Study.” *European Journal of Clinical Pharmacology* 75, no. 10 (October 2019): 1421–30. https://doi.org/10.1007/s00228-019-02707-z.

Foucault, Michel. *Discipline and Punish: The Birth of the Prison*. Translated by Alan Sheridan. New York: Pantheon Books, 1977.

Foucault, Michel. “The Subject and Power.” *Critical Inquiry* 8, no. 4 (1982): 777–95. http://www.jstor.org/stable/1343197.

Frakes, Michael, Jonathan Gruber, and Anupam Jena. “Is Great Information Good Enough? Evidence from Physicians as Patients.” *Journal of Health Economics* 75 (January 2021): 102406. https://doi.org/10.1016/j.jhealeco.2020.102406.

Frank, E. M. "Effect of Alzheimer's Disease on Communication Function." *Journal of the South Carolina Medical Association* 90, no. 9 (September 1994): 417–23.

Frates, Candace. "At Mayo Clinic, Sharing Patient Data with Companies Fuels AI Innovation—and Concerns about Consent." STAT. June 3, 2020. https://www.statnews.com/2020/06/03/mayo-clinic-patient-data-fuels-artificial-intelligence-consent-concerns/.

Freedman, Vicki, and Brenda Spillman. "Disability and Care Needs among Older Americans." *Milbank Quarterly* 92, no. 3 (2014): 509–41. https://doi.org/10.1111/1468-0009.12076.

Freeman, Karoline, Jacqueline Dinnes, Naomi Chuchu, Yemisi Takwoingi, Sue E. Bayliss, Rubeta N. Matin, Abhilash Jain, et al. "Algorithm Based Smartphone Apps to Assess Risk of Skin Cancer in Adults: Systematic Review of Diagnostic Accuracy Studies." *BMJ* 368 (February 2020): m127. https://doi.org/10.1136/bmj.m127.

Fricker, Miranda. "Epistemic Injustice and a Role for Virtue in the Politics of Knowing." *Metaphilosophy* 34, no. 1/2 (2003): 154–73. https://www.jstor.org/stable/24439230.

Fricker, Miranda. *Epistemic Injustice: Power and the Ethics of Knowing*. Oxford: Oxford University Press, 2007.

Friedman, Marilyn. *Autonomy, Gender, and Politics*. New York: Oxford University Press, 2003.

Furukawa, Toshi A., Stephen Z. Levine, Shiro Tanaka, Yair Goldberg, Myrto Samara, John M. Davis, Andrea Cipriani, and Stefan Leucht. "Initial Severity of Schizophrenia and Efficacy of Antipsychotics: Participant-Level Meta-Analysis of 6 Placebo-Controlled Studies." *JAMA Psychiatry* 72, no. 1 (January 2015): 14–21. https://doi.org/10.1001/jamapsychiatry.2014.2127.

Gagnon, Marilou, Jean Daniel Jacob, and Adrian Guta. "Treatment Adherence Redefined: A Critical Analysis of Technotherapeutics." *Nursing Inquiry* 20, no. 1 (March 2013): 60–70. https://doi.org/10.1111/j.1440-1800.2012.00595.x.

Galambos, Colleen, Marilyn Rantz, Andy Craver, Marie Bongiorno, Michael Pelts, Austin John Holik, and Jung Sim Jun. "Living with Intelligent Sensors: Older Adult and Family Member Perceptions." *CIN: Computers, Informatics, Nursing* 37, no. 12 (2019). https://journals.lww.com/cinjournal/Fulltext/2019/12000/Living_With_Intelligent_Sensors__Older_Adult_and.3.aspx.

Galozy, Alexander, and Slawomir Nowaczyk. "Prediction and Pattern Analysis of Medication Refill Adherence through Electronic Health Records and Dispensation Data." *Journal of Biomedical Informatics* 112S (2020): 100075. https://doi.org/10.1016/j.yjbinx.2020.100075.

Gao, Jing, Peng Li, Zhikui Chen, and Jianing Zhang. "A Survey on Deep Learning for Multimodal Data Fusion." *Neural Computation* 32, no. 5 (2020): 829–64. https://doi.org/10.1162/neco_a_01273.

García, Saínza, Mónica Martínez-Cengotitabengoa, Saioa López-Zurbano, Iñaki Zorrilla, Purificación López, Eduard Vieta, and Ana González-Pinto. "Adherence to Antipsychotic Medication in Bipolar Disorder and Schizophrenic Patients: A Systematic Review." *Journal of Clinical Psychopharmacology* 36, no. 4 (August 2016): 355–71. https://doi.org/10.1097/JCP.0000000000000523.

Gawande, Atul. "Why Doctors Hate Their Computers." *New Yorker*. November 5, 2018. https://www.newyorker.com/magazine/2018/11/12/why-doctors-hate-their-computers.

Gebhart, Andrew. "Nobi Will Watch over Your Grandparents, Literally, from a Ceiling Mounted Smart Lamp." CNET. January 12, 2021. https://www.cnet.com/home/smart-home/nobi-will-watch-over-your-grandparents-literally-from-a-ceiling-mounted-smart-lamp.

Gellad, Walid F., Jerry L. Grenard, and Zachary A. Marcum. "A Systematic Review of Barriers to Medication Adherence in the Elderly: Looking Beyond Cost and Regimen Complexity." *American Journal of Geriatric Pharmacotherapy* 9, no. 1 (February 2011): 11–23. https://doi.org/10.1016/j.amjopharm.2011.02.004.

Genin, Konstantin, and Thomas Grote. "Randomized Controlled Trials in Medical AI: A Methodological Critique." *Philosophy of Medicine* 2, no. 1 (2021). https://doi.org/10.5195/philmed.2021.27.

Genworth. "Cost of Care: Trends and Insights." Accessed February 8, 2022. https://www.genworth.com/aging-and-you/finances/cost-of-care/cost-of-care-trends-and-insights.html.

Gerke, Sara, Boris Babic, Theodoros Evgeniou, and I. Glenn Cohen. "The Need for a System View to Regulate Artificial Intelligence/Machine Learning-Based Software as Medical Device." *npj Digital Medicine* 3, no. 53 (April 2020). https://doi.org/10.1038/s41746-020-0262-2.

Germain, Thomas. "Mental Health Apps Aren't All as Private as You May Think." Consumer Reports. March 2, 2021. https://www.consumerreports.org/health-privacy/mental-health-apps-and-user-privacy/.

Giger, Jarod T., Natalie D. Pope, H. Bruce Vogt, Cassity Gutierrez, Lisa A. Newland, Jason Lemke, and Michael J. Lawler. "Remote Patient Monitoring Acceptance Trends among Older Adults Residing in a Frontier State." *Computers in Human Behavior* 44 (March 2015): 174–82. https://doi.org/10.1016/j.chb.2014.11.044.

Gigerenzer, Gerd, Wolfgang Gaissmaier, Elke Kurz-Milcke, Lisa M. Schwartz, and Steven Woloshin. "Helping Doctors and Patients Make Sense of Health Statistics." *Psychological Science in the Public Interest* 8, no. 2 (November 2007): 53–96. https://doi.org/10.1111/j.1539-6053.2008.00033.x.

Gilbert, Fiona J., Susan M. Astley, Maureen G. C. Gillan, Olorunsola F. Agbaje, Matthew G. Wallis, Jonathan James, Caroline R. M. Boggis, and Stephen W. Duffy. "Single Reading with Computer-Aided Detection for Screening

Mammography." *New England Journal of Medicine* 359, no. 16 (Oct. 2008): 1675–84. https://doi.org/10.1056/NEJMoa0803545.

Gillani, Nazia, and Tughrul Arslan. "Intelligent Sensing Technologies for the Diagnosis, Monitoring and Therapy of Alzheimer's Disease: A Systematic Review." *Sensors* 21, no. 12 (June 2021): 4249. https://doi.org/10.3390/s21124249.

Gilmer, Todd P., Christian R. Dolder, Jonathan P. Lacro, David P. Folsom, Laurie Lindamer, Piedad Garcia, and Dilip V. Jeste. "Adherence to Treatment with Antipsychotic Medication and Health Care Costs among Medicaid Beneficiaries with Schizophrenia." *American Journal of Psychiatry* 161, no. 4 (April 2004): 692–99. https://doi.org/10.1176/appi.ajp.161.4.692.

Glenn, Evelyn Nakano. *Forced to Care: Coercion and Caregiving in America.* Cambridge, MA: Harvard University Press, 2012.

Goff, Donald C., Michele Hill, and Oliver Freudenreich. "Strategies for Improving Treatment Adherence in Schizophrenia and Schizoaffective Disorder." *Journal of Clinical Psychiatry* 71, Suppl. 2 (2010): 20–26. https://doi.org/10.4088/JCP.9096su1cc.04.

Goldfine, Charlotte, Jeffrey T. Lai, Evan Lucey, Mark Newcomb, and Stephanie Carreiro. "Wearable and Wireless mHealth Technologies for Substance Use Disorder." *Current Addiction Reports* 7, no. 3 (September 2020): 291–300. https://doi.org/10.1007/s40429-020-00318-8.

Goodfellow, Ian, Yoshua Bengio, and Aaron Courville. *Deep Learning.* 1st ed. Cambridge, MA: MIT Press, 2016.

Gottliebsen, Kristian, and Göran Petersson. "Limited Evidence of Benefits of Patient Operated Intelligent Primary Care Triage Tools: Findings of a Literature Review." *BMJ Health & Care Informatics* 27, no. 1 (May 2020): e100114. https://doi.org/10.1136/bmjhci-2019-100114.

Gourlay, Douglas L., and Howard A. Heit. "Universal Precautions Revisited: Managing the Inherited Pain Patient." *Pain Medicine* 10, Suppl 2 (July 2009): S115–23. https://doi.org/10.1111/j.1526-4637.2009.00671.x.

Gourlay, Douglas L., Howard A. Heit, and Abdulaziz Almahrezi. "Universal Precautions in Pain Medicine: A Rational Approach to the Treatment of Chronic Pain." *Pain Medicine* 6, no. 2 (April 2005): 107–12. https://doi.org/10.1111/j.1526-4637.2005.05031.x.

Grenfell, Pippa, Nerissa Tilouche, Jill Shawe, and Rebecca S. French. "Fertility and Digital Technology: Narratives of Using Smartphone App 'Natural Cycles' while Trying to Conceive." *Sociology of Health & Illness* 43, no. 1 (January 2021): 116–32. https://doi.org/10.1111/1467-9566.13199.

Grippo, Karen P., and Melanie S. Hill. "Self-Objectification, Habitual Body Monitoring, and Body Dissatisfaction in Older European American Women: Exploring Age and Feminism as Moderators." *Body Image* 5, no. 2 (June 2008): 173–82. https://doi.org/10.1016/j.bodyim.2007.11.003.

Grote, Thomas, and Philipp Berens. "On the Ethics of Algorithmic Decision-Making in Healthcare." *Journal of Medical Ethics* 46, no. 3 (March 2020): 205. https://doi.org/10.1136/medethics-2019-105586.

Gulshan, Varun, Lily Peng, Marc Coram, Martin C. Stumpe, Derek Wu, Arunachalam Narayanaswamy, Subhashini Venugopalan, et al. "Development and Validation of a Deep Learning Algorithm for Detection of Diabetic Retinopathy in Retinal Fundus Photographs." *Journal of the American Medical Association* 316, no. 22 (2016): 2402–10. https://doi.org/10.1001/jama.2016.17216.

Guta, Adrian, Jijian Voronka, and Marilou Gagnon. "Resisting the Digital Medicine Panopticon: Toward a Bioethics of the Oppressed." *American Journal of Bioethics* 18, no. 9 (September 2018): 62–64. https://doi.org/10.1080/15265161.2018.1498936.

Haddad, Peter M., Cecilia Brain, and Jan Scott. "Nonadherence with Antipsychotic Medication in Schizophrenia: Challenges and Management Strategies." *Patient Related Outcome Measures* 5 (2014): 43–62. https://doi.org/10.2147/PROM.S42735.

Hamzelou, Jessica. "DNA Firms Are Set to Profit from Your Data as Testing Demand Falls." *New Scientist*, February 7, 2020. https://www.newscientist.com/article/2232770-dna-firms-are-set-to-profit-from-your-data-as-testing-demand-falls/.

Hancock, Black Hawk. "Michel Foucault and the Problematics of Power: Theorizing DTCA and Medicalized Subjectivity." *Journal of Medicine and Philosophy* 43, no. 4 (August 2018): 439–68. https://doi.org/10.1093/jmp/jhy010.

Hao, Karen. "AI is Sending People to Jail—and Getting It Wrong." MIT Technology Review. January 21, 2019. https://www.technologyreview.com/2019/01/21/137783/algorithms-criminal-justice-ai/.

Hartwig, Tilman, Yuko Ikkatai, Naohiro Takanashi, and Hiromi M. Yokoyama. "Artificial Intelligence ELSI Score for Science and Technology: A Comparison between Japan and the US." *AI & Society* (January 2022). https://doi.org/10.1007/s00146-021-01323-9.

Harwell, Drew. "Ring and Nest Helped Normalize American Surveillance and Turned Us into a Nation of Voyeurs." *Washington Post*. February 18, 2020. https://www.washingtonpost.com/technology/2020/02/18/ring-nest-surveillance-doorbell-camera/.

Hatch, Ainslie, John P. Docherty, Daniel Carpenter, Ruth Ross, and Peter J. Weiden. "Expert Consensus Survey on Medication Adherence in Psychiatric Patients and Use of a Digital Medicine System." *Journal of Clinical Psychiatry* 78, no. 7 (July 2017): e803–12. https://doi.org/10.4088/JCP.16m11252.

Hawkins, Alice K., and Anita Ho. "Genetic Counseling and the Ethical Issues around Direct-to-Consumer Genetic Testing." *Journal of Genetic Counseling* 21, no. 3 (June 2012): 367–73. https://doi.org/10.1007/s10897-012-9488-8.

Hawley-Hague, Helen, Elisabeth Boulton, Alex Hall, Klaus Pfeiffer, and Chris Todd. "Older Adults' Perceptions of Technologies Aimed at Falls Prevention, Detection or Monitoring: A Systematic Review." *International Journal of Medical Informatics* 83, no. 6 (2014): 416–26. https://doi.org/10.1016/j.ijmedinf.2014.03.002.

Häyry, Matti. "The Tension between Self Governance and Absolute Inner Worth in Kant's Moral Philosophy." *Journal of Medical Ethics* 31, no. 11 (2005): 645–47. https://doi.org/10.1136/jme.2004.010058.

Health Catalyst. "Machine Learning Tools Unlock the Most Critical Insights from Unstructured Health Data." December 6, 2019. https://www.healthcatalyst.com/insights/healthcare-machine-learning-unlocks-unstructured-data.

Heathfield, Heather. "The Rise and 'Fall' of Expert Systems in Medicine." *Expert Systems* 16, no. 3 (1999): 183–88. https://doi.org/10.1111/1468-0394.00107.

Henderson, Sara, and Alan Petersen, eds. *Consuming Health: The Commodification of Health Care*. London: Routledge, 2002.

Herrman, John. "Who's Watching Your Porch?" *New York Times*. January 19, 2020. https://www.nytimes.com/2020/01/19/style/ring-video-doorbell-home-security.html.

Hickner, J., D. G. Graham, N. C. Elder, E. Brandt, C. B. Emsermann, S. Dovey, and R. Phillips. "Testing Process Errors and Their Harms and Consequences Reported from Family Medicine Practices: A Study of the American Academy of Family Physicians National Research Network." *Quality and Safety in Health Care* 17, no. 3 (June 2008): 194. https://doi.org/10.1136/qshc.2006.021915.

Hill, Maureen V., Michelle L. McMahon, Ryland S. Stucke, and Richard J. Barth. "Wide Variation and Excessive Dosage of Opioid Prescriptions for Common General Surgical Procedures." *Annals of Surgery* 265, no. 4 (2016): 709–14. https://doi.org/10.1097/SLA.0000000000001993.

Hillcoat-Nallétamby, Sarah. "The Meaning of 'Independence' for Older People in Different Residential Settings." *Journals of Gerontology: Series B* 69, no. 3 (May 2014): 419–30. https://doi.org/10.1093/geronb/gbu008.

Hillman, Lisa A., Cynthia Peden-McAlpine, Djenane Ramalho-de-Oliveira, and Jon C. Schommer. "The Medication Experience: A Concept Analysis." *Pharmacy* 9, no. 1 (December 2020). https://doi.org/10.3390/pharmacy9010007.

Ho, Anita. "Are We Ready for Artificial Intelligence Health Monitoring in Elder Care?" *BMC Geriatrics* 20, no. 1 (September 2020): 358. https://doi.org/10.1186/s12877-020-01764-9.

Ho, Anita. "Can Public Health Investment and Oversight Save Digital Mental Health?" *AJOB Neuroscience* 13, no. 3 (July 2022): 201–3. https://doi.org/10.1080/21507740.2022.2082586.

Ho, Anita. "Deep Ethical Learning: Taking the Interplay of Human and Artificial Intelligence Seriously." *Hastings Center Report* 49, no. 1 (2019): 38–41. https://doi.org/10.1002/hast.977.

Ho, Anita. "Epistemic Injustice." In *Encyclopedia of Bioethics*, 4th ed., edited by Bruce Jennings. Belmont, CA: Wadsworth Publishing, 2014.

Ho, Anita. "The Individualist Model of Autonomy and the Challenge of Disability." *Bioethical Inquiry* 5 (2008): 193–207. https://doi.org/10.1007/s11673-007-9075-0.

Ho, Anita. "Reconciling Patient Safety and Epistemic Humility: An Ethical Use of Opioid Treatment Plans." *Hastings Center Report* 47, no. 3 (May 2017): 34–35. https://doi.org/10.1002/hast.703.

Ho, Anita. "Relational Autonomy or Undue Pressure? Family's Role in Medical Decision-Making." *Scandinavian Journal of Caring Sciences* 22, no. 1 (March 2008): 128–35. https://doi.org/10.1111/j.1471-6712.2007.00561.x.

Ho, Anita. "Trusting Experts and Epistemic Humility in Disability." *International Journal of Feminist Approaches to Bioethics* 4, no. 2 (September 2011): 102–23. https://doi.org/10.3138/ijfab.4.2.102.

Ho, Anita, and Daniel Buchman. "Pain." In *Encyclopedia of Global Bioethics*, edited by Henk ten Have. New York: Springer, 2015. https://doi.org/10.1007/978-3-319-05544-2_322-1.

Ho, Anita, Stephen J. Pinney, and Kevin Bozic. "Ethical Concerns in Caring for Elderly Patients with Cognitive Limitations: A Capacity-Adjusted Shared Decision-Making Approach." *Journal of Bone and Joint Surgery* 97, no. 3 (2015): e16. https://doi.org/10.2106/JBJS.N.00762.

Ho, Anita, and Oliver Quick. "Leaving Patients to Their Own Devices? Smart Technology, Safety and Therapeutic Relationships." *BMC Medical Ethics* 19 (2018). https://doi.org/10.1186/s12910-018-0255-8.

Ho, Anita, Anita Silvers, and Tim Stainton. "Continuous Surveillance of Persons with Disabilities: Conflicts and Compatibilities of Personal and Social Goods." *Journal of Social Philosophy* 45, no. 3 (2014): 348–68. https://doi.org/10.1111/josp.12067.

Hogan, Niamh M., and Michael J. Kerin. "Smart Phone Apps: Smart Patients, Steer Clear." *Patient Education and Counseling* 89, no. 2 (November 2012): 360–61. https://doi.org/10.1016/j.pec.2012.07.016.

Holmes, D. "From Iron Gaze to Nursing Care: Mental Health Nursing in the Era of Panopticism." *Journal of Psychiatric and Mental Health Nursing* 8, no. 1 (February 2001): 7–15. https://doi.org/10.1046/j.1365-2850.2001.00345.x.

Holstein, Martha B., and Meredith Minkler. "Critical Gerontology: Reflections for the 21st Century." In *Critical Perspectives on Ageing Societies*, edited by Miriam Bernard and Thomas Scharf. Bristol: Policy Press, 2007.

hooks, bell. "Homeplace: A Site of Resistance." In *Undoing Place? A Geographical Reader*, edited by Linda McDowell, 33–38. London: Routledge, 1997.

Hooten, W. Michael, Chad M. Brummett, Mark D. Sullivan, Jenna Goesling, Jon C. Tilburt, Jessica S. Merlin, Jennifer L. St. Sauver, et al. "A Conceptual

Framework for Understanding Unintended Prolonged Opioid Use." *Mayo Clinic Proceedings* 92, no. 12 (December 2017): 1822–30. https://doi.org/10.1016/j.mayocp.2017.10.010.

Huang, Hannah Chu-Han, and Dennis Ougrin. "Impact of the COVID-19 Pandemic on Child and Adolescent Mental Health Services." *BJPsych Open* 7, no. 5 (2021): e145. https://doi.org/10.1192/bjo.2021.976.

Huang, Jui-Chen. "Remote Health Monitoring Adoption Model Based on Artificial Neural Networks." *Expert Systems with Applications* 37, no. 1 (2010): 307–14. https://doi.org/10.1016/j.eswa.2009.05.063.

Huckvale, Kit, Samanta Adomaviciute, José Tomás Prieto, Melvin Khee-Shing Leow, and Josip Car. "Smartphone Apps for Calculating Insulin Dose: A Systematic Assessment." *BMC Medicine* 13, no. 1 (May 2015): 106. https://doi.org/10.1186/s12916-015-0314-7.

Huckvale, Kit, John Torous, and Mark E. Larsen. "Assessment of the Data Sharing and Privacy Practices of Smartphone Apps for Depression and Smoking Cessation." *JAMA Network Open* 2, no. 4 (April 2019): e192542. https://doi.org/10.1001/jamanetworkopen.2019.2542.

Hughson, Jo-Anne Patricia, J. Oliver Daly, Robyn Woodward-Kron, John Hajek, and David Story. "The Rise of Pregnancy Apps and the Implications for Culturally and Linguistically Diverse Women: Narrative Review." *JMIR mHealth and uHealth* 6, no. 11 (November 2018): e189. https://doi.org/10.2196/mhealth.9119.

Hugtenburg, Jacqueline G., Lonneke Timmers, Petra J. M. Elders, Marcia Vervloet, and Liset van Dijk. "Definitions, Variants, and Causes of Nonadherence with Medication: A Challenge for Tailored Interventions." *Patient Preference and Adherence* 7 (July 2013): 675–82. https://doi.org/10.2147/PPA.S29549.

Hurtado-de-Mendoza, Alejandra, Mark L. Cabling, and Vanessa B. Sheppard. "Rethinking Agency and Medical Adherence Technology: Applying Actor Network Theory to the Case Study of Digital Pills." *Nursing Inquiry* 22, no. 4 (December 2015): 326–35. https://doi.org/10.1111/nin.12101.

Hyer, J. Madison, Anghela Z. Paredes, Susan White, Aslam Ejaz, and Timothy M. Pawlik. "Assessment of Utilization Efficiency Using Machine Learning Techniques: A Study of Heterogeneity in Preoperative Healthcare Utilization among Super-Utilizers." *American Journal of Surgery* 220, no. 3 (2020): 714–20. https://doi.org/10.1016/j.amjsurg.2020.01.043.

Ibrahim, Hussein, Xiaoxuan Liu, Nevine Zariffa, Andrew D. Morris, and Alastair K. Denniston. "Health Data Poverty: An Assailable Barrier to Equitable Digital Health Care." *Lancet Digital Health* 3, no. 4 (April 2021): e260–65. https://doi.org/10.1016/S2589-7500(20)30317-4.

International Association for the Study of Pain. *Unrelieved Pain Is a Major Global Health-Care Problem*. Washington, DC: International Association for the Study of Pain, 2012.

IQVIA Institute. "Digital Health Trends, 2021." July 21, 2021. https://www.iqvia.com/insights/the-iqvia-institute/reports/digital-health-trends-2021.

Irving, Greg, Ana Luisa Neves, Hajira Dambha-Miller, Ai Oishi, Hiroko Tagashira, Anistasiya Verho, and John Holden. "International Variations in Primary Care Physician Consultation Time: A Systematic Review of 67 Countries." *BMJ Open* 7, no. 10 (2017): e017902. https://doi.org/10.1136/bmjopen-2017-017902.

Iuga, Aurel O., and Maura J. McGuire. "Adherence and Health Care Costs." *Risk Management and Healthcare Policy* 7 (2014): 35–44. https://doi.org/10.2147/RMHP.S19801.

Jenkinson, Bec, Sue Kruske, and Sue Kildea. "The Experiences of Women, Midwives and Obstetricians When Women Decline Recommended Maternity Care: A Feminist Thematic Analysis." *Midwifery* 52 (September 2017): 1–10. https://doi.org/10.1016/j.midw.2017.05.006.

Jercich, Kat. "Nurse Unions Slam Kaiser's Advanced Care at Home Strategy." Healthcare IT News. November 8, 2021. https://www.healthcareitnews.com/news/nurse-unions-slam-kaisers-advanced-care-home-strategy.

Jiang, Fei, Yong Jiang, Hui Zhi, Yi Dong, Hao Li, Sufeng Ma, Yilong Wang, et al. "Artificial Intelligence in Healthcare: Past, Present and Future." *Stroke and Vascular Neurology* 2, no. 4 (2017). https://doi.org/10.1136/svn-2017-000101.

Joannou, Simone Lee. "Toward an Account of Relational Autonomy in Healthcare and Treatment Settings." *Essays in the Philosophy of Humanism* 24, no. 1 (2016): 1–20.

Joint Commission. "Managing Patient Care via Telehealth (OME)." Standards FAQs. Last modified December 22, 2021. https://www.jointcommission.org/standards/standard-faqs/home-care/provision-of-care-treatment-and-services-pc/000002289/.

Joseph-Williams, Natalie, Glyn Elwyn, and Adrian Edwards. "Knowledge Is Not Power for Patients: A Systematic Review and Thematic Synthesis of Patient-Reported Barriers and Facilitators to Shared Decision Making." *Patient Education and Counseling* 94, no. 3 (March 2014): 291–309. https://doi.org/10.1016/j.pec.2013.10.031.

Jung, Beth, and Marcus M. Reidenberg. "Physicians Being Deceived." *Pain Medicine* 8, no. 5 (August 2007): 433–37. https://doi.org/10.1111/j.1526-4637.2007.00315.x.

Jutel, Annemarie, and Deborah Lupton. "Digitizing Diagnosis: A Review of Mobile Applications in the Diagnostic Process." *Diagnosis* 2, no. 2 (2015): 89–96. https://doi.org/10.1515/dx-2014-0068.

Kalantarian, Haik, Babak Motamed, Nabil Alshurafa, and Majid Sarrafzadeh. "A Wearable Sensor System for Medication Adherence Prediction." *Artificial Intelligence in Medicine* 69 (May 2016): 43–52. https://doi.org/10.1016/j.artmed.2016.03.004.

Kane, Sunanda, and Fadia Shaya. "Medication Non-Adherence Is Associated with Increased Medical Health Care Costs." *Digestive Diseases and Sciences* 53, no. 4 (April 2008): 1020–24. https://doi.org/10.1007/s10620-007-9968-0.

Kang, Hyun Gu, Diane F. Mahoney, Helen Hoenig, Victor A. Hirth, Paolo Bonato, Ihab Hajjar, and Lewis A. Lipsitz. "In Situ Monitoring of Health in Older Adults: Technologies and Issues." *Journal of the American Geriatrics Society* 58, no. 8 (August 2010): 1579–86. https://doi.org/10.1111/j.1532-5415.2010.02959.x.

Kannan, Anitha. "The Science of Assisting Medical Diagnosis: From Expert Systems to Machine-Learned Models." Medium. April 15, 2019. https://medium.com/curai-tech/the-science-of-assisting-medical-diagnosis-from-expert systems-to-machine-learned-models-cc2ef0b03098.

Kant, Immanuel. *Foundations of the Metaphysics of Morals*. Translated by Lewis White Beck. Indianapolis: Bobbs-Merrill, 1959.

Karlekar, Sweta, Tong Niu, and Mohit Bansal. "Detecting Linguistic Characteristics of Alzheimer's Dementia by Interpreting Neural Models." *Proceedings of the 2018 Conference of the North American Chapter of the Association for Computational Linguistics: Human Language Technologies, Volume 2 (Short Papers)* (June 2018): 701–7. https://doi.org/10.18653/v1/N18-2110.

Karpati, Adam, Sandro Galea, Tamara Awerbuch, and Richard Levins. "Variability and Vulnerability at the Ecological Level: Implications for Understanding the Social Determinants of Health." *American Journal of Public Health* 92, no. 11 (2002): 1768–72. https://doi.org/10.2105/ajph.92.11.1768.

Kass, Nancy E., and Ruth R. Faden. "Ethics and Learning Health Care: The Essential Roles of Engagement, Transparency, and Accountability." *Learning Health Systems* 2, no. 4 (2018): e10066. https://doi.org/10.1002/lrh2.10066.

Kass, Nancy E., Ruth R. Faden, Steven N. Goodman, Peter Pronovost, Sean Tunis, and Tom L. Beauchamp. "The Research-Treatment Distinction: A Problematic Approach for Determining Which Activities Should Have Ethical Oversight." *Hastings Center Report* 43, no. 1 (2013): S4–S15. https://doi.org/10.1002/hast.133.

Katz, Stephen. "Growing Older without Aging? Positive Aging, Anti-Ageism, and Anti-Aging." *Generations* 25 (2001/2002): 27–32.

Kennedy, Helen, Thomas Poell, and Jose van Dijck. "Data and Agency." *Big Data & Society* 2, no. 2 (December 2015). https://doi.org/10.1177/2053951715621569.

Kennedy-Hendricks, Alen, Andrea Gielen, Eileen McDonald, Emma E. McGinty, Wendy Shields, and Colleen L. Barry. "Medication Sharing, Storage, and Disposal Practices for Opioid Medications among U.S. Adults." *JAMA Internal Medicine* 176, no. 7 (2016): 1027–29. https://doi.org/10.1001/jamainternmed.2016.2543.

Kenner, Alison Marie. "Securing the Elderly Body: Dementia, Surveillance, and the Politics of 'Aging in Place.'" *Surveillance & Society* 5, no. 3 (2008). https://doi.org/10.24908/ss.v5i3.3423.

Kesselheim, Aaron S., and Jerry Avorn. "New '21st Century Cures' Legislation: Speed and Ease vs Science. *Journal of the American Medical Association* 317, no. 6 (February 14, 2017): 581–82. https://doi: 10.1001/jama.2016.20640. PMID: 28056124.

Kessels, Roy P. C. "Patients' Memory for Medical Information." *Journal of the Royal Society of Medicine* 96, no. 5 (May 2003): 219–22. https://doi.org/10.1258/jrsm.96.5.219.

Kikkert, Martijn J., and Jack Dekker. "Medication Adherence Decisions in Patients with Schizophrenia." *Primary Care Companion for CNS Disorders* 19, no. 6 (December 2017). https://doi.org/10.4088/PCC.17n02182.

Kleinschmidt, Thea K., Jonathan R. Bull, Vincenzo Lavorini, Simon P. Rowland, Jack T. Pearson, Elina Berglund Scherwitzl, Raoul Scherwitzl, and Kristina Gemzell Danielsson. "Advantages of Determining the Fertile Window with the Individualised Natural Cycles Algorithm over Calendar-Based Methods." *European Journal of Contraception & Reproductive Health Care* 24, no. 6 (November 2019): 457–63. https://doi.org/10.1080/13625187.2019.1682544.

Kliff, Sarah, and Aatish Bhatia. "When They Warn of Rare Disorders, These Prenatal Tests Are Usually Wrong." *New York Times*. January 1, 2022. https://www.nytimes.com/2022/01/01/upshot/pregnancy-birth-genetic-testing.html?action=click&module=Well&pgtype=Homepage&section=The%20Upshot.

Knapp, Martin, Derek King, Klaus Pugner, and Pablo Lapuerta. "Non-Adherence to Antipsychotic Medication Regimens: Associations with Resource Use and Costs." *British Journal of Psychiatry* 184 (June 2004): 509–16. https://doi.org/10.1192/bjp.184.6.509.

Knoppers, Bartha Maria, and Adrian Mark Thorogood. "Ethics and Big Data in Health." *Current Opinion in Systems Biology* 4 (August 2017): 53–57. https://doi.org/10.1016/j.coisb.2017.07.001.

Koesmahargyo, Vidya, Anzar Abbas, Li Zhang, Lei Guan, Shaolei Feng, Vijay Yadav, and Isaac R. Galatzer-Levy. "Accuracy of Machine Learning-Based Prediction of Medication Adherence in Clinical Research." *Psychiatry Research* 294 (December 2020): 113558. https://doi.org/10.1016/j.psychres.2020.113558.

Komorowski, Matthieu, and Leo Anthony Celi. "Will Artificial Intelligence Contribute to Overuse in Healthcare?" *Critical Care Medicine* 45, no. 5 (May 2017): 912–13. https://doi.org/10.1097/CCM.0000000000002351.

Korsgaard, Christine. *Self-Constitution: Agency, Identity, and Integrity*. Oxford: Oxford University Press, 2009.

Korsgaard, Christine. *The Sources of Normativity*. Cambridge: Cambridge University Press, 1996.

Kraft, Stephanie A. "Respect and Trustworthiness in the Patient-Provider-Machine Relationship: Applying a Relational Lens to Machine Learning Healthcare Applications." *American Journal of Bioethics* 20, no. 11 (2020): 51–53. https://doi.org/10.1080/15265161.2020.1820108.

Kraft, Stephanie A., Mildred K. Cho, Katherine Gillespie, Meghan Halley, Nina Varsava, Kelly E. Ormond, Harold S. Luft, et al. "Beyond Consent: Building Trusting Relationships with Diverse Populations in Precision Medicine Research." *American Journal of Bioethics* 18, no. 4 (2018): 3–20. https://doi.org/10.1080/15265161.2018.1431322.

Krebs, Paul, and Dustin T. Duncan. "Health App Use Among US Mobile Phone Owners: A National Survey." *JMIR mHealth and uHealth* 3, no. 4 (November 2015): e101. https://doi.org/10.2196/mhealth.4924.

Kroenke, Kurt, Daniel P. Alford, Charles Argoff, Bernard Canlas, Edward Covington, Joseph W. Frank, Karl J. Haake, et al. "Challenges with Implementing the Centers for Disease Control and Prevention Opioid Guideline: A Consensus Panel Report." *Pain Medicine* 20, no. 4 (April 2019): 724–35. https://doi.org/10.1093/pm/pny307.

Kroken, Rune A., Eirik Kjelby, Tore Wentzel-Larsen, Liv S. Mellesdal, Hugo A. Jørgensen, and Erik Johnsen. "Time to Discontinuation of Antipsychotic Drugs in a Schizophrenia Cohort: Influence of Current Treatment Strategies." *Therapeutic Advances in Psychopharmacology* 4, no. 6 (December 2014): 228–39. https://doi.org/10.1177/2045125314545614.

Krska, Janet, Charles W. Morecroft, Helen Poole, and Philip H. Rowe. "Issues Potentially Affecting Quality of Life Arising from Long-Term Medicines Use: A Qualitative Study." *International Journal of Clinical Pharmacy* 35, no. 6 (December 2013): 1161–69. https://doi.org/10.1007/s11096-013-9841-5.

Kvarnström, Kirsi, Aleksi Westerholm, Marja Airaksinen, and Helena Liira. "Factors Contributing to Medication Adherence in Patients with a Chronic Condition: A Scoping Review of Qualitative Research." *Pharmaceutics* 13, no. 7 (July 2021). https://doi.org/10.3390/pharmaceutics13071100.

Labovitz, Daniel L., Laura Shafner, Morayma Reyes Gil, Deepti Virmani, and Adam Hanina. "Using Artificial Intelligence to Reduce the Risk of Nonadherence in Patients on Anticoagulation Therapy." *Stroke* 48, no. 5 (2017): 1416–19. https://doi.org/10.1161/STROKEAHA.116.016281.

Lam, Wai Yin, and Paula Fresco. "Medication Adherence Measures: An Overview." *BioMed Research International* (2015): 217047. https://doi.org/10.1155/2015/217047.

Landi, Heather. "IBM Sells Watson Health Assets to Investment Firm Francisco Partners." Fierce Healthcare. January 21, 2022. https://www.fiercehealthcare.com/tech/ibm-sells-watson-health-assets-to-investment-firm-francisco-partners.

Landi, Heather. "Proteus Digital Health Was Once Valued at $1.5B. It May Be Acquired in a $15M 'Stalking Horse' Bid." Fierce Healthcare. July 27, 2020.

https://www.fiercehealthcare.com/tech/proteus-digital-health-could-exit-bankruptcy-15m-stalking-horse-from-otsuka.

Lanzing, Marjolein. "The Transparent Self." *Ethics and Information Technology* 18, no. 1 (March 2016): 9–16. https://doi.org/10.1007/s10676-016-9396-y.

Lee, Chaiwoo, and Joseph F. Coughlin. "Perspective: Older Adults' Adoption of Technology: An Integrated Approach to Identifying Determinants and Barriers." *Journal of Product Innovation Management* 32, no. 5 (September 2015): 747–59. https://doi.org/10.1111/jpim.12176.

Lee, Won-Suk, Sung Min Ahn, Jun-Won Chung, Kyoung Oh Kim, Kwang An Kwon, Yoonjae Kim, Sunjin Sym, et al. "Assessing Concordance with Watson for Oncology, a Cognitive Computing Decision Support System for Colon Cancer Treatment in Korea." *JCO Clinical Cancer Informatics* 2 (December 2018): 1–8. https://doi.org/10.1200/CCI.17.00109.

Lehane, Elaine, and Geraldine McCarthy. "Medication Non-Adherence—Exploring the Conceptual Mire." *International Journal of Nursing Practice* 15, no. 1 (February 2009): 25–31. https://doi.org/10.1111/j.1440-172X.2008.01722.x.

Lehoux, Pascale, Jocelyne Saint-Arnaud, and Lucie Richard. "The Use of Technology at Home: What Patient Manuals Say and Sell vs. What Patients Face and Fear." *Sociology of Health & Illness* 26, no. 5 (July 2004): 617–44. https://doi.org/10.1111/j.0141-9889.2004.00408.x.

Lemire, Marc. "What Can Be Expected of Information and Communication Technologies in Terms of Patient Empowerment in Health?" *Journal of Health Organization and Management* 24, no. 2 (January 2010): 167–81. https://doi.org/10.1108/14777261011047336.

Lemstra, Mark, Chijioke Nwankwo, Yelena Bird, and John Moraros. "Primary Nonadherence to Chronic Disease Medications: A Meta-Analysis." *Patient Preference and Adherence* 12 (2018): 721–31. https://doi.org/10.2147/PPA.S161151.

Lerman, Rachel, and Hamza Shaban. "Amazon Will See You Now: Tech Giant Buys Health-Care Chain for $3.9 Billion." *Washington Post*. July 21, 2022. https://www.washingtonpost.com/business/2022/07/21/amazon-health-care/.

Leslie, R. Scott, Breanne Tirado, Bimal V. Patel, and Philip J. Rein. "Evaluation of an Integrated Adherence Program Aimed to Increase Medicare Part D Star Rating Measures." *Journal of Managed Care Pharmacy* 20, no. 12 (December 2014): 1193–1203. https://doi.org/10.18553/jmcp.2014.20.12.1193.

Li, Yanping, Josje Schoufour, Dong D. Wang, Klodian Dhana, An Pan, Xiaoran Liu, Mingyang Song, et al. "Healthy Lifestyle and Life Expectancy Free of Cancer, Cardiovascular Disease, and Type 2 Diabetes: Prospective Cohort Study." *BMJ* 368 (January 2020): l6669. https://doi.org/10.1136/bmj.l6669.

Litchfield, Ian, Louise Bentham, Richard Lilford, Richard J. McManus, Ann Hill, and Sheila Greenfield. "Test Result Communication in Primary Care: A

Survey of Current Practice." *BMJ Quality & Safety* 24, no. 11 (November 2015): 691. https://doi.org/10.1136/bmjqs-2014-003712.

Lo-Ciganic, Wei-Hsuan, James L. Huang, Hao H. Zhang, Jeremy C. Weiss, Yonghui Wu, C. Kent Kwoh, Julie M. Donohue, et al. "Evaluation of Machine-Learning Algorithms for Predicting Opioid Overdose Risk among Medicare Beneficiaries with Opioid Prescriptions." *JAMA Network Open* 2, no. 3 (March 2019): e190968. https://doi.org/10.1001/jamanetworkopen.2019.0968.

Loeser, John D., and Michael E. Schatman. "Chronic Pain Management in Medical Education: A Disastrous Omission." *Postgraduate Medicine* 129, no. 3 (April 2017): 332–35. https://doi.org/10.1080/00325481.2017.1297668.

Lohr, Steve. "What Ever Happened to IBM's Watson?" *New York Times*. July 17, 2021. https://www.nytimes.com/2021/07/16/technology/what-happened-ibm-watson.html.

Lomas, Natasha. "Clue Gets FDA Clearance to Launch a Digital Contraceptive." TechCrunch. March 1, 2021. https://techcrunch.com/2021/03/01/clue-gets-fda-clearance-to-launch-a-digital-contraceptive/.

Long, Erping, Haotian Lin, Zhenzhen Liu, Xiaohang Wu, Liming Wang, Jiewei Jiang, Yingying An, et al. "An Artificial Intelligence Platform for the Multihospital Collaborative Management of Congenital Cataracts." *Nature Biomedical Engineering* 1 (2017). https://doi.org/10.1038/s41551-016-0024.

Longoni, Chiara, Andrea Bonezzi, and Carey K. Morewedge. "Resistance to Medical Artificial Intelligence." *Journal of Consumer Research* 46, no. 4 (December 2019): 629–50. https://doi.org/10.1093/jcr/ucz013.

Lordon, Ross J., Sean P. Mikles, Laura Kneale, Heather L. Evans, Sean A. Munson, Uba Backonja, and William B. Lober. "How Patient-Generated Health Data and Patient-Reported Outcomes Affect Patient-Clinician Relationships: A Systematic Review." *Health Informatics Journal* 26, no. 4 (December 2020): 2689–2706. https://doi.org/10.1177/1460458220928184.

Luo, Zelun, Jun-Ting Hsieh, Niranjan Balachandar, Serena Yeung, Guido Pusiol, Jay S. Luxenberg, Grace Li, et al. "Computer Vision-Based Descriptive Analytics of Seniors' Daily Activities for Long-Term Health Monitoring." *Proceedings of Machine Learning Research* 85 (2018): 1–18.

Lupton, Deborah. "The Digitally Engaged Patient: Self-Monitoring and Self-Care in the Digital Health Era." *Social Theory & Health* 11, no. 3 (August 2013): 256–70. https://doi.org/10.1057/sth.2013.10.

Lupton, Deborah. "The Diverse Domains of Quantified Selves: Self-Tracking Modes and Dataveillance." *Economy and Society* 45, no. 1 (January 2016): 101–22. https://doi.org/10.1080/03085147.2016.1143726.

Lupton, Deborah. "Health Promotion in the Digital Era: A Critical Commentary." *Health Promotion International* 30, no. 1 (March 2015):174–83. https://doi: 10.1093/heapro/dau091. PMID: 25320120.

Lupton, Deborah. "Quantified Sex: A Critical Analysis of Sexual and Reproductive Self-Tracking Using Apps." *Culture, Health & Sexuality* 17, no. 4 (April 2015): 440–53. https://doi.org/10.1080/13691058.2014.920528.

Lupton, Deborah. "Quantifying the Body: Monitoring and Measuring Health in the Age of mHealth Technologies." *Critical Public Health* 23, no. 4 (December 2013): 393–403. https://doi.org/10.1080/09581596.2013.794931.

Lupton, Deborah, and Annemarie Jutel. "'It's Like Having a Physician in Your Pocket!' A Critical Analysis of Self-Diagnosis Smartphone Apps." *Social Science & Medicine* 133 (2015): 128–35. https://doi.org/10.1016/j.socscimed.2015.04.004.

Lutfey, Karen. "On Practices of 'Good Doctoring': Reconsidering the Relationship between Provider Roles and Patient Adherence." *Sociology of Health & Illness* 27, no. 4 (May 2005): 421–47. https://doi.org/10.1111/j.1467-9566.2005.00450.x.

MacIntyre, Alasdair. *Dependent Rational Animals*. London: Duckworth, 1999.

Mack, Heather. "FDA Clears WellDoc's Non-RX Version of BlueStar, Its Mobile Diabetes Management Tool." MobiHealthNews. January 19, 2017. https://www.mobihealthnews.com/content/fda-clears-welldocs-non-rx-version-bluestar-its-mobile-diabetes-management-tool.

Mackenzie, Catriona. "Feminist Innovation in Philosophy: Relational Autonomy and Social Justice." *Women's Studies International Forum* 72 (2019): 144–51. https://doi.org/10.1016/j.wsif.2018.05.003.

Mackenzie, Catriona. "Relational Autonomy, Normative Authority and Perfectionism." *Journal of Social Philosophy* 39, no. 4 (December 2008): 512–33. https://doi.org/10.1111/j.1467-9833.2008.00440.x.

Mackenzie, Catriona. "Three Dimensions of Autonomy: A Relational Analysis." In *Autonomy, Oppression, and Gender*, edited by Andrea Veltman and Mark Piper, 15–41. New York: Oxford University Press, 2014.

Mackenzie, Catriona, and Natalie Stoljar, eds. *Relational Autonomy: Feminist Perspectives on Autonomy, Agency, and the Social Self*. New York: Oxford University Press, 2000.

Mahowald, Mary Briody. "To Be or Not Be a Woman: Anorexia Nervosa, Normative Gender Roles, and Feminism." *Journal of Medicine and Philosophy* 17, no. 2 (April 1992): 233–51. https://doi.org/10.1093/jmp/17.2.233.

Mamedova, Saida, and Emily Pawlowski. "A Description of U.S. Adults Who Are Not Digitally Literate." American Institutes for Research. May 1, 2018. https://www.air.org/resource/brief/description-us-adults-who-are-not-digitally-literate.

Mandl, Kenneth D., and Arjun K. Manrai. "Potential Excessive Testing at Scale: Biomarkers, Genomics, and Machine Learning." *Journal of the American Medical Association* 321, no. 8 (February 2019): 739–40. https://doi.org/10.1001/jama.2019.0286.

Marron, Jonathan M., Kaitlin Kyi, Paul S. Appelbaum, and Allison Magnuson. "Medical Decision-Making in Oncology for Patients Lacking Capacity." *American Society of Clinical Oncology Educational Book* 40 (May 2020): e186–96. https://doi.org/10.1200/EDBK_280279.

Martani, Andrea, Lester Darryl Geneviève, Christopher Poppe, Carlo Casonato, and Tenzin Wangmo. "Digital Pills: A Scoping Review of the Empirical Literature and Analysis of the Ethical Aspects." *BMC Medical Ethics* 21, no. 1 (January 2020): 3. https://doi.org/10.1186/s12910-019-0443-1.

Martinez-Aran, Anabel, Jan Scott, Francesc Colom, Carla Torrent, Rafael Tabares-Seisdedos, Claire Daban, Marion Leboyer, et al. "Treatment Nonadherence and Neurocognitive Impairment in Bipolar Disorder." *Journal of Clinical Psychiatry* 70, no. 7 (July 2009): 1017–23. https://doi.org/10.4088/JCP.08m04408.

Maturo, Antonio, and Francesca Setiffi. "The Gamification of Risk: How Health Apps Foster Self-Confidence and Why This Is Not Enough." *Health, Risk & Society* 17, no. 7–8 (February 2016): 477–94. https://doi.org/10.1080/13698575.2015.1136599.

McColl, Mary Ann. *Appreciative Disability Studies*. Concord, Ontario: Captus Press, 2019.

McConnell, Michael V., Anna Shcherbina, Aleksandra Pavlovic, Julian R. Homburger, Rachel L. Goldfeder, Daryl Waggot, Mildred K. Cho, et al. "Feasibility of Obtaining Measures of Lifestyle From a Smartphone App: The MyHeart Counts Cardiovascular Health Study." *JAMA Cardiology* 2, no. 1 (January 2017): 67–76. https://doi.org/10.1001/jamacardio.2016.4395.

McGrail, Samantha. "88% of Providers Investing in Remote Patient Monitoring Tech." mHealthIntelligence. Accessed February 9, 2022. https://mhealthintelligence.com/news/88-of-providers-investing-in-remote-patient-monitoring-tech.

McGraw, Deven, and Kenneth D. Mandl. "Privacy Protections to Encourage Use of Health-Relevant Digital Data in a Learning Health System." *npj Digital Medicine* 4, no. 1 (2021). https://doi.org/10.1038/s41746-020-00362-8.

McKinney, Scott Mayer, Marcin Sieniek, Varun Godbole, Jonathan Godwin, Natasha Antropova, Hutan Ashrafian, Trevor Back, et al. "International Evaluation of an AI System for Breast Cancer Screening." *Nature* 577 (2020): 89–94. https://doi.org/10.1038/s41586-019-1799-6.

McLeod, Carolyn. *Self-Trust and Reproductive Autonomy*. Cambridge, MA: MIT Press, 2002.

McLeod, Carolyn, and Susan Sherwin. "Relational Autonomy, Self-Trust, and Health Care for Patients Who Are Oppressed." In *Relational Autonomy: Feminist Perspectives on Autonomy, Agency, and the Social Self*, edited by Catriona Mackenzie and Natalie Stoljar, 259–79. New York: Oxford University Press, 2000. https://ir.lib.uwo.ca/philosophypub/345.

McMurray, Josephine, Gillian Strudwick, Cheryl Forchuk, Adam Morse, Jessica Lachance, Arani Baskaran, Lauren Allison, and Richard Booth. "The Importance of Trust in the Adoption and Use of Intelligent Assistive Technology by Older Adults to Support Aging in Place: Scoping Review Protocol." *JMIR Research Protocols* 6, no. 11 (2017). https://doi.org/10.2196/resprot.8772.

McQuaid, Elizabeth L., and Wendy Landier. "Cultural Issues in Medication Adherence: Disparities and Directions." *Journal of General Internal Medicine* 33, no. 2 (February 2018): 200–206. https://doi.org/10.1007/s11606-017-4199-3.

Medical Futurist. "FDA-Approved A.I.-Based Algorithms." Accessed January 6, 2022. https://medicalfuturist.com/fda-approved-ai-based-algorithms/.

Merrell, Ronald C. "Geriatric Telemedicine: Background and Evidence for Telemedicine as a Way to Address the Challenges of Geriatrics." *Healthcare Informatics Research* 21, no. 4 (2015): 223–29. https://doi.org/10.4258/hir.2015.21.4.223.

Meskó, Bertalan, and Marton Görög. "A Short Guide for Medical Professionals in the Era of Artificial Intelligence." *npj Digital Medicine* 3, no. 1 (December 2020): 126. https://doi.org/10.1038/s41746-020-00333-z.

Meskó, Bertalan, Gergely Hetényi, and Zsuzsanna Győrffy. "Will Artificial Intelligence Solve the Human Resource Crisis in Healthcare?" *BMC Health Services Research* 18 (2018). https://doi.org/10.1186/s12913-018-3359-4.

Metaxiotis, K. S., J.-E. Samouilidis, and J. E. Psarras. "Expert Systems in Medicine: Academic Illusion or Real Power?" *Journal of Innovation in Health Informatics* 9, no. 1 (February 2000): 3–8.

Mill, John Stuart. *On Liberty*. Peterborough, Ontario: Broadview, 1999.

Milligan, Christine. *There's No Place Like Home: Place and Care in an Ageing Society*. 1st ed. London: Routledge, 2009.

Miotto, Riccardo, Li Li, Brian A. Kidd, and Joel T. Dudley. "Deep Patient: An Unsupervised Representation to Predict the Future of Patients from the Electronic Health Records." *Scientific Reports* 6 (2016). https://doi.org/10.1038/srep26094.

Miotto, Riccardo, Fei Wang, Shuang Wang, Xiaoqian Jiang, and Joel T. Dudley. "Deep Learning for Healthcare: Review, Opportunities and Challenges." *Briefings in Bioinformatics* 19, no. 6 (2018): 1236–46. https://doi.org/10.1093/bib/bbx044.

Mittelstadt, Brent Daniel, Patrick Allo, Mariarosaria Taddeo, Sandra Wachter, and Luciano Floridi. "The Ethics of Algorithms: Mapping the Debate." *Big Data & Society* 3, no. 2 (December 2016). https://doi.org/10.1177/2053951716679679.

Mol, Annemarie, and John Law. "Embodied Action, Enacted Bodies: The Example of Hypoglycaemia." *Body & Society* 10, no. 2–3 (June 2004): 43–62. https://doi.org/10.1177/1357034X04042932.

Moncrieff, J., D. Cohen, and J. P. Mason. "The Subjective Experience of Taking Antipsychotic Medication: A Content Analysis of Internet Data." *Acta Psychiatrica Scandinavica* 120, no. 2 (August 2009): 102–11. https://doi.org/10.1111/j.1600-0447.2009.01356.x.

Morain, Stephanie R., Nancy E. Kass, and Ruth R. Faden. "Learning Is Not Enough: Earning Institutional Trustworthiness through Knowledge Translation." *American Journal of Bioethics* 18, no. 4 (2018): 31–34. https://doi.org/10.1080/15265161.2018.1431708.

Moreno, Jonathan D., Ulf Schmidt, and Steve Joffe. "The Nuremberg Code 70 Years Later." *Journal of the American Medical Association* 318, no. 9 (2017): 795–796. https://doi:10.1001/jama.2017.10265.

Mortenson, W. Ben, Andrew Sixsmith, and Robert Beringer. "No Place Like Home? Surveillance and What Home Means in Old Age." *Canadian Journal on Aging* 35, no. 1 (March 2016): 103–14. https://doi.org/10.1017/S0714980815000549.

Moyer, Dawn. "Your Fancy Proprietary AI Model Has No Value to Me." Medium. November 16, 2020. https://towardsdatascience.com/your-fancy-proprietary-ai-model-has-no-value-to-me-2a7d40dfd8ca.

Mullin, Emily. "Digital Pills Track How Patients Use Opioids." MIT Technology Review. December 11, 2017. https://www.technologyreview.com/2017/12/11/147144/digital-pills-track-how-patients-use-opioids/.

Nagendran, Myura, Yang Chen, Christopher A. Lovejoy, Anthony C. Gordon, Matthieu Komorowski, Hugh Harvey, Eric J. Topol, et al. "Artificial Intelligence versus Clinicians: Systematic Review of Design, Reporting Standards, and Claims of Deep Learning Studies." *BMJ* 368 (March 2020): m689. https://doi.org/10.1136/bmj.m689.

Nagy, Matthew, and Bryan Sisk. "How Will Artificial Intelligence Affect Patient–Clinician Relationships?" *AMA Journal of Ethics* 22, no. 5 (May 2020): E395–E400. https://doi.org/10.1001/amajethics.2020.395.

National Academies of Sciences, Engineering, and Medicine. *Families Caring for an Aging America*. Washington, DC: National Academies Press, 2016. https://www.ncbi.nlm.nih.gov/books/NBK396397/.

National Nurses United. "National Nurses United Condemns Industry Plans to Maximize Profit by Sending Patients Home All Alone, Replacing 24/7 Hands-on Nursing Care with Technology." November 4, 2021. https://www.nationalnursesunited.org/press/nnu-condemns-industry-plans-to-maximize-profit-by-sending-patients-home-alone.

Nayak, Rahul K., and Steven D. Pearson. "The Ethics of 'Fail First': Guidelines and Practical Scenarios for Step Therapy Coverage Policies." *Health Affairs (Millwood)* 33, no. 10 (October 2014): 1779–85. doi:10.1377/hlthaff.2014.0516. PMID: 25288422.

Nebeker, Camille, John Torous, and Rebecca J. Bartlett Ellis. "Building the Case for Actionable Ethics in Digital Health Research Supported by Artificial Intelligence." *BMC Medicine* 17, no. 1 (July 2019): 137. https://doi.org/10.1186/s12916-019-1377-7.

Nedelsky, Jennifer. *Law's Relations: A Relational Theory of Self, Autonomy, and Law*. New York: Oxford University Press, 2012.

Nelson, Hilde Lindemann. "Feminist Bioethics: Where We've Been, Where We're Going." *Metaphilosophy* 31, no. 5 (2000): 492–508. https://doi.org/10.1111/1467-9973.00165.

Nelson, Robert M., Tom Beauchamp, Victoria A. Miller, William Reynolds, Richard F. Ittenbach, and Mary Frances Luce. "The Concept of Voluntary Consent." *American Journal of Bioethics* 11, no. 8 (2011): 6–16. https://doi.org/10.1080/15265161.2011.583318.

Neven, Louis. "By Any Means? Questioning the Link between Gerontechnological Innovation and Older People's Wish to Live at Home." *Technological Forecasting and Social Change* 93 (April 2015): 32–43. https://doi.org/10.1016/j.techfore.2014.04.016.

Nield, David. "Employee Wellness Programs Now One of Fitbit's Fastest Growing Areas." Digital Trends. April 19, 2014. https://www.digitaltrends.com/mobile/employee-wellness-programs-now-one-fitbits-fastest-growing-areas/#!bDRFJr.

Nielsen-Bohlman, Lynn, Allison M. Panzer, and David A. Kindig, eds. *Health Literacy: A Prescription to End Confusion*. Washington, DC: National Academies Press, 2004. https://doi.org/10.17226/10883.

Nieuwlaat, Robby, Nancy Wilczynski, Tamara Navarro, Nicholas Hobson, Rebecca Jeffery, Arun Keepanasseril, Thomas Agoritsas, et al. "Interventions for Enhancing Medication Adherence." *Cochrane Database of Systematic Reviews* 11 (November 2014): CD000011. https://doi.org/10.1002/14651858.CD000011.pub4.

Noble, Meredith, Jonathan R. Treadwell, Stephen J. Tregear, Vivian H. Coates, Philip J. Wiffen, Clarisse Akafomo, Karen M. Schoelles, and Roger Chou. "Long-Term Opioid Management for Chronic Noncancer Pain." *Cochrane Database of Systematic Reviews* 1 (January 2010). https://doi.org/10.1002/14651858.CD006605.pub2.

Nutbeam, Don, and Jane E. Lloyd. "Understanding and Responding to Health Literacy as a Social Determinant of Health." *Annual Review of Public Health* 42 (April 2021): 159–73. https://doi.org/10.1146/annurev-publhealth-090419-102529.

Nys, Thomas. "Autonomy, Trust, and Respect." *Journal of Medicine and Philosophy* 41, no. 1 (2016): 10–24.

Obermeyer, Ziad, Brian Powers, Christine Vogeli, and Sendhil Mullainathan. "Dissecting Racial Bias in an Algorithm Used to Manage the Health of Populations." *Science* 366, no. 6464 (October 2019): 447–53. https://doi.org/10.1126/science.aax2342.

Office of U.S. Senator Bob Casey. "Disability Digest." *Aging Newsletter* 1, no. 1 (May 2020). https://www.aging.senate.gov/imo/media/doc/CASEY%20Aging%20Newsletter%20Issue%201.1.pdf.

Organization for Economic Cooperation and Development. "Trustworthy AI in Health: Background Paper for the G20 AI Dialogue, Digital Economy Task Force." April 2020. https://www.oecd.org/health/trustworthy-artificial-intelligence-in-health.pdf.

Oudshoorn, Nelly. "How Places Matter: Telecare Technologies and the Changing Spatial Dimensions of Healthcare." *Social Studies of Science* 42, no. 1 (2012): 121–42. https://www.doi.org/10.1177/0306312711431817.

Paasche-Orlow, Michael K., and Michael S. Wolf. "The Causal Pathways Linking Health Literacy to Health Outcomes." *American Journal of Health Behavior* 31, Suppl. 1 (October 2007): S19–S26. https://doi.org/10.5555/ajhb.2007.31.supp.S19.

Pancani, Luca, Marco Marinucci, Nicolas Aureli, and Paolo Riva. "Forced Social Isolation and Mental Health: A Study on 1,006 Italians under COVID-19 Lockdown." *Frontiers in Psychology* 12 (2021): 663799. https://doi.org/10.3389/fpsyg.2021.663799.

Panch, Trishan, and Nikhil Bhojwani. "How AI Vendors Can Navigate the Health Care Industry." *Harvard Business Review*. May 17, 2021. https://hbr.org/2021/05/how-ai-vendors-can-navigate-the-health-care-industry.

Paterson, David L., Susan Swindells, Jeffrey Mohr, Michelle Brester, Emanuel N. Vergis, Cheryl Squier, Marilyn M. Wagener, and Nina Singh. "Adherence to Protease Inhibitor Therapy and Outcomes in Patients with HIV Infection." *Annals of Internal Medicine* 133, no. 1 (July 2000): 21–30. https://doi.org/10.7326/0003-4819-133-1-200007040-00004.

Pelaccia, Thierry, Jacques Tardif, Emmanuel Triby, Christine Ammirati, Catherine Bertrand, Bernard Charlin, and Valérie Dory. "Do Emergency Physicians Trust Their Patients?" *Internal and Emergency Medicine* 11, no. 4 (June 2016): 603–8. https://doi.org/10.1007/s11739-016-1410-1.

Peters-Strickland, Timothy, Linda Pestreich, Ainslie Hatch, Shashank Rohatagi, Ross A. Baker, John P. Docherty, Lada Markovtsova, et al. "Usability of a Novel Digital Medicine System in Adults with Schizophrenia Treated with Sensor-Embedded Tablets of Aripiprazole." *Neuropsychiatric Disease and Treatment* 12 (2016): 2587–94. https://doi.org/10.2147/NDT.S116029.

Pierson, Emma, David M. Cutler, Jure Leskovec, Sendhil Mullainathan, and Ziad Obermeyer. "An Algorithmic Approach to Reducing Unexplained Pain Disparities in Underserved Populations." *Nature Medicine* 27, no. 1 (January 2021): 136–40. https://doi.org/10.1038/s41591-020-01192-7.

Pirzada, Pireh, Adriana Wilde, Gayle Helane Doherty, and David Harris-Birtill. "Ethics and Acceptance of Smart Homes for Older Adults." *Informatics for Health and Social Care* (July 2021): 1–28. https://doi.org/10.1080/17538157.2021.1923500.

Plowman, R. Scooter, Timothy Peters-Strickland, and George M. Savage. "Digital Medicines: Clinical Review on the Safety of Tablets with Sensors." *Expert Opinion on Drug Safety* 17, no. 9 (September 2018): 849–52. https://doi.org/10.1080/14740338.2018.1508447.

Pol, Margriet, Fenna van Nes, Margo van Hartingsveldt, Bianca Buurman, Sophia de Rooij, and Ben Kröse. "Older People's Perspectives Regarding the Use of Sensor Monitoring in Their Home." *Gerontologist* 56, no. 3 (2016): 485–93. https://doi.org/10.1093/geront/gnu104.

Pound, Pandora, Nicky Britten, Myfanwy Morgan, Lucy Yardley, Catherine Pope, Gavin Daker-White, and Rona Campbell. "Resisting Medicines: A Synthesis of Qualitative Studies of Medicine Taking." *Social Science & Medicine* 61, no. 1 (July 2005): 133–55. https://doi.org/10.1016/j.socscimed.2004.11.063.

Prayaga, Rena Brar, Ridhika Agrawal, Benjamin Nguyen, Erwin W. Jeong, Harmony K. Noble, Andrew Paster, and Ram S. Prayaga. "Impact of Social Determinants of Health and Demographics on Refill Requests by Medicare Patients Using a Conversational Artificial Intelligence Text Messaging Solution: Cross-Sectional Study." *JMIR mHealth and uHealth* 7, no. 11 (November 2019): e15771. https://doi.org/10.2196/15771.

Prendki, Jennifer. "Are You Spending Too Much Money Labeling Data?" Towards Data Science. March 24, 2020. https://towardsdatascience.com/are-you-spending-too-much-money-labeling-data-70a712123df1.

Pritchard-Jones, Laura. "Ageism and Autonomy in Health Care: Explorations Through a Relational Lens." *Health Care Analysis* 25, no. 1 (March 2017): 72–89. https://doi.org/10.1007/s10728-014-0288-1.

Putka, Sophie. "Meta, Hospitals Sued for Sharing Private Medical Info." Medpage Today. August 3, 2022. https://www.medpagetoday.com/special-reports/features/100050.

Rabiee, Parvaneh. "Exploring the Relationships between Choice and Independence: Experiences of Disabled and Older People." *British Journal of Social Work* 43, no. 5 (July 2013): 872–88. https://doi.org/10.1093/bjsw/bcs022.

Radin, Jennifer M., Steven R. Steinhubl, Andrew I. Su, Hansa Bhargava, Benjamin Greenberg, Brian M. Bot, Megan Doerr, and Eric J. Topol. "The Healthy Pregnancy Research Program: Transforming Pregnancy Research through a ResearchKit App." *npj Digital Medicine* 1 (2018): 45. https://doi.org/10.1038/s41746-018-0052-2.

Rajagopalan, Ramesh, Irene Litvan, and Tzyy-Ping Jung. "Fall Prediction and Prevention Systems: Recent Trends, Challenges, and Future Research Directions." *Sensors* 17, no. 11 (November 2017). https://doi.org/10.3390/s17112509.

Rajkomar, Alvin, Eyal Oren, Kai Chen, Andrew M. Dai, Nissan Hajaj, Michaela Hardt, Peter J. Liu, et al. "Scalable and Accurate Deep Learning with Electronic Health Records." *npj Digital Medicine* 1 (2018). https://doi.org/10.1038/s41746-018-0029-1.

Ranzijn, Rob. "Active Ageing—Another Way to Oppress Marginalized and Disadvantaged Elders? Aboriginal Elders as a Case Study." *Journal of Health*

Psychology 15, no. 5 (July 2010): 716–23. https://doi.org/10.1177/1359105310368181.

Rao, Maya E., and Dhananjai M. Rao. "The Mental Health of High School Students During the COVID-19 Pandemic." *Frontiers in Education* 6 (2021): 275. https://doi.org/10.3389/feduc.2021.719539.

Ravì, Daniele, Clarence Wong, Fani Deligianni, Melissa Berthelot, Javier Andreu-Perez, Benny Lo, and Guang-Zhong Yang. "Deep Learning for Health Informatics." *IEEE Journal of Biomedical and Health Informatics* 21, no. 1 (January 2017): 4–21. https://doi.org/10.1109/JBHI.2016.2636665.

Reddy, Nihaal, Neha Verma, and Kathleen Dungan. "Monitoring Technologies: Continuous Glucose Monitoring, Mobile Technology, Biomarkers of Glycemic Control." In *Endotext*, edited by Kenneth Feingold, Bradley Anawalt, Alison Boyce, George Chrousos, Keta Dhatariya, Kathleen Dungan, Hans Hofland, et al. South Dartmouth, MA: MDText.com, 2000. https://www.ncbi.nlm.nih.gov/books/NBK279046/.

Redfoot, Donald, Lynn Feinberg, and Ari Houser. "The Aging of the Baby Boom and the Growing Care Gap: A Look at Future Declines in the Availability of Family Caregivers." AARP Public Policy Institute. August 2013. https://www.aarp.org/home-family/caregiving/info-08-2013/the-aging-of-the-baby-boom-and-the-growing-care-gap-AARP-ppi-ltc.html.

Reindal, Solveig Magnus. "Independence, Dependence, Interdependence: Some Reflections on the Subject and Personal Autonomy." *Disability & Society* 14, no. 3 (1999), 353–67.

Reynoso, Rebecca. "A Complete History of Artificial Intelligence." G2. May 25, 2021. https://www.g2.com/articles/history-of-artificial-intelligence.

Rhodes, Rosamond. "When Is Participation in Research a Moral Duty?" *Journal of Law, Medicine & Ethics* 45, no. 3 (2017): 318–26. https://doi.org/10.1177/1073110517737529.

Rice, Louis, and Rachel Sara. "Updating the Determinants of Health Model in the Information Age." *Health Promotion International* 34, no. 6 (December 2019): 1241–49. https://doi.org/10.1093/heapro/day064.

Rich, B. A. "The Doctor as Double Agent." *Pain Medicine* 6, no. 5 (2005): 393–95.

Rich, Emma, and Andy Miah. "Mobile, Wearable and Ingestible Health Technologies: Towards a Critical Research Agenda." *Health Sociology Review* 26, no. 1 (January 2017): 84–97. https://doi.org/10.1080/14461242.2016.1211486.

Richardson, Jordan P., Cambray Smith, Susan Curtis, Sara Watson, Xuan Zhu, Barbara Barry, and Richard R. Sharp. "Patient Apprehensions about the Use of Artificial Intelligence in Healthcare." *npj Digital Medicine* 4, no. 1 (September 2021): 140. https://doi.org/10.1038/s41746-021-00509-1.

Riggare, Sara, and Maria Hägglund. "Precision Medicine in Parkinson's Disease—Exploring Patient-Initiated Self-Tracking." *Journal of Parkinson's Disease* 8, no. 3 (2018): 441–46. https://doi.org/10.3233/JPD-181314.

Rioux, Liliane. "The Well-Being of Aging People Living in Their Own Homes." *Journal of Environmental Psychology* 25, no. 2 (June 2005): 231–43. https://doi.org/10.1016/j.jenvp.2005.05.001.

Robbins, Rebecca. "An Experiment in End-of-Life Care: Tapping AI's Cold Calculus to Nudge the Most Human of Conversations." STAT. July 1, 2020. https://www.statnews.com/2020/07/01/end-of-life-artificial-intelligence/.

Robbins, Rebecca, and Erin Brodwin. "An Invisible Hand: Patients Aren't Being Told about the AI Systems Advising Their Care." STAT. July 15, 2020. https://www.statnews.com/2020/07/15/artificial-intelligence-patient-consent-hospitals/.

Roberts, Michael, Derek Driggs, Matthew Thorpe, Julian Gilbey, Michael Yeung, Stephan Ursprung, Angelica I. Aviles-Rivero, et al. "Common Pitfalls and Recommendations for Using Machine Learning to Detect and Prognosticate for COVID-19 Using Chest Radiographs and CT Scans." *Nature Machine Intelligence* 3 (2021): 199–217. https://doi.org/10.1038/s42256-021-00307-0.

Rockwell, Kimberly Lovett. "Direct-to-Consumer Medical Testing in the Era of Value-Based Care." *Journal of the American Medical Association* 317, no. 24 (June 2017): 2485–86. https://doi.org/10.1001/jama.2017.5929.

Rodriguez-Ruiz, Alejandro, Kristina Lång, Albert Gubern-Merida, Mireille Broeders, Gisella Gennaro, Paola Clauser, Thomas H. Helbich, et al. "Stand-Alone Artificial Intelligence for Breast Cancer Detection in Mammography: Comparison with 101 Radiologists." *Journal of the National Cancer Institute* 111, no. 9 (2019): 916–22. https://doi.org/10.1093/jnci/djy222.

Rogers, Wendy A. "Is There a Moral Duty for Doctors to Trust Patients?" *Journal of Medical Ethics* 28, no. 2 (April 2002): 77–80. https://doi.org/10.1136/jme.28.2.77.

Rogers, Wendy A., Heather Draper, and Stacy M. Carter. "Evaluation of Artificial Intelligence Clinical Applications: Detailed Case Analyses Show Value of Healthcare Ethics Approach in Identifying Patient Care Issues." *Bioethics* 35, no. 7 (September 2021): 623–33. https://doi.org/10.1111/bioe.12885.

Rolison, J. J., Y. Hanoch, and A. M. Freund. "Perception of Risk for Older Adults: Differences in Evaluations for Self versus Others and across Risk Domains." *Gerontology* 65, no. 5 (2019): 547–59. https://doi.org/10.1159/000494352.

Rosenbaum, Lisa. "Swallowing a Spy—The Potential Uses of Digital Adherence Monitoring." *New England Journal of Medicine* 378, no. 2 (January 2018): 101–3. https://doi.org/10.1056/NEJMp1716206.

Ross, Casey. "At Mayo Clinic, Sharing Patient Data with Companies Fuels AI Innovation—and Concerns about Consent." STAT. June 3, 2020. https://www.statnews.com/2020/06/03/mayo-clinic-patient-data-fuels-artificial-intelligence-consent-concerns/.

Roth, Carl B., Andreas Papassotiropoulos, Annette B. Brühl, Undine E. Lang, and Christian G. Huber. "Psychiatry in the Digital Age: A Blessing or a Curse?" *International Journal of Environmental Research and Public Health* 18, no. 16 (August 2021). https://doi.org/10.3390/ijerph18168302.

Rowland, Simon P., J. Edward Fitzgerald, Thomas Holme, John Powell, and Alison McGregor. "What Is the Clinical Value of mHealth for Patients?" *npj Digital Medicine* 3, no. 1 (January 2020): 4. https://doi.org/10.1038/s41746-019-0206-x.

Rubeis, Giovanni. "The Disruptive Power of Artificial Intelligence: Ethical Aspects of Gerontechnology in Elderly Care." *Archives of Gerontology and Geriatrics* 91 (November 2020): 104186. https://doi.org/10.1016/j.archger.2020.104186.

Ruckenstein, Minna, and Natasha Dow Schüll. "The Datafication of Health." *Annual Review of Anthropology* 46, no. 1 (October 2017): 261–78. https://doi.org/10.1146/annurev-anthro-102116-041244.

Rudin, Cynthia, and Joanna Radin. "Why Are We Using Black Box Models in AI When We Don't Need To? A Lesson from an Explainable AI Competition." *Harvard Data Science Review* 1, no. 2 (Fall 2019). https://doi.org/10.1162/99608f92.5a8a3a3d.

Rudman, Debbie Laliberte. "Shaping the Active, Autonomous and Responsible Modern Retiree: An Analysis of Discursive Technologies and Their Links with Neo-Liberal Political Rationality." *Ageing and Society* 26 (March 2006): 181–201. https://doi.org/10.1017/S0144686X05004253.

Sabaté, Eduardo, ed. *Adherence to Long-Term Therapies: Evidence for Action* . Geneva: World Health Organization, 2003. https://apps.who.int/iris/bitstream/handle/10665/42682/9241545992.pdf?sequence=1&isAllowed=y.

Sackett, D. L., R. B. Haynes, E. S. Gibson, D. W. Taylor, R. S. Roberts, and A. L. Johnson. "Patient Compliance with Antihypertensive Regimens." *Patient Counselling and Health Education* 1, no. 1 (January–March 1978): 18–21. https://doi.org/10.1016/s0738-3991(78)80033-0.

Sainato, Michael. "US Workers Who Risked Their Lives to Care for Elderly Demand Change." *The Guardian*. April 19, 2021. https://www.theguardian.com/us-news/2021/apr/19/nursing-home-care-workers-coronavirus.

Sapci, A. Hasan, and H. Aylin Sapci. "Innovative Assisted Living Tools, Remote Monitoring Technologies, Artificial Intelligence-Driven Solutions, and Robotic Systems for Aging Societies: Systematic Review." *JMIR Aging* 2, no. 2 (November 2019): e15429. https://doi.org/10.2196/15429.

Savage, Thomas Robert. "Artificial Intelligence in Medical Education." *Academic Medicine* 96, no. 9 (2021): 1229–30. https://doi.org/10.1097/ACM.0000000000004183.

Scher, Stephen, and Kasia Kozlowska. "The Rise of Bioethics: A Historical Overview." In *Rethinking Health Care Ethics*, edited by Stephen Scher and Kasia Kozlowska, 31–44. Singapore: Palgrave Pivot, 2018. https://doi.org/10.1007/978-981-13-0830-7_3.

Scherwitzl, E. Berglund, O. Lundberg, H. Kopp Kallner, K. Gemzell Danielsson, J. Trussell, and R. Scherwitzl. "Perfect-Use and Typical-Use Pearl Index of a Contraceptive Mobile App." *Contraception* 96, no. 6 (December 2017): 420–25. https://doi.org/10.1016/j.contraception.2017.08.014.

Schillinger, Dean. "The Intersections between Social Determinants of Health, Health Literacy, and Health Disparities." *Studies in Health Technology and Informatics* 269 (June 2020): 22–41. https://doi.org/10.3233/SHTI200020.

Schmietow, Bettina, and Georg Marckmann. "Mobile Health Ethics and the Expanding Role of Autonomy." *Medicine, Health Care, and Philosophy* 22, no. 4 (December 2019): 623–30. https://doi.org/10.1007/s11019-019-09900-y.

Schwab, Klaus. "The Fourth Industrial Revolution: What It Means and How to Respond." World Economic Forum. January 14, 2016. https://www.weforum.org/agenda/2016/01/the-fourth-industrial-revolution-what-it-means-and-how-to-respond/.

Secker, Jenny, Robert Hill, Louise Villeneau, and Sue Parkman. "Promoting Independence: But Promoting What and How?" *Ageing and Society* 23, no. 3 (2003): 375–91. https://doi.org/10.1017/S0144686X03001193.

Sedensky, Matt, and Bernard Condon. "Not Just COVID: Nursing Home Neglect Deaths Surge in Shadows." AP News. November 19, 2020. https://apnews.com/article/pandemics-us-news-coronavirus-pandemic-daac7f011bcf08747184bd851a1e1b8e.

Sharon, Tamar. "Self-Tracking for Health and the Quantified Self: Re-Articulating Autonomy, Solidarity, and Authenticity in an Age of Personalized Healthcare." *Philosophy & Technology* 30, no. 1 (March 2017): 93–121. https://doi.org/10.1007/s13347-016-0215-5.

Sheather, Julian. "Selling Sickness to the Worried Well." BMJ Opinion. February 12, 2010. https://blogs.bmj.com/bmj/2010/02/12/julian-sheather-selling-sickness-to-the-worried-well/.

Sherwin, Susan. "A Relational Approach to Autonomy in Health Care." In *The Politics of Women's Health: Exploring Agency and Autonomy*, edited by Susan Sherwin, 19–47. Philadelphia: Temple University Press, 1998.

Sidey-Gibbons, Jenni A. M., and Chris J. Sidey-Gibbons. "Machine Learning in Medicine: A Practical Introduction." *BMC Medical Research Methodology* 19 (2019). https://doi.org/10.1186/s12874-019-0681-4.

Siegler, Mark, "The Progression of Medicine: From Physician Paternalism to Patient Autonomy to Bureaucratic Parsimony." *Archives of Internal Medicine* 145, no. 4 (1985): 713–15. https://doi.org/10.1001/archinte.1985.00360040147031.

Silverstein, Matthew. "Agency and Normative Self-Governance." *Australasian Journal of Philosophy* 95, no. 3 (2017): 517–28. https://doi.org/10.1080/00048402.2016.1254263.

Sjoding, Michael W., Robert P. Dickson, Theodore J. Iwashyna, Steven E. Gay, and Thomas S. Valley. "Racial Bias in Pulse Oximetry Measurement." *New England Journal of Medicine* 383, no. 25 (2020): 2477–78. https://doi.org/10.1056/NEJMc2029240.

Skorburg, Joshua August, and Josephine Yam. "Is There an App for That?: Ethical Issues in the Digital Mental Health Response to COVID-19." *AJOB Neuroscience* 13, no. 3 (September 2022): 177–90. https://doi.org/10.1080/21507740.2021.1918284.

Snowden, Lonnie R., Ray Catalano, and Martha Shumway. "Disproportionate Use of Psychiatric Emergency Services by African Americans." *Psychiatric Services* 60, no. 12 (December 2009): 1664–71. https://doi.org/10.1176/ps.2009.60.12.1664.

Solaiman, Barry, and Mark G. Bloom, "AI, Explainability, and Safeguarding Patient Safety in Europe: Toward a Science-Focused Regulatory Model." In *The Future of Medical Device Regulation: Innovation and Protection*, edited by I. Glenn Cohen, Timo Minssen, W. Nicholson Price II, Christopher Robertson, and Carmel Shachar, 91–102. Cambridge: Cambridge University Press, 2022. doi:10.1017/9781108975452.008.

Spector-Bagdady, Kayte, and Jonathan Beever. "Rethinking the Importance of the Individual within a Community of Data." *Hastings Center Report* 50, no. 4 (July 2020): 9–11. https://doi.org/10.1002/hast.1112.

Spoel, Philippa, Roma Harris, and Flis Henwood. "The Moralization of Healthy Living: Burke's Rhetoric of Rebirth and Older Adults' Accounts of Healthy Eating." *Health* 16, no. 6 (April 2012): 619–35. https://doi.org/10.1177/1363459312441009.

Spoel, Philippa, Roma Harris, and Flis Henwood. "Rhetorics of Health Citizenship: Exploring Vernacular Critiques of Government's Role in Supporting Healthy Living." *Journal of Medical Humanities* 35, no. 2 (June 2014): 131–47. https://doi.org/10.1007/s10912-014-9276-6.

Sriram, Vimal, Crispin Jenkinson, and Michele Peters. "Informal Carers' Experience of Assistive Technology Use in Dementia Care at Home: A Systematic Review." *BMC Geriatrics* 19, no. 1 (2019): 160. https://doi.org/10.1186/s12877-019-1169-0.

Standing, Harriet, and Rob Lawlor. "Ulysses Contracts in Psychiatric Care: Helping Patients to Protect Themselves from Spiralling." *Journal of Medical Ethics* 45, no. 11 (November 2019): 693–99. https://doi.org/10.1136/medethics-2019-105511.

Stanford Medicine. *The Democratization of Health Care*. Stanford Medicine 2018 Health Trends Report. December 2018. https://med.stanford.edu/content/dam/sm/school/documents/Health-Trends-Report/Stanford-Medicine-Health-Trends-Report-2018.pdf.

Stein, Jeff. "'This Will Be Catastrophic': Maine Families Face Elder Boom, Worker Shortage in Preview of Nation's Future." *Washington Post*. August 14, 2019. https://www.washingtonpost.com/business/economy/this-will-be-catastrophic-maine-families-face-elder-boom-worker-shortage-in-preview-of-nations-future/2019/08/14/7cecafc6-bec1-11e9-b873-63ace636af08_story.html.

Stein, Natalie. "Leading Chronic Disease Management and Prevention—An Interview with Lark VP of Growth, Cameron D. Jacox and Research2Guidance." Lark. July 6, 2019. https://www.lark.com/blog/leading-chronic-disease-management-and-prevention-an-interview-with-lark-vp-of-growth-cameron-jacox-and-research2guidanc/.

Steiner, John F., and Mark A. Earnest. "The Language of Medication-Taking." *Annals of Internal Medicine* 132, no. 11 (June 2000): 926–30. https://doi.org/10.7326/0003-4819-132-11-200006060-00026.

Steiner, John F., P. Michael Ho, Brenda L. Beaty, L. Miriam Dickinson, Rebecca Hanratty, Chan Zeng, Heather M. Tavel, et al. "Sociodemographic and Clinical Characteristics Are Not Clinically Useful Predictors of Refill Adherence in Patients with Hypertension." *Circulation: Cardiovascular Quality and Outcomes* 2, no. 5 (September 2009): 451–57. https://doi.org/10.1161/CIRCOUTCOMES.108.841635.

Steinkamp, Jackson M., Nathaniel Goldblatt, Jacob T. Borodovsky, Amy LaVertu, Ian M. Kronish, Lisa A. Marsch, and Zev Schuman-Olivier. "Technological Interventions for Medication Adherence in Adult Mental Health and Substance Use Disorders: A Systematic Review." *JMIR Mental Health* 6, no. 3 (March 2019): e12493. https://doi.org/10.2196/12493.

Stenner, Paul, Tara McFarquhar, and Ann Bowling. "Older People and 'Active Ageing': Subjective Aspects of Ageing Actively." *Journal of Health Psychology* 16, no. 3 (April 2011): 467–77. https://doi.org/10.1177/1359105310384298.

Stirratt, Michael J., Jeffrey R. Curtis, Maria I. Danila, Richard Hansen, Michael J. Miller, and C. Ann Gakumo. "Advancing the Science and Practice of Medication Adherence." *Journal of General Internal Medicine* 33, no. 2 (February 2018): 216–22. https://doi.org/10.1007/s11606-017-4198-4.

Stirratt, Michael J., Jacqueline Dunbar-Jacob, Heidi M. Crane, Jane M. Simoni, Susan Czajkowski, Marisa E. Hilliard, James E. Aikens, et al. "Self-Report Measures of Medication Adherence Behavior: Recommendations on Optimal Use." *Translational Behavioral Medicine* 5, no. 4 (December 2015): 470–82. https://doi.org/10.1007/s13142-015-0315-2.

Stones, Damien, and Judith Gullifer. "'At Home It's Just So Much Easier to Be Yourself': Older Adults' Perceptions of Ageing in Place." *Ageing and Society* 36, no. 3 (2016): 449–81. https://doi.org/10.1017/S0144686X14001214.

Stonham, Scott. "AI, Wearable Tech and Mental Health Well-Being." Well, That's Interesting Tech. April 20, 2020. https://wellthatsinteresting.tech/ai-tech-mental-health-well-being/.

Storrs, Carina. "Patients Armed with Their Own Genetic Data Raise Tough Questions." *Health Affairs* 37, no. 5 (May 2018): 690–93. https://doi.org/10.1377/hlthaff.2018.0364.

Strickland, Eliza. "IBM Watson, Heal Thyself: How IBM Overpromised and Underdelivered on AI Health Care." *IEEE Spectrum* 56, no. 4 (April 2019): 24–31. https://doi.org/10.1109/MSPEC.2019.8678513.

SuperFlux Lab. "Uninvited Guests" [Short film]. Uploaded May 26, 2015. https://vimeo.com/128873380.

Sutton, Reed T., David Pincock, Daniel C. Baumgart, Daniel C. Sadowski, Richard N. Fedorak, and Karen I. Kroeker. "An Overview of Clinical Decision Support Systems: Benefits, Risks, and Strategies for Success." *npj Digital Medicine* 3, no. 1 (February 2020): 17. https://doi.org/10.1038/s41746-020-0221-y.

Suwanvecho, Suthida, Harit Suwanrusme, Montinee Sangtian, Andrew D. Norden, Alexandra Urman, Annette Hicks, Irene Dankwa-Mullan, et al. "Concordance Assessment of a Cognitive Computing System in Thailand." *Journal of Clinical Oncology* 35, no. 15_suppl (May 2017). https://doi.org/10.1200/JCO.2017.35.15_suppl.6589.

Swan, Melanie. "Health 2050: The Realization of Personalized Medicine through Crowdsourcing, the Quantified Self, and the Participatory Biocitizen." *Journal of Personalized Medicine* 2, no. 3 (September 2012): 93–118. https://doi.org/10.3390/jpm2030093.

Swartz, Anna K. "Smart Pills for Psychosis: The Tricky Ethical Challenges of Digital Medicine for Serious Mental Illness." *American Journal of Bioethics* 18, no. 9 (September 2018): 65–67. https://doi.org/10.1080/15265161.2018.1498948.

Szalavitz, Maia. "The Pain Was Unbearable. So Why Did Doctors Turn Her Away?" Wired. August 11, 2021. https://www.wired.com/story/opioid-drug-addiction-algorithm-chronic-pain/.

Tai-Seale, Ming, Thomas G. McGuire, and Weimin Zhang. "Time Allocation in Primary Care Office Visits." *Health Services Research* 42, no. 5 (October 2007): 1871–94. https://doi.org/10.1111/j.1475-6773.2006.00689.x.

Tangari, Gioacchino, Muhammad Ikram, Kiran Ijaz, Mohamed Ali Kaafar, and Shlomo Berkovsky. "Mobile Health and Privacy: Cross Sectional Study." *BMJ* 373 (June 2021): n1248. https://doi.org/10.1136/bmj.n1248.

Tanne, Janice Hopkins. "Direct to Consumer Medical Tests Are Offered in United States." *BMJ* 333, no. 7557 (July 2006): 12. https://doi.org/10.1136/bmj.333.7557.12-a.

Taquet, Maxime, John R. Geddes, Masud Husain, Sierra Luciano, and Paul J. Harrison. "6-Month Neurological and Psychiatric Outcomes in 236 379 Survivors of COVID-19: A Retrospective Cohort Study Using Electronic Health Records." *Lancet Psychiatry* 8, no. 5 (May 2021): 416–27. https://doi.org/10.1016/S2215-0366(21)00084-5.

Tariq, Soofia. "Nine out of 10 Health Apps Harvest User Data, Global Study Shows." *The Guardian*. June 17, 2021. https://www.theguardian.com/technology/2021/jun/17/nine-out-of-10-health-apps-harvest-user-data-global-study-shows.

Taylor, Danielle M. "Americans with Disabilities: 2014." United States Census Bureau. November 29, 2018. https://www.census.gov/library/publications/2018/demo/p70-152.html.

Teri, L., and A. W. Wagner. "Assessment of Depression in Patients with Alzheimer's Disease: Concordance among Informants." *Psychology and Aging* 6, no. 2 (June 1991): 280–85. https://doi.org/10.1037//0882-7974.6.2.280.

Thorne, Sally E., and Carole A. Robinson. "Reciprocal Trust in Health Care Relationships." *Journal of Advanced Nursing* 13, no. 6 (November 1988): 782–89. https://doi.org/10.1111/j.1365-2648.1988.tb00570.x.

Ti, Lianping, Anita Ho, and Rod Knight. "Towards Equitable AI Interventions for People Who Use Drugs: Key Areas That Require Ethical Investment." *Journal of Addiction Medicine* 15, no. 2 (April 2021): 96–98. https://doi.org/10.1097/ADM.0000000000000722.

Till, Chris. "Exercise as Labour: Quantified Self and the Transformation of Exercise into Labour." *Societies* 4, no. 3 (2014): 446–62. https://doi.org/10.3390/soc4030446.

Timmerman, L., D. L. Stronks, J. G. Groeneweg, and F. J. Huygen. "Prevalence and Determinants of Medication Non-Adherence in Chronic Pain Patients: A Systematic Review." *Acta Anaesthesiologica Scandinavica* 60, no. 4 (April 2016): 416–31. https://doi.org/10.1111/aas.12697.

Ting, Kai Ming. "Sensitivity and Specificity." In *Encyclopedia of Machine Learning*, edited by Claude Sammut and Geoffrey I. Webb. Boston: Springer, 2011. https://doi.org/10.1007/978-0-387-30164-8_752.

Tomlinson, Mandy. "Artificial General Intelligence (AGI) and Healthcare Adaptation." Isabel. February 17, 2016. https://info.isabelhealthcare.com/blog/artificial-general-intelligence-agi-and-healthcare-adaptation.

Tomlinson, Tom. "Getting Off the Leash." *American Journal of Bioethics* 18, no. 9 (September 2018): 48–49. https://doi.org/10.1080/15265161.2018.1498938.

Topol, Eric. "High-Performance Medicine: The Convergence of Human and Artificial Intelligence." *Nature Medicine* 25, no. 1 (January 2019): 44–56. https://doi.org/10.1038/s41591-018-0300-7.

Topol, Eric. *The Patient Will See You Now: The Future of Medicine Is in Your Hands*. New York: Basic Books, 2015.

"Tracking the States Where Abortion Is Now Banned." *New York Times*. Last modified July 27, 2022. https://www.nytimes.com/interactive/2022/us/abortion-laws-roe-v-wade.html.

Tran, Viet-Thi, Carolina Riveros, and Philippe Ravaud. "Patients' Views of Wearable Devices and AI in Healthcare: Findings from the ComPaRe e-Cohort." *npj Digital Medicine* 2, no. 1 (June 2019): 53. https://doi.org/10.1038/s41746-019-0132-y.

Trostle, J. A., W. A. Hauser, and I. S. Susser. "The Logic of Noncompliance: Management of Epilepsy from the Patient's Point of View." *Culture, Medicine and Psychiatry* 7, no. 1 (March 1983): 35–56. https://doi.org/10.1007/BF00249998.

Tseregounis, Iraklis Erik, and Stephen G. Henry. "Assessing Opioid Overdose Risk: A Review of Clinical Prediction Models Utilizing Patient-Level Data." *Translational Research* 234 (August 2021): 74–87. https://doi.org/10.1016/j.trsl.2021.03.012.

Tsigelny, Igor F. "Artificial Intelligence in Drug Combination Therapy." *Briefings in Bioinformatics* 20, no. 4 (2018): 1434–48. https://doi.org/10.1093/bib/bby004.

Tysnes, Ole-Bjørn, and Anette Storstein. "Epidemiology of Parkinson's Disease." *Journal of Neural Transmission* 124, no. 8 (August 2017): 901–5. https://doi.org/10.1007/s00702-017-1686-y.

University of Florida College of Pharmacy. "New AI Tool Will Predict Patients at High Risk for Opioid Use Disorder and Overdose." August 11, 2021. https://pharmacy.ufl.edu/2021/08/11/new-ai-tool-will-predict-patients-at-high-risk-for-opioid-use-disorder-and-overdose/.

U.S. Department of Health and Human Services. "Federal Policy for the Protection of Human Subjects ('Common Rule')." 2018. https://www.hhs.gov/ohrp/regulations-and-policy/regulations/common-rule/index.html.

U.S. Department of Health and Human Services. "Healthy Aging." Last modified May 2, 2022. https://www.hhs.gov/aging/healthy-aging/index.html.

U.S. Department of Health and Human Services. "HHS Awards Nearly $55 Million to Increase Virtual Health Care Access and Quality Through Community Health Centers." February 14, 2022. https://www.hhs.gov/about/news/2022/02/14/hhs-awards-nearly-55-million-increase-virtual-health-care-access-quality-through-community-health-centers.html.

U.S. Department of Health and Human Services, Administration for Community Living. "2020 Profile of Older Americans." Last modified November 24, 2021. https://acl.gov/aging-and-disability-in-america/data-and-research/profile-older-americans.U.S. Department of Health and Human Services, Health Resources and Services Administration, Bureau of Health Workforce, and National Center for Health Workforce Analysis. *National and Regional Projections of Supply and Demand for Geriatricians: 2013–2025*. Rockville, MD, 2017. https://bhw.hrsa.gov/sites/default/files/bureau-health-workforce/data-research/geriatrics-report-51817.pdf.

U.S. Department of Health and Human Services, Office of Disease Prevention and Health Promotion. "Healthy Aging." Last modified September 24, 2021. https://health.gov/our-work/national-health-initiatives/healthy-aging.

U.S. Food and Drug Administration. "Artificial Intelligence/Machine Learning (AI/ML)-Based Software as a Medical Device (SaMD) Action Plan." January 2021. https://www.fda.gov/media/145022/download.

U.S. Food and Drug Administration. "Clinical Review: Aripiprazole + MIND1 System (Abilify Mycite)." Center for Drug Evaluation and Research. April 21, 2017. https://www.accessdata.fda.gov/drugsatfda_docs/nda/2017/207202Orig1s000MedR.pdf.

U.S. Food and Drug Administration. "De Novo Classification Request." Last modified January 3, 2022. https://www.fda.gov/medical-devices/premarket-submissions/de-novo-classification-request.

U.S. Food and Drug Administration. "FDA Allows Marketing of First Direct-to-Consumer App for Contraceptive Use to Prevent Pregnancy." August 10, 2018. https://www.fda.gov/news-events/press-announcements/fda-allows-marketing-first-direct-consumer-app-contraceptive-use-prevent-pregnancy.

U.S. Food and Drug Administration. "Marketing Authorization for Irregular Rhythm Notification Feature DEN180042." September 11, 2018. https://www.accessdata.fda.gov/cdrh_docs/pdf18/DEN180042.pdf.

U.S. Food and Drug Administration. "Policy for Device Software Functions and Mobile Medical Applications: Guidance for Industry and Food and Drug Administration Staff." September 27, 2019. https://www.fda.gov/media/80958/download.

U.S. Food and Drug Administration. "Premarket Approval (PMA)." Last modified May 16, 2019. https://www.fda.gov/medical-devices/premarket-submissions-selecting-and-preparing-correct-submission/premarket-approval-pma.

U.S. Food and Drug Administration. "Premarket Approval for Guardian Connect System." Last modified January 3, 2022. https://www.accessdata.fda.gov/scripts/cdrh/cfdocs/cfpma/pma.cfm?id=P160007.

U.S. Food and Drug Administration. "Premarket Notification 510(k)." Last modified March 13, 2020. https://www.fda.gov/medical-devices/premarket-submissions-selecting-and-preparing-correct-submission/premarket-notification-510k.

U.S. Food and Drug Administration. "Pulse Oximeter Accuracy and Limitations: FDA Safety Communication." February 19, 2021. https://www.fda.gov/medical-devices/safety-communications/pulse-oximeter-accuracy-and-limitations-fda-safety-communication.

U.S. Food and Drug Administration. "Statement from FDA Commissioner Scott Gottlieb, M.D. on Steps toward a New, Tailored Review Framework for Artificial Intelligence-Based Medical Devices." April 2, 2019. https://www.fda.gov/news-events/press-announcements/statement-fda-commissioner-scott-gottlieb-md-steps-toward-new-tailored-review-framework-artificial.

Vallor, Shannon. *Technology and the Virtues: A Philosophical Guide to a Future Worth Wanting*. New York: Oxford University Press, 2016.

Vandemeulebroucke, Tijs, Bernadette Dierckx de Casterlé, and Chris Gastmans. "The Use of Care Robots in Aged Care: A Systematic Review of Argument-Based Ethics Literature." *Archives of Gerontology and Geriatrics* 74 (January 2018): 15–25. https://doi.org/10.1016/j.archger.2017.08.014.

van der Weele, Simon, Femmianne Bredewold, Carlo Leget, and Evelien Tonkens. "What Is the Problem of Dependency? Dependency Work

Reconsidered." *Nursing Philosophy* 22, no. 2 (April 2021): e12327. https://doi.org/10.1111/nup.12327.

van de Schoot, Rens, Sarah Depaoli, Ruth King, Bianca Kramer, Kaspar Märtens, Mahlet G. Tadesse, Marina Vannucci, et al. "Bayesian Statistics and Modelling." *Nature Reviews Methods Primers* 1, no. 1 (January 2021): 1. https://doi.org/10.1038/s43586-020-00001-2.

van Hoof, J., H. Kort, P. Rutten, and M. Duijnstee. "Ageing-in-Place with the Use of Ambient Intelligence Technology: Perspectives of Older Users." *International Journal of Medical Informatics* 80, no. 5 (2011): 310–31. http://doi.org/10.1016/j.ijmedinf.2011.02.010.

van Kolfschooten, Hannah. "The mHealth Power Paradox: Improving Data Protection in Health Apps through Self-Regulation in the European Union." In *The Future of Medical Device Regulation: Innovation and Protection*, edited by I. Glenn Cohen, Timo Minssen, W. Nicholson Price II, Christopher Robertson, and Carmel Shachar, 63–76. Cambridge: Cambridge University Press, 2022. https://doi:10.1017/9781108975452.006.

Van Noorden, Richard. "The Ethical Questions That Haunt Facial-Recognition Research." *Nature* 587, no. 7834 (November 2020): 354–58. https://doi.org/10.1038/d41586-020-03187-3.

Velligan, Dawn I., Yui-Wing Francis Lam, David C. Glahn, Jennifer A. Barrett, Natalie J. Maples, Larry Ereshefsky, and Alexander L. Miller. "Defining and Assessing Adherence to Oral Antipsychotics: A Review of the Literature." *Schizophrenia Bulletin* 32, no. 4 (October 2006): 724–42. https://doi.org/10.1093/schbul/sbj075.

Velligan, Dawn I., Mei Wang, Pamela Diamond, David C. Glahn, Desiree Castillo, Scott Bendle, Y. W. Francis Lam, et al. "Relationships among Subjective and Objective Measures of Adherence to Oral Antipsychotic Medications." *Psychiatric Services* 58, no. 9 (September 2007): 1187–92. https://doi.org/10.1176/ps.2007.58.9.1187.

Victor, Lisa, and Steven H. Richeimer. "Trustworthiness as a Clinical Variable: The Problem of Trust in the Management of Chronic, Nonmalignant Pain." *Pain Medicine* 6, no. 5 (October 2005): 385–91. https://doi.org/10.1111/j.1526-4637.2005.00063.x.

Vines, John, Stephen Lindsay, Gary W. Pritchard, Mabel Lie, David Greathead, Patrick Olivier, and Katie Brittain. "Making Family Care Work: Dependence, Privacy and Remote Home Monitoring Telecare Systems." *Proceedings of the 2013 ACM International Joint Conference on Pervasive and Ubiquitous Computing* (September 2013): 607–16. https://doi.org/10.1145/2493432.2493469.

Viswanathan, Meera, Carol E. Golin, Christine D. Jones, Mahima Ashok, Susan J. Blalock, Roberta C. M. Wines, Emmanuel J. L. Coker-Schwimmer, et al. "Interventions to Improve Adherence to Self-Administered Medications for Chronic Diseases in the United States: A Systematic Review." *Annals of*

Internal Medicine 157, no. 11 (2012): 785–95. https://doi.org/10.7326/0003-4819-157-11-201212040-00538.

Vlasnik, Jon J., Sherry L. Aliotta, and Bonnie DeLor. "Medication Adherence: Factors Influencing Compliance with Prescribed Medication Plans." *Case Manager* 16, no. 2 (March 2005): 47–51. https://doi.org/10.1016/j.casemgr.2005.01.009.

Wachter, Robert. *The Digital Doctor: Hope, Hype, and Harm at the Dawn of Medicine's Computer Age*. New York: McGraw Hill, 2017.

Wagner, Jennifer K. "The Federal Trade Commission and Consumer Protections for Mobile Health Apps." *Journal of Law, Medicine & Ethics* 48, no. 1_suppl (March 2020): 103–14. https://doi.org/10.1177/1073110520917035.

Wali, Huda, and Kelly Grindrod. "Don't Assume the Patient Understands: Qualitative Analysis of the Challenges Low Health Literate Patients Face in the Pharmacy." *Research in Social & Administrative Pharmacy* 12, no. 6 (December 2016): 885–92. https://doi.org/10.1016/j.sapharm.2015.12.003.

Wardrope, Alistair. "Relational Autonomy and the Ethics of Health Promotion." *Public Health Ethics* 8, no. 1 (April 2015): 50–62. https://doi.org/10.1093/phe/phu025.

Wartman, Steven A., and C. Donald Combs. "Medical Education Must Move from the Information Age to the Age of Artificial Intelligence." *Academic Medicine* 93, no. 8 (August 2018): 1107–9. https://doi.org/10.1097/ACM.0000000000002044.

Weiss, Anthony P., and Barak D. Richman, "Professional Self-Regulation in Medicine: Will the Rise of Intelligent Tools Mean the End of Peer Review?" In *The Future of Medical Device Regulation: Innovation and Protection*, edited by I. Glenn Cohen, Timo Minssen, W. Nicholson Price II, Christopher Robertson, and Carmel Shachar, 244–255. Cambridge: Cambridge University Press, 2022. https://doi:10.1017/9781108975452.019.

Werling, Anna Maria, Susanne Walitza, Stephan Eliez, and Renate Drechsler. "The Impact of the COVID-19 Pandemic on Mental Health Care of Children and Adolescents in Switzerland: Results of a Survey among Mental Health Care Professionals after One Year of COVID-19." *International Journal of Environmental Research and Public Health* 19, no. 6 (March 2022). https://doi.org/10.3390/ijerph19063252.

Westlund, Andrea C. "Rethinking Relational Autonomy." *Hypatia* 24, no. 4 (2009): 26–49.

Wetsman, Nicole. "Birth Control Apps Show the Contradictions in FDA Device Oversight." The Verge. March 17, 2021. https://www.theverge.com/22335858/birth-control-app-clue-natural-cycles-fda.

Wexler, Anna, and Steven Joffe. "5 Ways to Address the Challenges of Direct-to-Consumer Health Products." STAT. April 2, 2019. https://www.statnews.com/2019/04/02/address-challenges-direct-to-consumer-health-products/.

White House Office of Science and Technology Policy. "Blueprint for an AI Bill of Rights." October 2022. https://www.whitehouse.gov/ostp/ai-bill-of-rights/.

Wiles, Janine L., Annette Leibing, Nancy Guberman, Jeanne Reeve, and Ruth E. S. Allen. "The Meaning of 'Aging in Place' to Older People." *Gerontologist* 52 (2012): 357–66. https://doi.org/10.1093/geront/gnr098.

Winder, Davey. "How to Stop Your Smart Home Spying on You." *The Guardian*. March 8, 2020. https://www.theguardian.com/technology/2020/mar/08/how-to-stop-your-smart-home-spying-on-you-lightbulbs-doorbell-ring-google-assistant-alexa-privacy.

Wisconsin Department of Health Services. "Differences in Crisis Services and Psychiatric Hospitalizations across Race and Ethnicity." Last modified February 4, 2021. https://www.dhs.wisconsin.gov/library/p-02904.htm.

Wisniewski, Pamela, Celia Linton, Aditi Chokshi, Brielle Perlingieri, Varadraj Gurupur, and Meghan Gabriel. "We Have Built It, But They Have Not Come: Examining the Adoption and Use of Assistive Technologies for Informal Family Caregivers." In *Advances in Usability, User Experience and Assistive Technology*, edited by Tareq Z. Ahram and Christianne Falcão, 824–36. Cham: Springer International Publishing, 2019.

Woliver, Laura R. *The Political Geographies of Pregnancy*. Urbana: University of Illinois Press, 2002.

Wu, Eric, Kevin Wu, Roxana Daneshjou, David Ouyang, Daniel E. Ho, and James Zou. "How Medical AI Devices Are Evaluated: Limitations and Recommendations from an Analysis of FDA Approvals." *Nature Medicine* 27, no. 4 (April 2021): 582–84. https://doi.org/10.1038/s41591-021-01312-x.

Yadav, Arvind Kumar, Rohit Shukla, and Tiratha Raj Singh. "Machine Learning in Expert Systems for Disease Diagnostics in Human Healthcare." In *Machine Learning, Big Data, and IoT for Medical Informatics*, edited by Pardeep Kumar, Yugal Kumar, and Mohamed A. Tawhid, 179–200. Cambridge, MA: Academic Press, 2021. https://doi.org/10.1016/B978-0-12-821777-1.00022-7.

Yap, Angela Frances, Thiru Thirumoorthy, and Yu Heng Kwan. "Systematic Review of the Barriers Affecting Medication Adherence in Older Adults." *Geriatrics & Gerontology International* 16, no. 10 (October 2016): 1093 1101. https://doi.org/10.1111/ggi.12616.

Yeung, Serena, N. Lance Downing, Li Fei-Fei, and Arnold Milstein. "Bedside Computer Vision—Moving Artificial Intelligence from Driver Assistance to Patient Safety." *New England Journal of Medicine* 378, no. 14 (April 2018): 1271–73. https://doi.org/10.1056/NEJMp1716891.

Yobo, Peter. "How DTC Is Disrupting Health Care." Credera. May 1, 2020. https://www.credera.com/insights/how-dtc-is-disrupting-health-care.

You, Yue, and Xinning Gui. "Self-Diagnosis through AI-Enabled Chatbot-Based Symptom Checkers: User Experiences and Design Considerations." *AMIA Annual Symposium Proceedings 2020* (January 2021): 1354–63. https://www.ncbi.nlm.nih.gov/pmc/articles/PMC8075525/.

Young, Iris Marion. *Justice and the Politics of Difference*. Princeton, NJ: Princeton University Press, 1990.

Young, Mark A., and Lauren DiMartino. "The Emergence of Trackable Pill Technology: Hype or Hope?" *Practical Pain Management* 18, no. 4 (April 2019). https://www.practicalpainmanagement.com/treatments/pharmacological/opioids/editorial-emergence-trackable-pill-technology-hype-hope.

Zhou, Na, Chuan-Tao Zhang, Hong-Ying Lv, Chen-Xing Hao, Tian-Jun Li, Jing-Juan Zhu, Hua Zhu, et al. "Concordance Study Between IBM Watson for Oncology and Clinical Practice for Patients with Cancer in China." *Oncologist* 24, no. 6 (June 2019): 812–19. https://doi.org/10.1634/theoncologist.2018-0255.

Ziefle, Martina, Carsten Rocker, and Andreas Holzinger. "Medical Technology in Smart Homes: Exploring the User's Perspective on Privacy, Intimacy and Trust." *2011 IEEE 35th Annual Computer Software and Applications Conference Workshops* (2011): 410–15. https://doi.org/10.1109/COMPSACW.2011.75.

Index

For the benefit of digital users, indexed terms that span two pages (e.g., 52–53) may, on occasion, appear on only one of those pages.